Blood
Physiology and Pathophysiology

Chris Pallister MSc, FIBMS, CBic
Senior Lecturer in Haematology
Faculty of Applied Sciences
University of the West of England
Bristol, UK

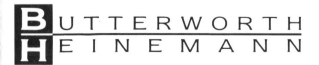

Butterworth-Heinemann
Linacre House, Jordan Hill, Oxford OX2 8DP
A division of Reed Educational and Professional Publishing Ltd

A member of the Reed Elsevier plc group

OXFORD   BOSTON   JOHANNESBURG
MELBOURNE   NEW DELHI   SINGAPORE

First published 1994
Reprinted 1997

British Library Cataloguing in Publication Data
A catalogue record for this book is available from the British Library

Library of Congress Cataloguing in Publication Data
A catalogue record for this book is available from the Library of Congress

ISBN 0 7506 0581 2

Printed and bound in Great Britain by Bookcraft, Avon

Contents

Contributors

Haemoglobin Synthesis, Structure and Function
Structural Haemoglobinopathies

M S Watson
Senior Lecturer in Haematology and Physiology
University of the West of England
Bristol

The Acute Leukaemias
The Chronic Leukaemias

D M Reardon & S O'Connor
Principal Technologist & Senior Technologist
Department of Haematology
Addenbrookes Hospital
Cambridge

The Myelodysplastic Syndromes

N R Porter
Senior Chief MLSO
Department of Haematology
Royal Hallamshire Hospital
Sheffield

Haemostasis: an Overview

J Francis
Principal Scientist
University Department of Haematology
Southampton General Hospital
Southampton

Hereditary Disorders of Haemostasis
Acquired Disorders of Haemostasis

R Luddington
Senior Technologist
Department of Haematology
Addenbrookes Hospital
Cambridge

Preface

The science of haematology occupies a privileged position among the biomedical sciences. Because of the relative ease with which blood and blood-forming tissue can be obtained and studied in the laboratory, it has become perhaps the most intensively studied organ of the body. Much of what we currently know about biochemistry, cell biology, genetics and molecular biology has been learned by study of the blood in health and disease.

The approach adopted in this book is deliberately idiosyncratic and non-traditional. Instead of the traditional emphasis on practical laboratory or clinical aspects of haematology, I have chosen to emphasise the *science* and fundamental concepts which underpin our current knowledge and understanding of the blood and its diseases. Only a basic knowledge of biochemistry, cell biology and genetics is assumed. This approach has imposed certain constraints on the ordering and grouping of material within the book. Experienced readers of haematology texts will find certain differences in the way in which disease states are grouped and described. For example, the chapter on structural haemoglobinopathies emphasises the reasons *why* amino acid substitutions cause altered behaviour of the haemoglobin molecule and how this is manifest. This reflects my belief that it is far better to understand than to know. Each chapter on normal physiology is followed by one or more chapters on pathophysiology. The latter chapters assume knowledge and understanding of the former.

This book is intended primarily for undergraduates in the life sciences and medicine, but I hope that it will also be valuable to practising haematologists as a refresher and to post-graduate students as a basis for advanced study.

I am grateful to the contributing authors for making time in their busy lives to write their chapters and for their patience with my inept editorship. I am also very grateful to Caroline Makepeace and Tim Brown of Butterworth-Heinemann for believing that this book would one day be finished (despite all of the evidence to the contrary!). Finally, my heartfelt thanks must go to my wife, Maddalena and to my children Kevin and Donna without whose help, patience and understanding this book would never have seen the light of day.

Chris Pallister
August 1994

Blood Physiology: an Introduction

Blood has always been a source of great fascination. Over the centuries, it has occupied the minds of scientists, philosophers, scribes and artists. The importance of the blood in the preservation of life appears to have been recognised as early as Paleolithic times. Cave paintings often depict the hunting and killing of animals such as mammoth for food. In some of these paintings, dying animals are portrayed with their hearts exposed and their life-blood issuing forth. The earliest known example of the use of a symbol for blood in written language dates from about 3,000 years BC: the ancient Sumerian pictograph for blood was shaped like an inverted Y.

From the time of Hippocrates (460-375 BC), curiosity about the blood and its functions combined with ignorance and mysticism to produce a plethora of mistaken beliefs, myths and legends. The aura of mystery which surrounds the blood still has not completely been dispelled. Examples of the vestiges of primitive belief abound in the work of poets, playwrights and authors. Obvious examples include tales of vampires who must regularly imbibe the blood of virgins to sustain life and the constant reference to blood to symbolise murder and the pangs of conscience of the anguished Lord and Lady Macbeth following the murder of Duncan (see sidebox). Our everyday language is enriched by expressions such as "hot-blooded" which denotes passion or "venting of the spleen" which indicates an outburst of bad temper. Both of these expressions have their roots in mediaeval belief about the power and properties of the blood.

This apparently excessive regard and reverence for the blood is not entirely inappropriate, however. The blood is one of the largest organs of the body. In an average 70 kg man the blood has a total volume of about 5 litres and weighs about 5.5 kg. If the blood-forming or **haemopoietic** organs of bone marrow, spleen, liver and lymphatic system are included, the haemopoietic system assumes pre-eminence among organs of the body. Blood circulates throughout the body and supports the function of all other body tissues. The blood is, in turn, dependent for its function on the activities of a number of other organs including the heart, lungs and kidneys.

> *Macbeth:* Will all great Neptune's ocean wash this blood clean from my hand? No, this my hand will rather the multitudinous seas incarnadine. Making the green one red. **II**.ii.61
>
> *Lady Macbeth:* Out damned spot! Out I say! **V**.i.38
>
> *Lady Macbeth:* What! Will these hands ne'er be clean? **V**.i.47
>
> *Lady Macbeth:* Here's the smell of the blood still: all the perfumes of Arabia will not sweeten this little hand. **V**.i.55

Because blood and bone marrow are easily sampled, the haemopoietic system probably is the most intensively studied organ of the body. This has led to an explosion of knowledge about blood and blood-forming tissue in both health and disease. The scientific study of the blood has contributed greatly to the expansion of knowledge and development of techniques in many other fields of scientific endeavour. Certainly, recent progress in the field of molecular genetics would have been hampered greatly if fresh blood and bone marrow had been difficult to obtain.

Content of the Blood

Normal peripheral blood is composed of three types of cell, **red cells**, **white cells** and **platelets**, suspended in a pale yellow fluid called **plasma**. The cells occupy about 40% of the total blood volume.

Red Cells

Mature red cells, or **erythrocytes**, are the most numerous of the blood cells: about 5×10^{12} normally are present in each litre of blood. The red cell count is regulated by a feedback control mechanism which is based upon oxygen delivery to the tissues. Briefly, the development of tissue hypoxia stimulates the synthesis and release of a regulatory hormone called **erythropoietin** which elicits an increase in erythropoietic activity within the bone marrow. As the circulating red cell count rises, oxygen delivery to the tissues increases and the stimulus for erythropoietin synthesis diminishes. Red cells survive in the circulation for about 120 days before being sequestered in the spleen and consumed by the phagocytic cells of the reticuloendothelial system.

During its 120 days in the circulation, the average red cell travels about 300 miles around the body. The senescent red cells that are destroyed within the spleen are constantly replaced by juvenile cells synthesised and released by the bone marrow. An average 70 kg adult male produces about 2.3×10^6 red cells every second!

The normal red cell is a biconcave discoid shape with a diameter of about 8.4 μm and a volume of about 88 fl. Its primary function is the transport of oxygen from the lungs to the tissues. This characteristic shape imparts flexibility to the cell allowing it to traverse the

Erythropoietin is coded for by a gene on the long arm of chromosome 7. It is a glycoprotein of molecular weight 30,400 which is synthesised mainly by renal tubular and peritubular cells. Small amounts are synthesised in the liver and also by macrophages.

The human erythropoietin gene has been cloned and recombinant erythropoietin (r-HuEPO) is now used successfully in the treatment of the anaemia of end-stage renal disease. It is likely that r-HuEPO will prove useful in the treatment of other conditions such as some cases of aplastic anaemia, the anaemia of prematurity and the anaemia of chronic inflammatory conditions such as rheumatoid arthritis.

smallest blood vessels which may have a diameter of only 3 μm and also maximises the surface area:volume ratio thereby facilitating gaseous exchange across the cell membrane. The oxygen-carrying pigment **haemoglobin** is present in high concentration within mature red cells and is responsible for the characteristic red colour of the blood.

The peculiar shape of the mature red cell largely is determined by the properties of the cytoskeletal proteins and the manner in which they associate. Assembly of the cytoskeleton requires energy which is derived within the red cell by the breakdown of glucose, a process known as **glycolysis**.

The physiology and pathophysiology of the red cell are described in detail in Chapters 3-12 of this book.

Platelets

The second most numerous type of cell in the blood is the platelet or **thrombocyte**: about 250×10^9 platelets are present in each litre of blood. The circulating platelet count is maintained within narrow limits by a feedback control mechanism similar to that for red cells. The platelet analogue of erythropoietin is called **thrombopoietin**. Platelets are produced by fragmentation of the peripheral cytoplasm of large multinucleate cells in the bone marrow called **megakaryocytes**.

Normal peripheral blood platelets are discoid, anucleate cells with a granular cytoplasm. They have a volume of about 7 fl, a diameter of about 3 μm and are about 1 μm thick. Platelets survive in the circulation for about 10-12 days.

The primary role of the blood platelet is in haemostasis: they stick to the edges of wounds and form a plug which arrests blood loss. Adequate numbers of functionally normal platelets are essential for optimal haemostasis. A drop in the circulating platelet count or an abnormality of platelet function can cause bleeding problems. Platelets are also involved in the development of atherosclerosis which can lead to thrombosis.

The role of platelets in normal and deranged haemostasis is described in Chapters 21-23.

White Cells

The least numerous of the blood cells is the white cell or **leucocyte**: about 5×10^9 white cells are present in each litre of blood. There are 5 different types of white cell normally present in the peripheral blood, viz **neutrophils**, **eosinophils**, **basophils**, **monocytes** and **lymphocytes**. The neutrophils, eosinophils and basophils form a group of white cells called the **granulocytes**. The lymphocytes and monocytes are sometimes known as **mononuclear leucocytes**. In contrast to red cells and platelets, all of the white cells have a nucleus.

Neutrophils

The neutrophil is the most numerous white cell in adults: about 60% of circulating white cells are neutrophils. The nucleus of the neutrophil is divided into a varying number of lobes which are joined by a thin chromatin strand. Because of this, the neutrophil is sometimes called a **polymorphonuclear leucocyte**, or **polymorph**. The cytoplasm of the neutrophil contains numerous fine granules which stain pale pink with Romanowsky dyes. It is the appearance of these cytoplasmic granules which distinguish the neutrophil from its granulocytic cousins, the eosinophil and basophil.

Neutrophils exist in two pools in the blood: the **marginated pool** which is in loose contact with the walls of the blood vessels and the **circulating pool** which circulates freely. Normally, there is a rapid and unrestricted exchange of cells between these two pools.

Neutrophils spend about 8-10 hours in the circulation before they exit to the tissues where they are responsible for non-specific defence against bacterial and fungal infection. Neutrophils are attracted to sites of infection by a process known as **chemotaxis**. Once at the site of an infection, the neutrophil engulfs the invading microbes, a process known as **phagocytosis**. The ingested organism is then killed by a variety of toxic substances stored within the cytoplasmic granules of the neutrophil. Once a neutrophil has left the bloodstream, it does not re-enter.

The physiology and pathophysiology of neutrophils are described in Chapters 13-14.

The importance of neutrophils in the defence against microbial infection is underlined by the nature, frequency and severity of such infections observed in neutropaenic individuals. A similar predisposition to infection is seen in dysfunctional states such as chronic granulomatous disease.

For example, patients undergoing chemotherapy for leukaemia frequently develop neutropaenia and are then susceptible to repeated and severe bacterial and fungal infections with organisms normally considered to be of low pathogenicity eg *P aeruginosa, Klebsiella sp, S epidermidis, S viridans, Candida sp* and *Aspergillus sp.*

Eosinophils

About 1% of the circulating white cells are eosinophils and are characterised by their large cytoplasmic granules which stain strongly with the acidic dye eosin. Typically the eosinophil nucleus is bilobed.

Eosinophils circulate in the bloodstream for about 4-5 hours before they exit to the tissues where they are responsible for defence against parasitic infestation and also help to dampen the allergic response. Tissue eosinophils also are capable of responding, albeit inefficiently, to bacterial and fungal infection in a similar manner to neutrophils.

Basophils

Basophils are the least numerous white cell in the blood: less than 1% of circulating white cells are basophils. The large cytoplasmic granules are characterised by their avidity for the basic dye methylene blue. Basophils are involved in anaphylactic, hypersensitivity and inflammatory reactions. For example, when IgE immunoglobulin binds to basophil surface receptors, the cell degranulates thereby releasing inflammatory mediators such as heparin, histamine and platelet activating factor to the surrounding tissue.

Monocytes

About 5% of circulating white cells are monocytes. The blood monocyte is a large cell (16-22 μm in diameter) with a kidney-shaped or distinctly cleft nucleus and a scattering of delicate azurophilic granules in the cytoplasm. Blood monocytes circulate for about 10 hours before they exit to the tissues where they mature into the actively phagocytic **tissue macrophages** which are responsible for the removal and processing of aged red cells and other debris. Tissue macrophages also play an important role in the processing and presentation of antigen to T lymphocytes as described in Chapter 13.

> The characteristic colours of the granules of neutrophils, eosinophils and basophils described opposite are imparted by staining of a methanol-fixed blood or bone marrow smear with Romanowsky dyes.
>
> Romanowsky dyes are mixtures of eosin and oxidised, or polychromed, methylene blue. Using this mixture, basic structures attract eosin and therefore stain a bright orange colour, while acidic structures attract methylene blue and therefore appear blue. A range of other colours are also produced eg nuclear chromatin stains purple, by various molecular interactions between dye molecules, a phenomenon known as **metachromasia**.
>
> Commonly used versions of Romanowsky dyes are named after their originators eg May-Grunwald, Giemsa, Wright and Lieshman.

Lymphocytes

Lymphocytes are the second most common white cell in the peripheral blood: about 33% of circulating white cells are lymphocytes. Typically, lymphocytes are much smaller than monocytes (10-12 μm in diameter) and have much less cytoplasm. In contrast to the monocyte, the lymphocyte nucleus is round and almost fills the cell. A proportion of lymphocytes have more abundant cytoplasm. Lymphocytes have a variable lifespan of between a few days and many years.

There are many different types of lymphocytes which play distinct roles in specific, or acquired, immunity. **T lymphocytes** account for 40-80% of the blood lymphocytes and are responsible for **cell-mediated immunity**. **B lymphocytes** normally account for 10-30% of the blood lymphocytes and are responsible for **humoral immunity**.

Plasma

Plasma occupies about 60% of the total blood volume. It is a pale yellow aqueous solution of electrolytes, proteins and small organic molecules such as glucose.

Plasma Electrolytes

The major extracellular cation is Na^+ which has a concentration of about 140 meq per litre of plasma. Other important plasma cations include K^+, Ca^{2+}, Fe^{2+} and Mg^{2+} but these are all found at much lower concentration. The relative concentrations of Na^+ and K^+ in the plasma contrast with their intracellular concentrations where K^+ is present at a higher concentration.

The major plasma anions are Cl^- and HCO_3^- although SO_4^{2-} and HPO_4^{2-} ions are also present at lower concentration. The concentrations of anions and cations in the plasma are always such that the total number of negative charges and positive charges exactly balance ie plasma is always electrically neutral.

Plasma Proteins

A large number of different plasma proteins exist but they fall into four distinct families viz haemostatic proteins, immunoglobulins, Complement and plasma transport proteins.

Haemostatic Proteins

The major haemostatic proteins are the **coagulation factors** most of which circulate in the blood as **pro-enzymes** or **zymogens** ie they circulate in an inactive form but are capable of conversion into active enzymes called **serine proteases**. The exceptions to this rule are factors V, VIII and high molecular weight kininogen (HMWK) which act as cofactors and potentiate the activity of the serine proteases, factor XIII which carries a cysteine rather than a serine residue at its active site and fibrinogen which is the substrate for thrombin. The coagulation factors are activated via a stepwise series of reactions which culminate in the formation of a solid fibrin clot. Fibrin deposition acts to strengthen and stabilise the platelet plug which is formed at the site of injury.

Protection against inappropriate clot formation, or **thrombosis**, is afforded by a second series of haemostatic proteins which form the **fibrinolytic system**. Effective haemostasis can be viewed as a precarious equilibrium between coagulant mechanisms which act to prevent blood loss and anticoagulant mechanisms which act to prevent inappropriate clot formation.

Maintenance of the haemostatic equilibrium is aided by a series of protein inhibitors of the coagulation and fibrinolytic systems. These should not be confused with the pathological inhibitors which can arise spontaneously eg in auto-immune disease.

The physiology and pathophysiology of haemostasis are described in Chapters 21-23 of this book.

Immunoglobulins

The immunoglobulins are antibody molecules which are synthesised by plasma cells. There are five different classes of immunoglobulin which are structurally related but perform distinct biological functions. These are designated as **IgA**, **IgD**, **IgE**, **IgG** and **IgM**. Antibodies which are produced in response to foreign

Plasma proteins can be classified according to their electrophoretic mobility at pH 8.6. At this pH, proteins are negatively charged and migrate towards the anode, forming seven groups of proteins with similar mobilities viz albumin, α_1-globulin, α_2-globulin, β-globulin, fibrinogen, γ_1-globulin and γ_2-globulin.

Using this system, the immunoglobulins are all γ-globulins, coagulation factors V, VIII, IX, XI, XII and XIII and haemopexin are all β-globulins and coagulation factors II and X, transcobalamin I and III and haptoglobin are α-globulins.

antigen are specific for that antigen. The structure and function of immunoglobulins are described in Chapter 13.

Complement

The Complement system is a family of plasma proteins which are important in the induction of inflammation and immunity against microbial infection. Complement proteins circulate in an inactive form and are activated via a cascading series of reactions in much the same way as the coagulation factors. Activation of Complement can proceed via two different pathways depending upon the initiator involved. The physiology of Complement activation is described in Chapter 13.

Transport Proteins

One of the many functions of the blood is to act as a transport system for nutrients and waste products. This function is mediated by carrier proteins in the plasma.

Some important substances have specific carrier proteins. For example, iron is transported in the plasma to developing erythroid precursors in the bone marrow by the specific iron-binding protein **transferrin**. Similarly, vitamin B_{12} is transported by a small family of carrier proteins known as the **transcobalamins**. These transport proteins are described in Chapter 3.

Intravascular haemolysis results in liberation of haemoglobin into the plasma. This free haemoglobin complexes rapidly with a specific transport protein called **haptoglobin**. The haptoglobin:haemoglobin complex is transported to the liver where it is metabolised and the iron and protein it contains are released for re-utilisation by the body. This represents an important mechanism for the prevention of loss of iron from the body. A similar function is performed by the haem-binding transport protein **haemopexin**.

Plasma transport is not always mediated by specific carrier proteins, however. Plasma **albumin** is an important non-specific binder of a wide range of substances such as bilirubin, folate and, once haemopexin has been exhausted, haem.

Functions of the Blood

Blood performs a number of vital physiological functions:

- **respiratory gas transport**. Perhaps the most important function of the blood is the transport of oxygen bound to haemoglobin from the lungs to the tissues and the carriage of waste carbon dioxide on the return journey.

- **transport of nutrients and waste products**. The blood circulatory system provides an efficient means of transporting nutrients absorbed from the gut to their site of storage or utilisation. The waste products of metabolism are similarly transported to their sites of excretion or reutilisation. The regulatory activities of endocrine hormones would be impossible without the efficient transport mechanism provided by the blood circulatory system.

- **thermoregulation**. Metabolic reactions produce heat energy. The blood plays two important roles in the handling and distribution of heat energy by the body. Because it is composed largely of water, blood is capable of absorbing a relatively large amount of heat energy for only a small rise in temperature. This stored heat is distributed throughout the body via the blood circulatory system. Control over blood flow via vasoconstriction and vasodilatation provides one means by which body temperature and heat loss are regulated.

- **haemostasis**. Maintenance of normal blood flow requires that the blood should remain fluid at all times. Conversely, staunching of blood loss following injury requires that the blood should also be capable of forming a solid plug rapidly. These conflicting demands are met by the many complex interactions of the blood vessel wall with platelets and the various haemostatic proteins which circulate in the blood.

- **immunity**. The blood plays an important part in immunity, principally by acting as a source of, and transport system for, immunocompetent cells and the effector substances of the immune system.

Suggested Further Reading

Wintrobe, M.M. (1980). *Blood, Pure and Eloquent.* New York: McGraw-Hill.

Blood Cell Formation

Under normal physiological conditions, the number of circulating blood cells is maintained within remarkably narrow limits. Since all blood cells have a limited life span, a dynamic equilibrium must exist between cell loss due to senescence or normal function and the synthesis and release of their replacements. Maintenance of this dynamic equilibrium requires a capacity for production of blood cells of astonishing fecundity coupled with exquisite responsiveness to the changing needs of the body for blood cells.

An average 70 kg adult male has a total blood volume of about 5 litres which contains a total of about 25×10^{12} red cells. Since normal red cells survive for an average of 120 days, maintenance of a constant cell number requires the replacement of more than 2×10^{11} red cells every day! If the destruction and replacement of the other blood cells is taken into account, the total daily requirement for new blood cells is about 5×10^{11}. This rate of production must be maintained without pause for an average of 70 years, during which time the bone marrow will have released more than 1×10^{16} mature blood cells!

Ontogeny of Haemopoiesis

Haemopoiesis is conducted at a number of different anatomical sites during the process of development from embryo to adult, as shown in Figure 2.1. Changes in the primary site of haemopoiesis are accompanied by simultaneous changes in the morphology of the cells produced and also in the types of haemoglobin molecule synthesised within the red cell precursors. The changes in globin chain synthesis are described in Chapter 6.

Embryonic Haemopoiesis

The earliest recognisable blood cell precursors are demonstrable in 2-week-old embryos. At this stage of development, the embryo consists of little more than two sacs - the **amniotic sac** and the **yolk sac** - separated by a wedge of tissue called the **embryonic plate**. As the

The fact that the bone marrow is the site of synthesis of blood cells after birth was first recognised independently by Ernst Neumann in Germany and Giulio Bizzozero in Italy in 1868.

Opposition to this idea was fierce because several other prominent investigators had conflicting ideas about the origins of red cells. These ranged from the suggestion that red cells were derived from the disintegrated nuclei of white cells to the idea that fat globules were transformed into red cells by the liver! Although these ideas are preposterous in the light of modern knowledge, they were serious contenders at the time.

I wonder what the haematologist of the 22nd century will make of the concepts and "facts" detailed in this book?

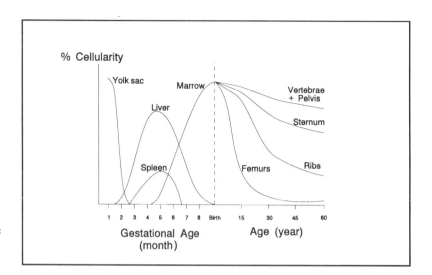

Figure 2.1 *Sites of haemopoiesis throughout life*

embryo develops, the amniotic sac expands greatly to fill the entire uterus and the placenta is formed. The yolk sac becomes compressed by the expanding amniotic sac into a narrow stalk which forms the core of the umbilical cord. The embryo develops from the embryonic plate.

The earliest haemopoietic cells to be produced are primitive erythroid precursors which can be seen in the yolk sac of 2-week-old embryos. At this stage, these erythroid cells are macrocytic relative to normal adult cells and retain their nucleus. The major haemoglobin present in these cells is haemoglobin Gower I ($\zeta_2\varepsilon_2$).

Leucopoiesis and thrombopoiesis do not commence until about 6 weeks gestation when megakaryocytes and granulocytes can be seen in the yolk sac. In contrast to other blood cells, lymphocytes are not formed in the yolk sac, but in the lymph sacs which begin to develop at about 7 weeks gestation.

Foetal Haemopoiesis

The role of the yolk sac as the primary source of blood cells is short-lived. Its early haemopoietic activity rapidly diminishes until, by about 10 weeks gestation, it has ceased to produce blood cells. The rapid demise of the yolk sac as a haemopoietic organ is accompanied by a rapid increase in the relative importance of the foetal liver in this role. Haemopoietic activity is first demonstrable in the foetal liver at about 6 weeks gestation. In the ensuing weeks, this organ quickly becomes established as the primary source of blood cells; a position it holds until about 30 weeks gestation. The major haemoglobin synthesised during the hepatic phase of foetal haemopoiesis is haemoglobin F ($\alpha_2\gamma_2$). Hepatic haemopoietic activity ceases just before normal, full-term delivery ie at about 40 weeks gestation.

The foetal spleen commences production of blood cells at about 10 weeks gestation and continues throughout the second trimester of pregnancy. However, even at the height of its activity, the foetal spleen is of secondary importance as a haemopoietic organ.

Bone cavities begin to form at about 20 weeks gestation and provide such an ideal environment for haemopoietic activity that the bone marrow rapidly becomes the sole source of blood cells in humans. The rise of the bone marrow to this exalted position is complete by 40 weeks gestation. Replacement of the liver as the primary haemopoietic organ is associated with a gradual replacement of haemoglobin F by haemoglobin A ($\alpha_2\beta_2$).

Haemopoiesis in the Developing Child and Adult

At birth, haemopoietically active, or red, marrow fills completely the available marrow space. This means that infants have no reserve haemopoietic capacity which can be called upon in times of increased demand. The only response open to a neonate in such circumstances is to expand the marrow volume. This is the cause of the skeletal deformities which develop in severe dyserythropoietic states such as thalassaemia.

During early childhood, marrow volume increases in parallel with the increased marrow space made available by growth. The bone marrow volume in an average 3 year old child has expanded to about 1500 ml (Figure 2.2). This is still entirely composed of active red marrow and is sufficient to meet the normal physiological demands for blood cells of an adult. Thus, as the child grows into an adult, and the available bone marrow space expands, there is no requirement for a concurrent increase in volume of active red marrow. The expanding marrow space becomes progressively filled with inactive, or yellow, marrow. This process begins in the peripheral diaphyses of the long bones and continues until, in an adult, three quarters of the red marrow is found in the pelvis, vertebrae and sternum (Figure 2.2).

SAQ 1

What is the major site of haemopoiesis in a baby born 13 weeks prematurely?

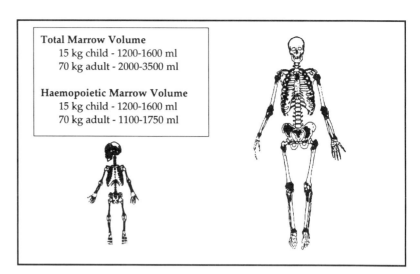

Total Marrow Volume
    15 kg child - 1200-1600 ml
    70 kg adult - 2000-3500 ml

Haemopoietic Marrow Volume
    15 kg child - 1200-1600 ml
    70 kg adult - 1100-1750 ml

Figure 2.2 *Total and haemopoietic bone marrow volume in the child and adult. Shaded areas represent haemopoietic marrow*

Yellow marrow can readily be converted into its active counterpart during periods of increased demand for blood cells. This means that adults have a potential reserve haemopoietic capacity of about six times normal.

In conditions where the bone marrow is unable to meet the demands of the body for blood cells, for example when much of the bone marrow space is occupied by metastatic carcinoma deposits, haemopoiesis may revert to foetal sites viz the spleen and liver. This phenomenon is known as **extramedullary haemopoiesis**.

Anatomy of Haemopoietic Bone Marrow

Knowledge of the structural organisation of haemopoietic bone marrow is essential for an adequate understanding of the processes involved in blood cell synthesis, maturation and release. The various structures present combine to form an ideal microenvironment for haemopoiesis. Disruption of this microenvironment is thought to be the cause of some cases of aplastic anaemia.

A schematic diagram of the gross anatomy of a typical long bone from an adult is shown in Figure 2.3. The main shaft of the bones is supplied with blood by one or more large **nutrient arteries** which penetrate the bony **cortex** and enter the **medullary cavity**. Within the medullary cavity, the nutrient artery branches repeatedly, forming the **epiphyseal**, **metaphyseal** and **periosteal capillaries**, which

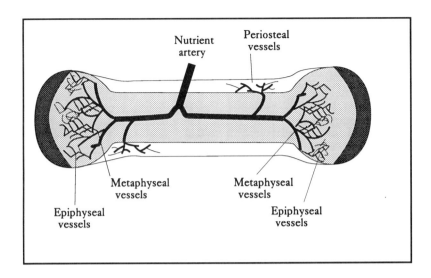

Figure 2.3 *Gross anatomy of a typical long bone*

supply the bony cortex and bone marrow with oxygen and nutrients. The periosteal capillaries empty into the **venous sinuses** (Figure 2.4) which, in turn, drain into the **emissary vein**. The emissary vein forms the route along which newly released blood cells join the systemic circulation.

In common with other veins, the venous sinuses are composed of three concentric layers. The central or medial layer of discontinuous basement membrane is covered on its inner or intimal face by a single layer of vascular endothelium while on its outer, or adventitial, face it is covered by a layer of reticular macrophages. These adventitial reticular cells send out numerous processes which divide the

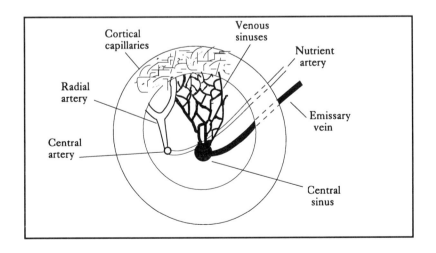

Figure 2.4 *Cross section of bone shown in Figure 2.3*

blood-forming cavity into separate compartments which the dividing and maturing blood cell precursors occupy.

The disposition of the different blood cell precursors within the blood-forming cavity is not random: each type occupies a specific position. Platelet-producing megakaryocytes are lodged adjacent to the venous sinus with their cytoplasmic processes projecting directly into the lumen of the sinus. Thus, the platelets which form at the tips of these processes are "washed away" into the systemic circulation. Platelets are also formed from megakaryocytes which reside in the lungs. Red cell precursors also lie adjacent to the venous sinus in groups called **erythroblastic islands**, each associated with its own macrophage or "nurse" cell. Granulocyte and monocyte precursors tend to lie more deeply within the blood-forming cavity. As these cells mature, they develop the capability of independent movement whereupon they crawl towards the venous sinus.

The timing of release of mature blood cells from the marrow space is influenced by a family of related adhesive proteins which bind the maturing cells to the stromal matrix. For example, early red cell precursors carry large numbers of specific receptors for the adhesive protein fibronectin on their surfaces, and so are tightly bound to the stromal matrix. As these precursors mature, the number of fibronectin receptors present decreases sharply, thereby facilitating the selective release of more mature cells.

Sequence of Differentiation of Blood Cells

Blood cells are produced in vast numbers throughout life, with no apparent sign of exhaustion of their source. This requires the existence of a population of precursor cells which are capable of both self-renewal and differentiation - the **stem cell compartment**. The theoretical necessity for such a pool of cells has been accepted for over a century but the nature of the stem cell compartment was the subject of fierce debate in the early decades of the 20th century. The debate centred on whether stem cells were **totipotential** ie capable of differentiation to form any mature blood cell type - the **monophyletic theory** or whether separate stem cells existed for each cell line - the **polyphyletic theory**. As so often in science, the truth of the matter turned out to be a synthesis of elements of both theories: both pluripotential and unipotential or committed stem cells are now known to exist.

The first unequivocal demonstration of the existence of pluripotential stem cells came in 1961 when Till and McCulloch performed experiments to determine the sensitivity of mouse bone marrow to damage by irradiation. Briefly, mice were subjected to a dose of ionising radiation sufficient to destroy their haemopoietic capacity and bone marrow cells from genetically identical mice were immediately transfused. After about 7 days the spleens of these mice had developed numerous macroscopic nodules which consisted of haemopoietic tissue. Subsequent experiments showed that these nodules were clonal in nature ie each was derived from a single stem cell which was given the name **colony forming unit-spleen** or **CFU-S**. Under different experimental conditions, CFU-S could be influenced to produce **granulocyte-macrophage colony forming units (CFU-GM), erythroid colony forming units (CFU-E)** or **megakaryocyte colony forming units (CFU-Meg)** or a mixture of more than one cell line.

Till, J.E. and McCulloch, E.A., Direct measurement of the radiation sensitivity of normal mouse bone marrow cells. *Radiat. Res.*, **14**: 213-222, 1961.

The results of many related experiments using human bone marrow cells in tissue culture have enabled the construction of the lineage tree shown in Figure 2.5. The common ancestral cell of all mature blood cells in man is the totipotential stem cell. This cell can differentiate to form either a **lymphoid stem cell (CFU-L)** or a **non-lymphoid stem cell (CFU-GEMM).** These cells are said to be **pluripotential** ie they have the capacity to differentiate along several different cell lines but their choice is limited, as shown. These stem cells retain the dual capacity for self-renewal and differentiation. Pluripotential stem cells are capable of differentiating into a number of different **unipotential** stem cells which are committed to differentiation along a single cell line eg BFU-E can only differentiate into mature red cells, they cannot be influenced to become any other cell type.

Control of Haemopoiesis

Our current understanding of the mechanisms which regulate haemopoiesis *in vivo* is far from complete. Advances in semi-solid cell culture techniques have led to the identification of a series of glycoproteins which are required for optimal growth and differentiation of haemopoietic progenitor cells. The structure, synthesis and mode(s) of action of these **haemopoietic growth factors** have been studied intensively, and an overall picture of the complex regulatory mechanisms involved in the control of haemopoiesis is beginning to emerge.

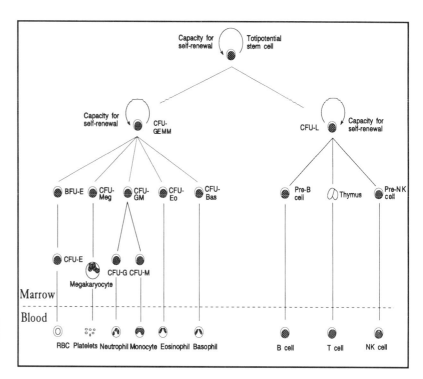

Figure 2.5 *Haemopoietic lineage tree showing the lines along which blood cells are produced*

Interleukin Trivial Names

IL-1 Lymphocyte activating factor
IL-2 T cell growth factor
IL-3 Multi-CSF
IL-4 B cell growth factor
IL-6 B cell stimulating factor
IL-7 Lymphopoietin

The concept of haemopoietic progenitor cells as colony-forming units has been extended to encompass the nomenclature of the haemopoietic growth factors. They are designated as **colony-stimulating factors** (CSFs), and each is prefixed with the initial letter of the type of colony whose production it stimulates. Thus, the growth factor which influences CFU-GM to produce granulocytes is known as G-CSF. Similarly, M-CSF and GM-CSF stimulate the production of monocytes and both granulocytes and monocytes respectively. Multi-CSF, now known as interleukin 3 (IL-3), regulates the proliferation and differentiation of a wide range of myeloid progenitor cells. Erythropoiesis is regulated by the action of another growth factor, known as **erythropoietin** (Epo). The main sites of action of these growth factors is depicted in Figure 2.6, and their most important properties are summarised in Table 2.1.

Recombinant human haemopoietic growth factors have considerable potential as therapeutic agents. Recombinant erythropoietin has been demonstrated to be effective in the control of chronic anaemia in anephric patients and preliminary results with r-HuGM-CSF and r-HuG-CSF suggest that they promote accelerated recovery of peripheral leucocyte counts in leukaemia patients

Growth Factor	Source	Major Functions
GM-CSF	T lymphocytes endothelial cells fibroblasts	Stimulates production of neutrophils, eosinophils, monocytes, red cells and platelets
G-CSF	Monocytes fibroblasts	Stimulates production of neutrophils
M-CSF	Macrophages endothelial cells	Stimulates production of monocytes
Erythropoietin	Peritubular cells liver ? macrophages	Stimulates production of red cells
IL-1	Macrophages activated lymphs endothelial cells	Cofactor for IL-3 and IL-6. Activates T cells
IL-2	Activated T cells	T cell growth factor. Stimulates IL-1 synthesis. Activates B cells and NK cells
IL-3	T cells	Stimulates production of all non-lymphoid cells
IL-4	Activated T cells	Growth factor for activated B cells, resting T cells and mast cells
IL-5	T cells	Induces differentiation of activated B cells and eosinophils
IL-6	T cells	Stimulates CFU-GEMM. Stimulates Ig synthesis
IL-7	T cells fibroblasts endothelial cells	Growth factor for pre-B cells

Table 2.1 *Human haemopoietic growth factors*

SAQ 2

Why is anaemia a common complication of chronic renal failure?

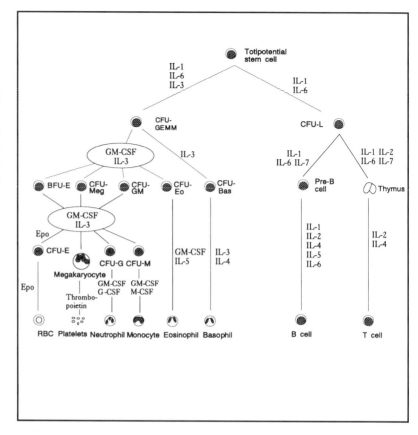

Figure 2.6 *Main sites of action of the human haemopoietic growth factors*

following cytoreductive chemotherapy or bone marrow transplant. Use of these growth factors may permit the use of more aggressive chemotherapy protocols.

The control mechanisms which inhibit haemopoiesis are even less well understood than those which promote growth and differentiation, although a number of potential inhibitory mechanisms have been proposed:

- **lactoferrin**, an iron-chelating protein present in neutrophil secondary granules, has been shown to inhibit release of GM-CSF. Thus, where neutrophil counts are high, further granulopoiesis is suppressed.

- **α and γ interferon** have been shown to inhibit growth of a wide range of haemopoietic progenitor cells *in vitro*.

- **transforming growth factor β** (TGF-β) is a multifunctional cytokine which is synthesised by platelets. It is a potent inhibitor of primitive haemopoietic progenitor cells.

- **peptide inhibitors**. A number of small peptides have been discovered which inhibit haemopoietic activity *in vitro*. For example, pGlu-Glu-Asp-Cys-Lys is synthesised by mature granulocytes and may be involved in some form of feedback inhibition of CFU-GM.

- **macrophage inflammatory protein 1a** (MIP-1a) is synthesised by activated macrophages and T lymphocytes and appears to regulate stem cell proliferation.

However, the physiological significance of these observations remains unclear.

Erythropoiesis

As already mentioned, the circulating red cell mass is maintained within remarkably narrow limits under normal physiological conditions. Maintenance of such a balance requires the existence of a feedback mechanism which can sense whether body oxygen demands are being met and adjust the rate of erythropoiesis accordingly. The mediator of this feedback mechanism is a glycoprotein hormone called erythropoietin.

The existence of erythropoietin was first demonstrated in the early 1950s when plasma from acutely bled animals was shown to elicit a reticulocyte response when transfused into normal animals. Briefly, the feedback mechanism operates in the following manner:

- a fall in the circulating red cell mass leads directly to a decreased delivery of oxygen to the tissues and hypoxia develops.

- tissue hypoxia is sensed by an ill-defined mecha-

> **SAQ 3**
>
> In which of the following circumstances would the plasma erythropoietin level be raised?
>
> A. A mountain-dweller
> B. Normal pregnancy
> C. Following acute blood loss
> D. Polycythaemia rubra vera

nism in the kidney which is thought to involve a haem-containing protein. This sensor stimulates synthesis of erythropoietin by the peritubular endothelial cells of the kidney. Small amounts of erythropoietin are also synthesised by the liver and other tissues.

- erythropoietin occupies specific receptor sites on the membranes of BFU-E and CFU-E, resulting in a shortening of cell-cycle time, an increased rate of maturation and an increased rate of release of red cells from the bone marrow.

- the increased red cell mass thus produced results in increased delivery of oxygen to the tissues, effectively removing the stimulus for erythropoietin synthesis. The rate of erythropoiesis therefore returns to normal.

A lineage tree for normal erythropoiesis and the effect of erythropoietin is shown in Figure 2.7.

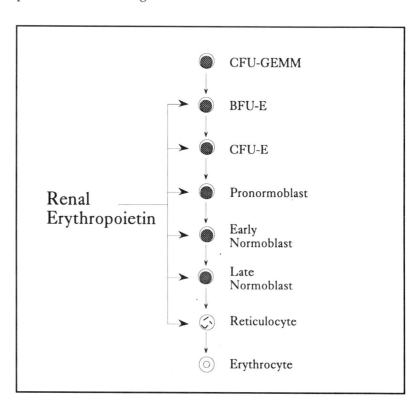

Figure 2.7 *Lineage tree for normal erythropoiesis showing the sites of action of erythropoietin*

Granulopoiesis and Monopoiesis

The regulation of granulocyte and monocyte production is incompletely understood, at present. The size of the circulating granulocyte pool is thought to be regulated by maintenance of a homeostatic balance between a number of different stimulatory and inhibitory influences. The main stimulatory factors are the haemopoietic growth factors described above, although oestrogen has also been shown to stimulate granulopoiesis. A number of substances which are produced by mature granulocytes and monocytes have been shown to be inhibitory *in vitro*. The concentration of these inhibitory substances such as the inhibitory pentapeptide described above and lactoferrin increases as the circulating neutrophil and monocyte counts increase, and thus may form the basis of a negative feedback system.

In circumstances where a rapid increase in neutrophil count is required, large numbers of mature cells can be recruited from the marginated to the circulating pool. A lineage tree for normal granulopoiesis and monopoiesis is shown in Figure 2.8.

SAQ 4

Which of the following are haemopoietic growth factors?

A. IL-6
B. TGF-β
C. G-CSF
D. BFU-E
E. γ interferon

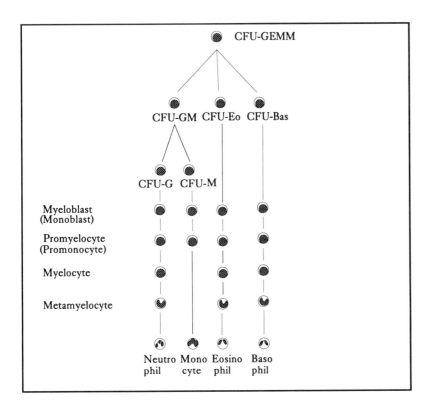

Figure 2.8 *Lineage tree for normal granulopoiesis and monopoiesis*

Thrombopoiesis

Megakaryoblasts are formed from CFU-Meg by a unique process called **endomitotic replication**. In this process, DNA replication and expansion of cytoplasmic volume occur but not cellular division. Thus, with each complete cycle of endomitosis, the cell becomes progressively larger and increasingly polyploid. Morphologically recognisable megakaryocytes may have up to 64n DNA content (ie 32 times the normal diploid (2n) content). Once endomitotic replication has ceased, the megakaryocyte nucleus becomes lobulated and the cytoplasm matures, with the formation of the structures which form the platelets and, finally, shedding of the platelets into the venous sinus. This process is estimated to take from 2 to 3 days. Each megakaryocyte is capable of producing between 2000 and 7000 platelets.

The regulation of thrombopoiesis is analogous to that for erythropoiesis in that it appears to be under feedback control based on the circulating platelet count. A transfusion of plasma from thrombocytopaenic animals stimulates thrombopoiesis in normal animals. The humoral regulatory factor is called **thrombopoietin**.

A lineage tree for normal thrombopoiesis is shown in Figure 2.9.

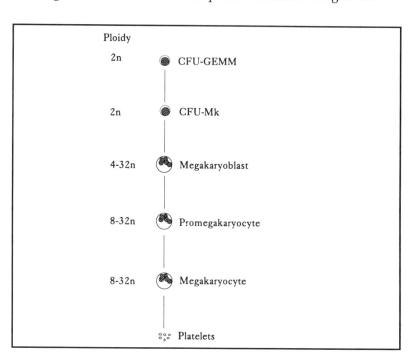

Figure 2.9 *Lineage tree for normal thrombopoiesis*

Lymphopoiesis

Lymphopoiesis occurs in two distinct phases:

- the lymphoid stem cell differentiates to form mature antigen-committed lymphocytes. This process occurs in the **primary lymphoid organs**. T lymphocyte differentiation occurs in the **thymus gland** while B lymphocyte differentiation takes place in the foetal liver and adult bone marrow.

- antigen-dependent proliferation and development of T and B lymphocytes occurs in the **secondary lymphoid organs** such as the **spleen, lymph nodes** and **mucosa-associated lymphoid tissue**.

Anatomy of Lymphatic Organs

The Thymus Gland

The thymus gland is the site of T lymphocyte differentiation. It is most active during foetal life when it becomes populated with committed lymphoid stem cells. Its task of populating secondary lymphoid tissue with mature antigen-committed T lymphocytes is largely complete within the first months of life following which thymic activity diminishes rapidly. Removal of the thymus gland from an adult (thymectomy) has no significant impact upon immune function whereas removal in the neonatal period induces a severe immunological deficit.

The thymus gland is a bilobed organ which is located in the anterior mediastinum. Each lobe is divided into a number of lobules by fibrous septa which branch off from the surrounding capsule as shown in Figure 2.10. The subcapsular region is populated by proliferating T lymphoid stem cells. The progeny of these stem cells pass through the cortical and medullary regions of the thymus and, from there, enter the circulation as mature T lymphocytes. During their journey, the T lymphocytes acquire surface receptors which are responsible for the specificity of their function. The processes involved in T cell maturation and differentiation are described further below and in more detail in Chapter 13.

The essential role of the thymus gland in immunity was demonstrated unequivocally in 1961 when it was shown that thymectomy of newborn mice greatly diminished their capacity to combat infection.

Miller J.F.A.P., Immunological function of the thymus. *Lancet*, **ii**: 748-749, 1961.

Miller J.F.A.P., Effect of neonatal thymectomy on the immunological responsiveness of the mouse. *Proc. R. Soc. Lond. (Biol.)*, **156**: 410-428, 1962.

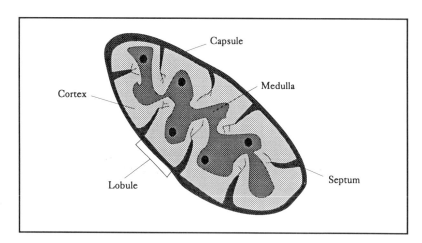

Figure 2.10 *The structure of the thymus gland*

Bone Marrow

In birds, the primary lymphoid organ responsible for the maturation and differentiation of B lymphocytes is known as the **Bursa of Fabricius**. In humans, induction of B lymphocyte differentiation is one of the many functions of the bone marrow. The processes involved in B cell maturation and differentiation are described further below and in more detail in Chapter 13.

The Spleen

The spleen is the largest of the lymphoid organs and is situated in the left hypochondrium, behind the stomach. It performs a number of important functions:

- **blood filtration**. The spleen selectively removes senescent or antibody-coated red cells from the circulation. Inclusions such as Heinz bodies also are selectively removed from red cells during their passage through the spleen.

- **blood pooling**. About one third of the total platelet mass is held in the spleen. The splenic platelet pool is in dynamic equilibrium with the circulating platelet pool. About 5% of the total red cell mass is present in the spleen. In severe splenomegaly, splenic sequestration of red cells can account for more than one third of the total red cell mass.

- **immune function.** The filtering action of the spleen collects and concentrates blood-borne foreign antigen for processing by the immune system. It is the major site of antibody synthesis within the body.

- **haemopoietic function.** As described earlier, the spleen normally is a haemopoietic organ *in utero* and, *in extremis*, can resume this function.

The spleen is enclosed by a fibrous capsule from which numerous trabeculae branch off, partitioning the interior parenchyma. Blood enters the spleen via the **splenic artery** which branches repeatedly to form the **trabecular arteries**, **central arteries** and then the **penicillary arteries** and **sheathed capillaries**. The central arteries are surrounded by lymphoid tissue called **white pulp** while the penicillary arteries drain into the **splenic cords** of the **red pulp** and, from there, into the **trabecular veins** and, finally, into the **splenic vein**. Most of the blood which flows through the spleen follows this route which is known as the **open circulation**. A proportion of the penicillary arteries drain directly into splenic venous sinuses, forming an alternative **closed circulation**.

There are two types of lymphoid masses within the white pulp: a sheath of T lymphocytes (mainly T_H lymphocytes) which surrounds the central arteries, and lymphoid follicles which are often found near arteriolar branches. The lymphoid follicles contain germinal centres which are rich in B lymphocytes surrounded by a mantle of T lymphocytes and antigen-presenting cells. About 50% of spleen cells are B lymphocytes; about 35% are T lymphocytes.

The boundary between the white pulp and the red pulp is known as the **marginal zone** and is rich in dendritic antigen-presenting cells which serve to capture, process and present foreign antigen in a form suitable for T lymphocyte stimulation.

The splenic cords consist of a loose arrangement of sponge-like cavities, supported by a framework of reticular cells. Because the gaps between the reticular cells are extremely narrow, poorly deformable or similarly defective red cells cannot pass and are trapped within the splenic cords. Trapped cells are consumed by splenic macrophages. Those cells which successfully traverse the splenic cords enter venous sinuses which drain into the **trabecular vein** and, from there, leave the spleen via the **splenic vein**. The structure of the spleen is shown schematically in Figure 2.11.

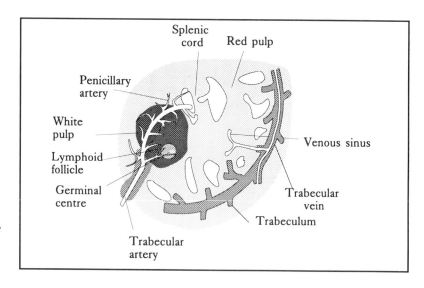

Figure 2.11 *The structure of the spleen*

The characteristics of blood flow within the spleen are such that the plasma and leucocytes flow preferentially through the white pulp while the red cells flow preferentially though the red pulp.

Lymph Nodes

The lymphatic circulatory system acts as a drainage system for excess interstitial fluid or **lymph** and bears many structural similarities to the blood circulatory system:

- the smallest lymphatic vessels are known as **lymphatic capillaries** and penetrate deep into almost all tissues of the body. These vessels are permeable to fluids, dissolved substances and lymphocytes.

- lymphatic capillaries drain into larger vessels which are the equivalent of veins.

- the largest lymphatic vessels, like arteries, are muscular and actively pump lymph into the **thoracic duct** and the **right main lymphatic duct** which drain into the left and right subclavian veins respectively.

SAQ 5

Why are the following changes commonly seen immediately post-splenectomy?

A. Thrombocytosis
B. Howell-Jolly bodies (red cell inclusions)

Lymph nodes are small bean-shaped structures which are found in clusters at junctions in the lymphatic circulatory system. The positions of some of the more important lymph nodes are shown in Figure 2.12.

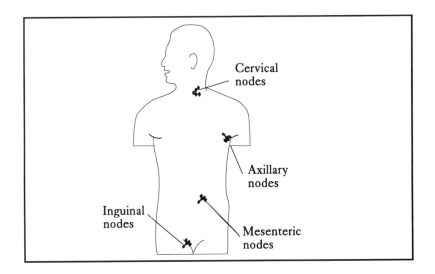

Figure 2.12 *The positions of some important lymph nodes*

Lymph enters the lymph node via a number of **afferent lymphatic vessels** and leaves via a single **efferent lymphatic vessel** as shown in Figure 2.13. The cortex of the lymph node contains numerous clusters of B lymphocytes called **lymphoid follicles**. Some of the lymphoid follicles contain a **germinal centre** where activated B lymphocytes proliferate in response to contact with foreign antigen.

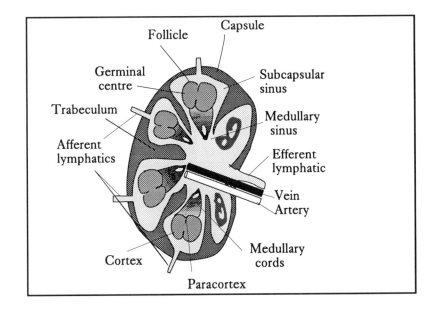

Figure 2.13 *The structure of a lymph node*

The paracortical region of the lymph node is populated by T lymphocytes which enter the node from the bloodstream. T lymphocytes leave the lymph node within a few hours unless they are activated by contact with antigen. The paracortical region is also rich in antigen-presenting cells. The medulla of the lymph node is rich in antibody-secreting plasma cells and macrophages.

Ontogeny of B Lymphocytes

The first step in the differentiation of a stem cell along the B lymphocyte line is the rearrangement of the immunoglobulin heavy chain genes as described in detail in Chapter 13. Successful rearrangement of the heavy chain genes permits the synthesis of IgM chains in the cytoplasm of the cell. As shown in Figure 2.14, the presence of **cytoplasmic μ chains** is the distinguishing feature of a

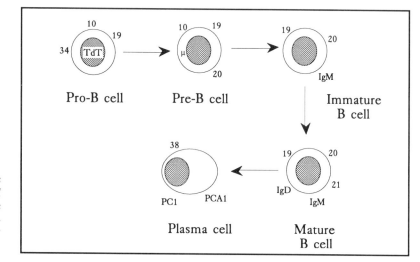

Figure 2.14 *B lymphocyte ontogeny. The numbers relate to surface markers which are detectable using monoclonal antibodies and have been codified as clusters of differentiation (CD) antigens eg CD19 is restricted to pre-B and mature B lymphocytes*

pre-B lymphocyte. Rearrangement of the immunoglobulin light chain genes permits the expression of monomeric IgM on the cell surface (sIgM). At this stage, the **immature B lymphocyte** is able to recognise and respond to antigen bound to its surface receptor. The **mature B lymphocyte** expresses both IgM and IgD receptors of identical specificity on its surface. Differentiation into a mature B lymphocyte occurs in the absence of antigenic stimulation. Contact with specific antigen triggers the activated B lymphocyte to proliferate and differentiate into **plasma cells** which synthesise and secrete monoclonal antibody of the specificity of the inducing antigen. A small number of lymphocytes revert to the quiescent state but are capable of mounting an extremely rapid response following further contact with the inducing antigen. These are known as **memory cells**. As described in Chapter 13, antigen dependent proliferation of B lymphocytes is accompanied by a phenomenon known as **class switching** ie the plasma cells are stimulated to synthesise immunoglobulin of identical antigenic specificity but of IgG, IgA or IgE subtype. Which immunoglobulin type is synthesised is regulated by T lymphocytes. Class switching results in the production of a range of immunoglobulins of identical antigenic specificity but varying biological function.

Ontogeny of T Lymphocytes

During foetal development, T lymphoid stem cells populate the subcapsular region of the thymus gland where, under the influence of epithelial nurse cells they proliferate and differentiate. The progeny of these lymphoid stem cells progress through the cortical and medullary regions of the thymus and, from there, enter the circulation as mature T lymphocytes. During their journey, the T lymphocytes acquire surface receptors which are responsible for the specificity of their function. The processes involved in T cell maturation and differentiation are described further below and in more detail in Chapter 13.

As shown in Figure 2.15, in the process of differentiation into a fully mature T lymphocyte, cortical T lymphoblasts progress through four distinct phases. The most primitive cortical T lymphoblasts

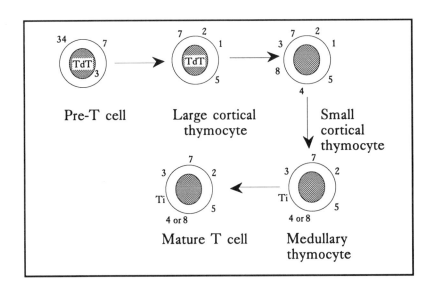

Figure 2.15 *T lymphocyte ontogeny. The numbers relate to surface markers which are detectable using monoclonal antibodies and have been codified as clusters of differentiation (CD) antigens eg CD7 is restricted to the T lymphocyte series*

possess the intranuclear enzyme TdT and express the surface marker CD7. The earliest events in the process of differentiation are the rearrangement of the T cell receptor genes and the expression of the adhesive molecule CD2. These markers of differentiation are associated with large cortical thymocytes. The next stage of differentiation involves the acquisition and expression of the **accessory molecules** CD4 and CD8. CD4 is responsible for recognition of MHC class II molecules while CD8 recognises MHC class I molecules. These accessory molecules play an important role in the selection of T lymphocytes within the thymus gland, a process explained in Chapter 13. Immature T lymphocytes in the thymic medulla express the antigen-specific T cell receptor complex (TiCD3) and therefore are capable of responding to foreign antigen which has been suitably processed and presented by macrophages. The final stage of maturation is marked by the loss of either CD4 or CD8 surface markers. Circulating T lymphocytes express either CD4 or CD8, never both.

Suggested Further Reading

Wickramasinghe, S.M. (1986). *Blood and Bone Marrow.* Edinburgh: Churchill Livingstone.

Hoffbrand, A.V. and Lewis, S.M. (1989) *Postgraduate Haematology.,* 3rd ed. Oxford: Butterworth-Heinemann.

Roitt, I.M. (1988) *Essential Immunology.* 6th ed. Oxford: Blackwell

Answers to Self-Assessment Questions

1. The liver. The bone marrow does not assume pre-eminence until 30 weeks gestation.

2. Erythropoietin synthesis is reduced in chronic renal failure.

3. B and C. Mountain dwellers do not have raised erythropoietin levels.

4. A and C. TGF–β and γ interferon are inhibitory. BFU-E is a red cell precursor.

5. Splenectomy causes the loss of the pooling and grooming functions of the spleen.

Nutritional Requirements for Haemopoiesis

Adequate nutrition is an essential requirement for the maintenance of normal bodily function, growth and repair. The nutritional requirements for optimal haemopoiesis generally coincide with those of the other cells of the body: there is no nutrient uniquely required for blood cell production. This chapter concentrates, however, on haematological aspects of nutrition.

Protein

Proteins are essential components of nearly all animal tissue. All of the huge variety of proteins found in living tissue are synthesised from the same twenty amino acids. Humans are incapable of synthesising nine of these amino acids and so must obtain these from the diet. In addition to its primary role, protein also provides about 10% of the daily requirement for energy. Diets which are extremely restricted in energy content eventually lead to loss of lean body mass as a result of protein oxidation.

Severe protein-energy malnutrition results in a condition called **kwashiorkor** which is characterised by oedema, hepatomegaly caused by fatty infiltration, cracking of the skin and hair loss or discolouration. The condition is most frequently seen nowadays in the Third World where drought and starvation unfortunately are still commonplace. Anaemia commonly is present in this condition but its aetiology is complex. Because kwashiorkor results from starvation conditions, deficiency of a wide range of other essential nutrients such as iron and folate almost always is present. The picture is complicated further by the presence of infections such as malaria which may have a haemolytic component.

Vitamins

Vitamin B_1 (Thiamine)

Thiamine is present naturally in products such as milk and eggs and is added to flour and breakfast cereals during their manufacture. The vitamin is involved in the extraction of energy by carbohydrate metabolism. The effects of vitamin B_1 deficiency are primarily neurological. In the absence of accompanying nutrient deficiency, anaemia seldom occurs. The only readily discernible haematological effect of vitamin B_1 deficiency is a rise in the levels of the enzyme transketolase and of pyruvate in red cells.

Vitamin B_2 (Riboflavin)

The most important natural dietary sources of vitamin B_2 are pulses, legumes, liver and kidney. Breakfast cereals commonly are fortified with the vitamin during their manufacture. Deficiency of vitamin B_2 is seen most commonly in severe malnutrition and is usually accompanied by other nutrient deficiencies. The haematological manifestations of vitamin B_2 deficiency include normocytic, normochromic anaemia, reduced red cell glutathione reductase activity, leucopaenia and, in severe cases, thrombocytopaenia.

Vitamin B_6 (Pyridoxine)

Vitamin B_6 occurs naturally in a variety of forms but all are derivatives of 2-methyl-3-hydroxy-5-hydroxymethylpyridine. It is widely distributed in foods of both plant and animal origin. The daily requirement for the vitamin is about 1.5 mg. Vitamin B_6 is required as a coenzyme in the synthesis of δ aminolaevulinic acid which is the first and rate-determining step in the synthesis of haem. Not surprisingly, therefore, deficiency of vitamin B_6 is associated with microcytic, hypochromic anaemia. Because of its widespread distribution in food, dietary deficiency of vitamin B_6 is rare.

Vitamin B_{12} (Cobalamin) and Folic Acid

The importance of vitamin B_{12} and folic acid in relation to haemopoiesis is described later in this chapter.

Vitamin C (Ascorbic Acid)

The most important sources of vitamin C are citrus fruits, potatoes, green vegetables and fortified fruit drinks. Vitamin C deficiency is called **scurvy** and, in developed countries, is seen mainly in association with a restricted diet eg in the elderly and in infants. In severe cases, anaemia, leucopaenia and, occasionally, thrombocytopaenia may be present. Vitamin C acts as a reducing agent and so increases

As described in the text, breakfast cereals commonly are fortified with vitamins and minerals during their manufacture. For example, an average (30 g) serving of corn flakes provides 30% of the recommended daily amount of vitamins B_1 (thiamine), B_2 (riboflavin), B_6 (pyridoxine), B_{12} (cobalamin), C (ascorbic acid) and iron.

iron absorption and also preserves folate during food preparation. Reduced plasma iron and folate deficiency commonly accompany deficiency of vitamin C.

Vitamin E (α Tocopherol)

Vitamin E is a lipid-soluble vitamin which is present in vegetable oils, eggs, whole-grain cereals and margarine. Deficiency is associated with low birth-weight or premature babies and malabsorptive states such as coeliac disease. Dietary deficiency is uncommon. Vitamin E acts as an antioxidant within the body; deficiency permits peroxidation of membrane lipids and results in red cell lysis.

Minerals

Iron

The importance of iron metabolism in the economy of the body is described later in this chapter.

Copper

Copper is widely distributed in food and is absorbed readily from the small intestine. The daily requirement for copper is about 2 mg and the typical United Kingdom diet contains at least 5 mg. Copper deficiency interferes with iron metabolism and leads to hypoferraemia.

Cobalt

Cobalt is required for the synthesis of vitamin B_{12} by bacteria. The element is present in most foods and is absorbed readily from the diet. Deficiency of cobalt is not a significant problem in man but causes a variety of neurological problems in farm animals.

Zinc

Zinc is present in both red cells and leucocytes. It probably is involved in free radical scavenging but its precise role remains obscure. Zinc deficiency is not associated with the development of anaemia but may predispose to bacterial and fungal infection.

Iron

The Role of Iron Within the Body

Iron is vital to the normal function of every cell of the body. Iron-containing compounds can be divided into two groups according to their role within the body: those which play a role in cellular metabolism and those which are required for iron transport and storage. Most of the iron-containing compounds which play a role in cellular metabolism contain the iron in the form of a haem group. The haem-containing compounds include **haemoglobin** and **myoglobin**, the oxygen carrying pigments of red cells and muscle respectively and the cytochromes which are a family of electron transport enzymes which play a variety of roles in oxidative metabolism. Iron compounds which do not contain a haem group also are important in cellular metabolism. Examples of such compounds include the enzymes nicotinamide adenine dinucleotide dehydrogenase (NADH) and succinic dehydrogenase.

Body Iron Distribution

A normal 70 kg male has a total body iron content of about 4 g. Almost three quarters of this is found in the form of the oxygen carriers haemoglobin and myoglobin, while most of the remainder is held in reserve in the body stores. The tiny proportion of total body iron which is found in the cytochromes belies their pivotal role in oxidative metabolism within the body. The approximate distribution of body iron is shown in Table 3.1.

Source	% of Total
Circulating haemoglobin	60
Body stores	25
Myoglobin	10
Bone marrow erythroblasts	4
Enzymes	1
Plasma iron	<0.1

Table 3.1 *Distribution of iron within the body*

Daily Iron Requirements

Iron has been described as a "one-way element" within the body. This means that iron is absorbed by the body from the diet but that no substantial mechanism for iron excretion exists. On the contrary, the body possesses elaborate mechanisms to prevent loss of iron. The level of body iron is maintained within normal limits by feedback control of absorption: absorption is increased in iron deficiency but decreased when body stores are replete.

In the normal steady state, daily iron requirements consist of the amount required to replace the small amount lost in sweat, tears, urine and faeces plus the amount required for expansion of the blood volume with growth. The actual requirement varies considerably with age, sex and body weight as shown in Table 3.2. The greatest daily iron requirement is found in menstruating females and during pregnancy. Menstruating females shed between 30 and 60 ml of blood in each cycle. This contains between 15 and 30 mg of iron and so imposes considerable strain on body iron stores, especially in adolescence when growth requirements are also high. The very high iron requirement in pregnancy consists of three components: the growth requirement of the foetus and placenta; the expansion in maternal blood volume; and haemorrhage at delivery. The figure quoted is an average value though, clearly, actual daily requirements vary according to the stage of pregnancy.

SAQ 1
Why is red meat a rich dietary source of iron?

	Daily Losses	Growth Req.	Total (mg)
Infant <1 year	0.5	0	0.5
Child <12 years	0.5	0.5	1.0
Male <18 years	0.9	0.9	1.8
Mens. female	1.9	0.5	2.4
Male >18 years	0.9	0	0.9
Pregnancy	0.9	2.6	3.5
Post-menopause	0.9	0	0.9

Table 3.2 *Daily iron requirements at different stages of life*

Iron Absorption

A normal, mixed daily diet in the United Kingdom contains about 18 mg of iron, far in excess of normal body requirements. The main dietary sources are liver, red meat, some green vegetables such as

Only about 10% of dietary iron is absorbed, mainly because much of the digestion of bound iron does not occur until the site of iron absorption has been passed.

Iron can only cross cell membranes as Fe^{2+} but is stored and transported as Fe^{3+}. Thus, a double redox reaction ($Fe^{3+} \rightarrow Fe^{2+} \rightarrow Fe^{3+}$) is required during iron absorption, transport and storage.

SAQ 2

What is the approximate iron content of a unit of blood for transfusion (volume 400 ml)?

spinach, cereals (which are often supplemented with iron during processing) and fish. Dietary iron falls into one of two categories: inorganic iron which mainly is present in cereals and vegetables and haem iron which is found in the haemoglobin and myoglobin of meat products.

Inorganic iron in food is released by the action of proteolytic enzymes and hydrochloric acid in the stomach. The low pH environment of the stomach encourages reduction of ferric ions (Fe^{3+}) to ferrous ions (Fe^{2+}), which are absorbed more readily. Iron is absorbed maximally from the duodenum and upper jejunum as shown in Figure 3.1. Absorption of inorganic iron is enhanced by any factor which increases its solubility. For example, ferrous compounds are generally more soluble than their ferric counterparts, so the presence of reducing agents such as ascorbic acid (vitamin C) improve absorption. Similarly, chelating agents such as fructose, glucose and succinate which form soluble complexes with iron also increase absorption. Conversely, inorganic iron absorption is retarded by the presence of substances which tend to decrease its solubility such as phosphates and phytates which are present in cereal products and also by alkaline pancreatic secretions.

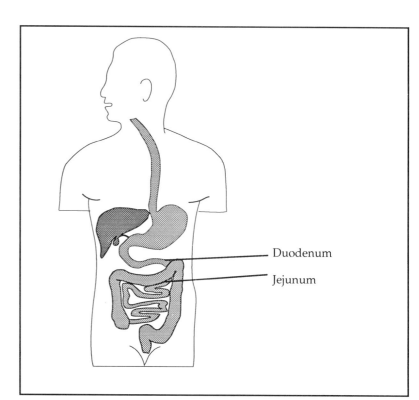

Figure 3.1 *Site of maximal absorption of iron from the diet under physiological conditions*

The iron in animal products is absorbed by a different, and as yet improperly understood, mechanism. The luminal factors described above have much less influence on the absorption of haem iron. Haem groups are absorbed intact by the intestinal mucosal cell, and subsequently broken down for release into the portal circulation.

Control of Iron Absorption

As already described, the body possesses no substantial physiological mechanism for the excretion of excess iron. Toxic accumulation of iron is prevented by careful regulation of iron absorption from the gut. The precise mechanism of this regulation remains controversial, but the most widely accepted model is the **mucosal block theory**.

When the intestinal mucosal cell is formed in the crypts of Lieberkühn, ferritin - a storage form of iron - is incorporated within the cell. The amount of ferritin incorporated is directly proportional to the body stores of iron at the time of synthesis of the mucosal cell. The intracellular ferritin is thought either to block absorption of iron from the gut or to interfere with the release of absorbed iron into the bloodstream. Thus, when body iron stores are low, the mucosal cells contain relatively little ferritin and absorption of iron from the gut is uninhibited. Conversely, in the presence of iron overload, high ferritin levels within the intestinal mucosae result in gross inhibition of absorption (Figure 3.2). Intestinal mucosal cells are relatively short-lived: they are constantly sloughed off into the

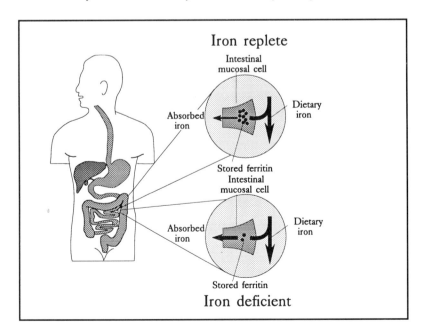

Figure 3.2 *The mucosal block model for the control of the rate of iron absorption from the diet*

faeces and replaced. This process provides a constantly updated indicator of body iron stores and acts as an effective and sensitive control mechanism for absorption of iron from the gut.

The rate of iron absorption also is augmented in response to the increased red cell turnover in haemolytic conditions irrespective of the state of the body iron stores. The mechanism of this response is unknown.

Absorption of iron from the diet in physiological amounts is an active, energy-consuming process. Control of absorption is only effective in the presence of physiological amounts of iron. In the presence of much higher iron concentrations such as those encountered during iron replacement therapy, iron absorption occurs by passive diffusion across the gut wall and is not dependent upon body iron status. For this reason, iron tablets which are often thought of as innocuous can be deadly if ingested in large amounts, for example by an inquisitive toddler.

Iron Transport

Iron absorbed from the duodenum is released into the bloodstream where it is bound to a specific carrier protein called **transferrin.** Transferrin is a β globulin with a molecular weight of 74,000 which can carry up to two ferric ions (Fe^{3+}) per molecule. Iron is transported to the bone marrow bound to transferrin where it is transferred to developing erythroblasts which carry specific transferrin receptors on their surfaces. The receptor-transferrin complex is internalised by the erythroblast, the iron is removed for utilisation in haem synthesis and the receptor and **apotransferrin** returned to the cell surface. Diferric transferrin binds with greater affinity than monoferric transferrin to the specific surface receptors and so delivers iron more effectively to developing erythroblasts. Ferrokinetic studies have shown that transferrin-bound iron has a rapid turnover (half-life of about 90 minutes).

Normal plasma contains sufficient transferrin to bind about 300 μg of iron per dl. This figure is called the **total iron binding capacity (TIBC)** and is one of the useful measures in the assessment of iron status. Typically, plasma transferrin is about 33% saturated with iron. The relationship between TIBC and % saturation in various disease states is described in Chapter 5.

Newly absorbed iron represents only about 5% of the iron utilised by developing erythroblasts for haem synthesis. About 90% of the iron required each day for this purpose is derived by recycling iron from the haemoglobin of senescent red cells. The shortfall in iron requirement is met by continuous slow release from the body iron stores.

It was once believed that an important ancillary method of iron acquisition in erythroblasts involved the direct "feeding" of ferritin to the cell by adjacent macrophages, a phenomenon known as **rhopheocytosis**. This phenomenon is now considered to be of doubtful physiological relevance.

Iron Storage

About one quarter of the total body iron is in storage and is found mainly in the liver, tissue macrophages and developing marrow erythroblasts. Storage iron is present in two forms: **ferritin** and **haemosiderin**. Ferritin is formed by the combination of ferric ions and the protein apoferritin and has a molecular weight of about 450,000. The molecule is composed of 24 polypeptide subunits which are clustered together to form a hollow spherical structure with a diameter of about 5 nm. The stored iron is present as hydrated ferric phosphate and forms a central core in the hollow of the protein sphere. Typically, ferritin contains about 25% of iron by weight. About two thirds of body iron stores are present as ferritin. Different tissues are associated with slightly different forms of ferritin or **isoferritins** which vary somewhat in their chemical and physical properties. The differences are explained by the fact that there are three different types of polypeptide subunit, and the relative proportion of each varies between the different isoferritins. All isoferritins share the same basic molecular shape, however. Plasma ferritin is thought to be derived from tissue macrophages and its estimation provides the single most useful indicator of iron status.

The other form of storage iron, haemosiderin, is not a single substance but a variety of different, amorphous, iron-protein complexes. Typically, it contains about 37% of iron by weight. Haemosiderin may represent ferritin in various stages of degradation.

The most common method of assessing body iron stores involves the measurement of serum ferritin concentration. This provides an adequate guide to the state of the iron stores in most cases. However, serum ferritin is an **acute phase protein** ie its concentration may be markedly increased in the presence of conditions such as rheumatoid arthritis and malignancy. In such cases, the serum ferritin concentration no longer reflects body iron stores accurately.

A definitive estimation of body iron stores requires a liver biopsy. The iron content of the biopsy sample can be assessed by dehydration and acid digestion of the tissue, followed by colorimetric assay using bathophenanthroline sulphonate. This technique is reserved for suspected cases of iron-overload when it can be combined with microscopic examination to assess tissue damage.

Vitamin B$_{12}$

Vitamin B$_{12}$ was isolated and crystallised from the liver for the first time as cyanocobalamin in 1948. The vitamin can exist in a variety of different chemical forms which, together, constitute the family of **cobalamins**. The cobalamins are organometallic complexes comprising three major structures: a corrin nucleus and, bound at right angles to the nucleus, a nucleotide and a variable chemical group. The structure of the corrin nucleus bears comparison with that of haem as shown in Figure 3.3. It consists of four pyrrole rings with a cobaltous ion (Co$^+$) instead of a ferrous ion (Fe^{2+}) at the centre. The nucleotide comprises a base (5,6-dimethylbenzimidazole) bound to a phosphorylated sugar (ribose-3-phosphate). The differences between the various cobalamins lie with the variable chemical group which is bound to the central cobalt ion (designated X in Figure 3.3).

In the physiologically active cobalamins, the variant chemical group is either a 5′-deoxyadenosyl group or a methyl group and the cobalt ion is in the Co(I) oxidation state. **5′-deoxyadenosylcobalamin** is the predominant form of the vitamin encountered in the liver while **methylcobalamin** predominates in the plasma. Both 5′-deoxyadenosylcobalamin and methylcobalamin are unstable compounds which, on exposure to light, rapidly denature to form **hydroxocobalamin** which contains a cobalt ion in the Co(III) oxidation state. Hydroxocobalamin is the main dietary form of the vitamin. **Cyanocobalamin** is a stable synthetic form of the vitamin.

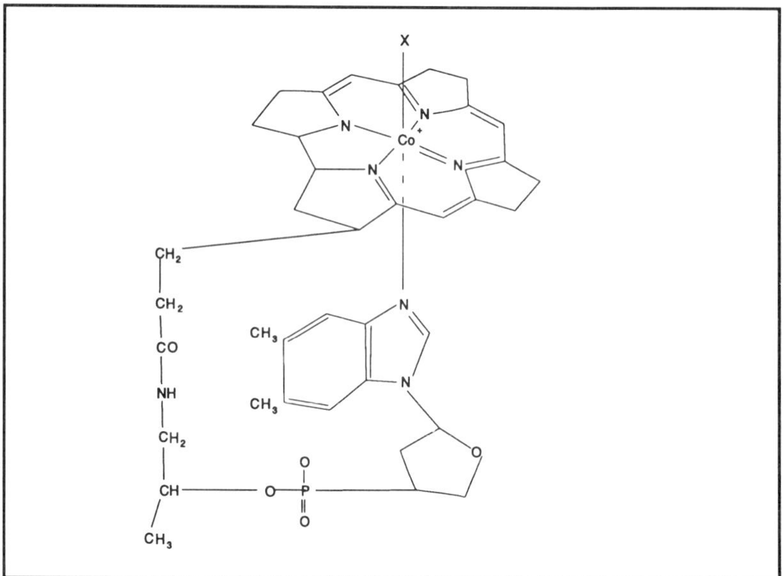

Certain microorganisms have an absolute requirement for exogenous vitamin B$_{12}$ for growth. This fact has been exploited in the microbiological assay of the vitamin in serum. If growth conditions are arranged in such a way that the only source of vitamin B$_{12}$ is that from the test serum, then the rate of microbial growth must be proportional to the concentration of vitamin B$_{12}$ in the test serum.

Examples of suitable test organisms include *Lactobacillus leichmannii* and *Euglena gracilis*.

This method of assay has been almost completely replaced by radio-isotopic methods.

Figure 3.3 *Chemical structure of the cobalamins*

The Role of Vitamin B$_{12}$ Within the Body

In bacteria, vitamin B$_{12}$ is involved in a relatively large number of metabolic reactions but, in humans, it is required as coenzyme for only two:

- **conversion of L-methylmalonyl Coenzyme A to succinyl Coenzyme A.** 5'-deoxyadenosylcobalamin is required as a coenzyme in this isomerisation reaction which is involved in the catabolism of a wide range of substances such as cholesterol, odd chain fatty acids, the amino acids methionine and threonine and the pyrimidines uracil and thymine.

- **methylation of homocysteine to methionine.** This reaction requires both methylcobalamin as a co-enzyme and N-5-methyltetrahydrofolate as the methyl donor, and is important in the intracellular synthesis of folate coenzymes.

Daily Vitamin B$_{12}$ Requirements and Body Stores

Vitamin B$_{12}$ is synthesised exclusively by microorganisms, the only source available to man is dietary. The main dietary sources are animal products such as liver, kidney, red meat, eggs, shellfish and dairy products. A typical mixed UK diet contains between 5 and 30 µg of vitamin B$_{12}$ per day, depending on the quantity of meat included. Diets which exclude all animal products contain no intrinsic vitamin B$_{12}$. However, even strict vegans obtain small amounts of vitamin B$_{12}$ from their diet as a result of bacterial contamination of their food. Vitamin B$_{12}$ is relatively heat-stable; little loss occurs in cooking.

Typical daily losses of vitamin B$_{12}$ are between 1 µg and 4 µg. The vitamin is lost primarily in the urine and faeces. Since, normally, there is no consumption of vitamin B$_{12}$ within the body, the daily requirement matches daily losses. Thus, a typical UK mixed diet provides more than enough vitamin B$_{12}$ to meet requirements.

Normally, the body stores about 3-4 mg of vitamin B$_{12}$, primarily in the liver. This would be sufficient to meet the requirement for vitamin B$_{12}$ for about 3 years if dietary intake ceased or if the ability to absorb the vitamin was lost.

Vitamin B$_{12}$ Absorption

There are two mechanisms for the absorption of vitamin B$_{12}$, although one is of far greater physiological importance than the other.

The more important mechanism is an active process which occurs in the ileum (Figure 3.4). Vitamin B$_{12}$ in food is liberated by gastric and duodenal proteolytic enzymes and rapidly complexes in a 1:1 ratio with a substance called **intrinsic factor.** Intrinsic factor is a glycoprotein of molecular weight 45,000 which is synthesised and secreted by gastric parietal cells. The IF:B$_{12}$ complex then progresses to the ileum where it attaches to specific receptors on the brush border of the ileal mucosal cells in the terminal ileum. Binding of the IF:B$_{12}$ complex to its specific receptor is via the intrinsic factor part of the complex and requires the presence of calcium ions and a neutral pH. The vitamin B$_{12}$ is internalised by the ileal mucosal cell and released from its complex with intrinsic factor. After a delay of about 6 hours, the newly absorbed vitamin B$_{12}$ is

One of the key experiments in the discovery of the aetiology of pernicious anaemia was performed in 1927 in Boston, Massachusetts, by William Castle. The experiment was divided into two phases:

In phase one, pernicious anaemia patients were fed on a diet of lean beef steak as the only source of animal protein. In phase two, lean beef steak was fed to healthy volunteers, their stomach contents recovered, and then administered to the test subjects. Lean beef steak fed directly had no effect on the anaemia whereas the partly digested stomach contents elicited a reticulocyte response.

Castle concluded from this experiment that some **intrinsic factor** in the gastric juice was acting in concert with some **extrinsic factor** in the beef steak. The extrinsic factor is now known as vitamin B$_{12}$, the name intrinsic factor is still in use today.

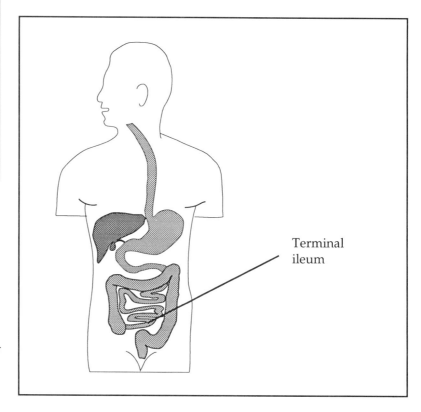

Terminal ileum

Figure 3.4 *Site of maximal absorption of vitamin B$_{12}$. For the purposes of clarity, the ileum is shown considerably shorter and less convoluted than reality*

released into the portal circulation. The intrinsic factor probably is digested within the ileal mucosal cells: it certainly is not recirculated and does not appear in the portal circulation. Because of the finite number of $IF:B_{12}$ receptors, absorption of vitamin B_{12} by this mechanism is saturable: a maximum of about 2 µg can be absorbed from one meal, regardless of its vitamin B_{12} content. After each exposure to vitamin B_{12}, ileal cells are unresponsive to further exposure for up to 6 hours.

The other mechanism for the absorption of dietary vitamin B_{12} is a passive process and is not restricted to the terminal ileum: it occurs along the entire length of the jejunum and ileum. This mechanism does not make a major contribution to total intestinal absorption of vitamin B_{12} under physiological conditions.

Excretion of vitamin B_{12} occurs mainly via the biliary system. A proportion of this vitamin is reabsorbed from the bile during its passage through the gut. This salvage mechanism is known as the **enterohepatic circulation** of vitamin B_{12}.

Vitamin B_{12} Transport

There are three specific vitamin B_{12} transport proteins normally present in plasma which are known as the **transcobalamins** (TCI-TCIII).

The physiologically important transcobalamin is TCII which is a β globulin with a molecular weight of 38,000. It is synthesised primarily in the liver and ileum and binds to vitamin B_{12} in a 1:1 ratio. The $TCII:B_{12}$ complex binds to specific surface receptors on developing blood cells in the bone marrow. The receptor:$TCII:B_{12}$ complex is internalised by endocytosis and the vitamin B_{12} released by hydrolysis. The TCII is not reutilised. A similar process for obtaining vitamin B_{12} is known to occur in other tissues. The vitamin B_{12} binding capacity of TCII is about 1 mg/l but normally it circulates with only about 3-4% of its binding sites occupied. Typically, TCII binds newly absorbed vitamin B_{12} and delivers it rapidly to developing tissues such as the bone marrow. The plasma half-life of the TCII:vitamin B_{12} complex is about 12 hours. Congenital absence of TCII causes a severe megaloblastic anaemia within weeks of birth.

Transcobalamins I and III are α globulins which are synthesised by granulocytes and have a molecular weight of about 58,000. They belong to a family of vitamin B_{12}-binding proteins known as **R-binders** which are present in a range of body secretions such as gastric juice, milk, bile and saliva. There is an increasing body of evidence which suggests that the R-binders are isoproteins which differ from each other only in their carbohydrate content and degree of saturation with vitamin B_{12}. In contrast to TCII, TCI and TCIII do not readily release vitamin B_{12} to developing cells. The plasma half-life of the TCI:vitamin B_{12} complex is about 9-12 days. The physiological function of TCI remains to be determined. R-binders have been shown to promote uptake of cobalamins by mitochondria and may also have a role in the binding of physiologically inert cobalamins in the plasma. About 80-90% of the vitamin B_{12} present in plasma circulates bound to TCI. Congenital absence of TCI causes no physiological impairment.

> **SAQ 3**
>
> Why is a markedly raised serum vitamin B_{12} concentration a common finding at presentation in chronic myeloid leukaemia (CML)?

Folates

The parent of the folate family of compounds is folic acid (pteroylglutamic acid) which has the basic structure shown in Figure 3.5. Humans are incapable of synthesising pteridine rings so all of the requirement for folate must be met from the diet. The most common dietary forms of folate differ from the parent compound in three important respects:

- they exist in reduced form as dihydro- or tetrahydrofolates. The additional hydrogen atoms are carried by the pteridine rings in positions 5-8 as shown in Figure 3.5.

- they carry a single-carbon group bonded to either the N5 or N10 nitrogen atom. This single-carbon group can exist in three different oxidation states: as a fully reduced methyl group (CH_3), as an oxidised formyl group (CHO) or formimino group (CHNH) or as an intermediate oxidation state methylene group (CH_2).

- most are conjugated with a series of glutamate residues, and are known as folate polyglutamates.

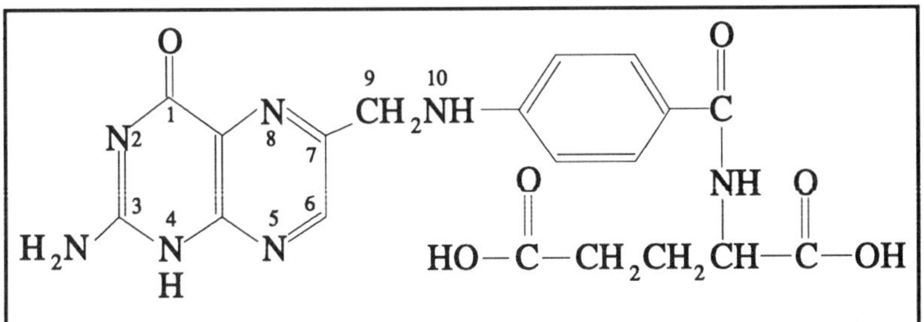

Figure 3.5 *The chemical structure of folic acid*

The Role of Folates Within the Body

The various forms of folate function as single-carbon group donor-acceptors in a variety of biosynthetic reactions as shown below. Many of these reactions are involved in the synthesis of DNA and RNA as discussed later in this chapter.

- **synthesis of methionine**. The regeneration of methionine from homocysteine involves the donation of a methyl group from N-5-methyl-tetrahydrofolate and requires the presence of vitamin B_{12} as methylcobalamin as coenzyme.

- **pyrimidine synthesis**. The methylation of deoxy-uridine-5'-monophosphate (dUMP) to thymidine-5'-monophosphate (dTMP) is the rate-limiting step in DNA synthesis and requires the presence of the folate coenzyme N-5,10-methylenetetrahydrofolate.

- **purine synthesis**. The synthesis of the purine ring is a multi-step affair. Two of the required reactions are formylations which provide the carbon atoms C2 and C8. The formyl group donor in each case is a folate coenzyme (N-5,10-methylenetetrahydrofolate or N-10-formyltetrahydrofolate).

- **conversion of serine into glycine**. This reaction differs from the above reactions in that tetrahydrofolate acts as an *acceptor* of a single-carbon group, and is converted into the folate coenzyme N-5,10-methylenetetrahydrofolate in the process.

SAQ 4

Which of the following substances are purines and which are pyrimidines?

A. Adenine
B. Cytosine
C. Uracil
D. Guanine
E. Thymine

- **histidine catabolism**. The catabolism of histidine involves its conversion into N-formiminoglutamic acid (FIGLU) which is subsequently converted into glutamate by the donation of the formimino group to tetrahydrofolate. This reaction was the basis for the now obsolete FIGLU test for folate deficiency.

Daily Folate Requirements and Body Stores

Losses of folate amount to about 100 µg per day, mainly in the faeces, urine, sweat and desquamated skin cells. Faeces contain a relatively large amount of both vitamin B_{12} and folate but these represent the biosynthetic activities of the microbial flora of the gut, rather than losses from body stores. In order to maintain body stores, the total daily requirement must match losses. Thus, the normal adult daily requirement for folate is about 100 µg.

Folates are present to some extent in most foods but liver, eggs, leafy vegetables, whole grains and yeast are particularly rich sources. Folate in food is extremely sensitive to heat: cooking can reduce the folate content of food by as much as 95%! Losses are particularly severe when cooking involves prolonged boiling in a relatively large volume of water. A typical UK mixed diet may contain as much as 700 µg of folate per day but injudicious food preparation can reduce this amount to perilously close to the minimum required to meet the daily requirement.

Typical body stores of folate in a normal, healthy adult are about 10 mg and are located mainly in the liver. Thus, if dietary folate intake or intestinal absorption ceased, the body stores would become exhausted in between three and four months.

Folate Absorption and Transport

Folates are absorbed maximally from the upper jejunum (Figure 3.1) but probably are absorbed to some extent throughout the small intestine. Folate polyglutamates must be digested to form monoglutamates before absorption. This digestion is mediated by the enzyme **γ-glutamyl conjugase** which is present in jejunal mucosal cells. Absorption of folic acid or folate monoglutamates is efficient and rapid. Within the jejunal mucosal cells, absorbed folates are

> In much the same way as *Lactobacillus leichmannii* can be used to assay serum vitamin B_{12} concentration, *Lactobacillus casei* can be used to determine the concentration of folate in serum.

converted into N-5-methyltetrahydrofolate and released into the portal bloodstream. Plasma folate circulates freely or loosely bound to a variety of plasma proteins. There is some evidence that a specific plasma folate transport protein exists and that its concentration is increased by folate deficiency but its physiological significance is unknown.

Once inside the developing blood cell, N-5-methyltetrahydrofolate is converted to tetrahydrofolate and reconjugated to the polyglutamate form. Conjugation facilitates the metabolic activities of folates and prevents leakage back into the plasma.

Role of Vitamin B_{12} and Folate in DNA and RNA Synthesis

Optimal DNA and RNA synthesis requires a ready supply of the purines adenosine-5′-diphosphate (ADP) and guanosine-5′-diphosphate (GDP) and the pyrimidines cytidine-5′-diphosphate (CDP) and uridine-5′-diphosphate (UDP) as shown in Figure 3.6.

Purines and pyrimidines are nitrogenous **bases**. The attachment of a β-D-ribose or β–D-2-deoxyribose sugar group to one of the nitrogen atoms of the base results in the formation of a **nucleoside**. The addition of one or more phosphate groups to the sugar group of a nucleoside results in the formation of a **nucleotide**.

Base	Nucleoside	Nucleotide
adenine	adenosine	AMP, ADP, ATP
guanine	guanosine	GMP, GDP, GTP
cytosine	cytidine	CMP, CDP, CTP
uracil	uridine	UMP, UDP, UTP
thymine	thymidine	dTMP, dTTP
orotic acid	orotidine	OMP

Nucleotides which include deoxyribose are designated with a d eg dTMP. The monophosphate form of a nucleotide can be designated as an -ylic acid eg UMP is also known as uridylic acid or uridylate.

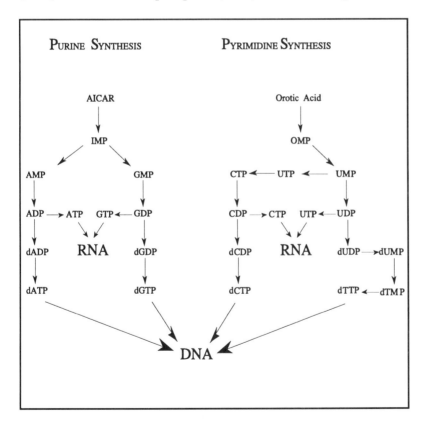

Figure 3.6 *DNA and RNA synthesis.*
AICAR - amino imidazole carboxamide ribotide
IMP - inosine monophosphate
AMP - adenosine-5′-monophosphate
(D - diphosphate, T - triphosphate)
GMP - gaunosine-5′–monophosphate
UMP - uridine-5′-monophosphate
CDP - cytidine-5′-diphosphate
dADP - deoxyadenosine-5′-diphosphate
dTMP - deoxythymidine-5′-monophosphate

As described earlier, two of the steps involved in purine synthesis are formylation reactions which require the presence of the folate coenzymes N-5,10-methylenetetrahydrofolate and 10-formyl-tetrahydrofolate. The methylation of deoxyuridine-5'-mono-phosphate (deoxyuridylate, dUMP) to form deoxythymidine-5'-monophosphate (deoxythymidylate, dTMP) is the rate-limiting reaction in DNA synthesis and requires the presence of the folate coenzyme N-5,10-methylenetetrahydrofolate.

It is the cycling of folic acid between its various coenzyme forms which unifies the seemingly disparate biochemical reactions in which vitamin B_{12} and folic acid are involved within the body as shown in Figure 3.7 and described in detail below.

SAQ 5

Why is liver a rich dietary source of vitamin B_{12}, folic acid and iron?

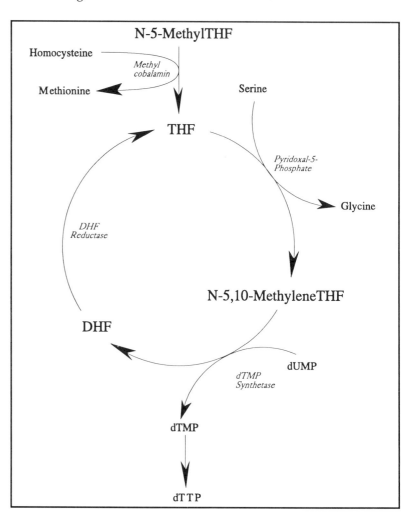

Figure 3.7 *The role of vitamin B_{12} and folic acid coenzymes in DNA synthesis*

As described above, dietary folate is absorbed in the jejunum and released into the portal circulation as N-5-methyltetrahydrofolate monoglutamate. This form is taken up by dividing cells and reconjugated to the polyglutamate form. N-5-methyltetrahydrofolate cannot be conjugated with glutamate, first it must donate its methyl group for the methylation of homocysteine to yield methionine and, in the process, form tetrahydrofolate monoglutamate. The methylation of homocysteine requires the presence of methylcobalamin as a coenzyme. In the absence of vitamin B_{12}, absorbed folate cannot be converted to a metabolically active form. The result is failure of DNA synthesis and the development of megaloblastic anaemia as described in Chapter 4. This is known as the **methyltetrahydrofolate trap.**

The tetrahydrofolate formed as a by-product of the above reaction acts as a cofactor with pyridoxal-5'-phosphate in the conversion of serine into glycine. The role of the tetrahydrofolate is to act as an acceptor of a single carbon unit (a methylene group) from the serine. The methylene group forms a bridge between the two nitrogen atoms at positions 5 and 10 on the tetrahydrofolate, forming N-5,10-methylenetetrahydrofolate.

N-5,10-methylenetetrahydrofolate acts as a methyl donor for the methylation of dUMP to form dTMP and, in the process, is converted to dihydrofolate. Deficiency of folate also results in impaired DNA synthesis and the development of megaloblastic anaemia.

The folate cycle is completed by the reduction of dihydrofolate to tetrahydrofolate by the enzyme dihydrofolate reductase.

Suggested Further Reading

Chaney, S.G. (1992). Principles of Nutrition I: Macronutrients. In Devlin, T.M. (ed.) *Textbook of Biochemistry with Clinical Correlations.* New York: Wiley-Liss.

Chaney, S.G. (1992). Principles of Nutrition II: Micronutrients. In Devlin, T.M. (ed.) *Textbook of Biochemistry with Clinical Correlations.* New York: Wiley-Liss.

Tomkins, A. (1990). Nutrition in Clinical Medicine. In Souhami, R.L. and Moxham, J. (eds.) *Medicine.* Edinburgh: Churchill Livingstone.

Answers to Self-Assessment Questions

1. Red meat is rich in myoglobin.

2. 400 ml of blood contains about 200 mg of iron.

3. The massive granulocytosis of chronic myeloid leukaemia causes an increased release of transcobalamin I and III.

4. Adenine and guanine are purines. Cytosine, uracil and thymine are pyrimidines.

5. Liver is the major storage organ for all three nutrients.

Megaloblastic Anaemias

The term megaloblastic anaemia refers to a group of panhypoplastic disorders which are characterised by retardation of DNA synthesis. RNA synthesis, however, proceeds at a normal rate. The resulting asynchrony between nuclear and cytoplasmic maturation in developing cells is responsible for the distinctive morphological and biochemical features of the megaloblastic anaemias.

The name megaloblastic anaemia is a misleading title for this group of disorders because all dividing cells are afflicted: anaemia is but one of a wide range of manifestations of this group of disorders. However, the term is well established and so will continue to be used in this book.

Most megaloblastic anaemias are caused by a deficiency of either vitamin B_{12} or folic acid or sometimes both. A number of uncommon exceptions exist where the cause of the disorder is not attributable to haematinic deficiency.

Vitamin B_{12} Deficiency

Causes of Vitamin B_{12} Deficiency

Deficiency of vitamin B_{12}, in common with deficiency of all nutrients, can result from inadequate dietary intake, intestinal malabsorption, increased requirements which cannot be met from the diet or failure of utilisation of absorbed vitamin.

Inadequate Dietary Intake

Deficiency of vitamin B_{12} attributable solely to inadequate dietary intake is uncommon for three main reasons:

- vitamin B_{12} is present in a wide range of readily available foodstuffs.

Anaemia can be defined as a reduced oxygen-carrying capacity due to a fall in the haemoglobin concentration.

The reference ranges for haemoglobin concentration and red cell count vary with age and sex:

Full-term cord blood

RBC	$4.0\text{-}5.6 \times 10^{12}/l$
Hb	13.6-19.6 g/dl

10 year old child

RBC	$4.2\text{-}5.2 \times 10^{12}/l$
Hb	11.5-14.8 g/dl

Adult male

RBC	$4.6\text{-}6.5 \times 10^{12}/l$
Hb	13.5-17.5 g/dl

Adult female

RBC	$3.9\text{-}5.6 \times 10^{12}/l$
Hb	11.5-16.0 g/dl

Other important causes of variation in these parameters include ethnic origin, geographic location, diurnal variation, pregnancy, exercise, smoking and alcohol.

- vitamin B_{12} is relatively heat-stable: it is not destroyed by injudicious cooking.

- body stores of vitamin B_{12} are sufficient to meet the needs of the body for at least 3 years following complete cessation of dietary intake or intestinal absorption.

Dietary deficiency of vitamin B_{12} is restricted to vegans who eschew all animal and dairy products. Inadequate diet, however, frequently contributes to the rapid development of vitamin B_{12} deficiency attributable mainly to other causes.

Malabsorption of Vitamin B_{12}

Malabsorption of vitamin B_{12} is the most common cause of deficiency. A wide range of abnormalities exist which cause malabsorption of this vitamin:

- lack of intrinsic factor

- gastrointestinal disease

- drug-induced malabsorption

Lack of Intrinsic Factor

The most common cause of vitamin B_{12} deficiency in Northern Europeans is **pernicious anaemia** which is characterised by achlorhydria and a failure of gastric parietal cells to synthesise intrinsic factor. The disease is uncommon below the age of 45 years except, for as yet unexplained reasons, in black American and South African women in whom earlier onset is relatively frequent. The disease is more common in women than in men and shows an association with blood group A.

About 90% of individuals with pernicious anaemia have cytotoxic IgG antibodies directed against gastric parietal cells or intrinsic factor demonstrable in their serum. In about 75% of these the antibody also is present in gastric juice. Polyclonal IgG or IgA antibodies directed against intrinsic factor are demonstrable in the serum and gastric juice of about 50% of cases of pernicious anaemia. These

The value of many haematological parameters fluctuates within an individual during the course of the day. This phenomenon is entirely normal and is known as **diurnal variation**.

The haemoglobin concentration and red cell count tend to be higher in the morning than in the evening. The platelet count and neutrophil count peak in the middle of the afternoon. The eosinophil count is at its lowest in the late morning and peaks just after midnight. Interestingly, these trends tend to be reversed in night-shift workers.

anti-intrinsic factor antibodies act in one of two ways: they either prevent the binding of vitamin B_{12} to intrinsic factor (type I antibody) or they inhibit absorption of the intrinsic factor:vitamin B_{12} complex (type II antibody). Type II antibodies are only found in association with type I antibodies.

Antibodies directed against gastric parietal cells are demonstrable in a wide range of autoimmune conditions. About 30% of close relatives of people with pernicious anaemia also have these antibodies. Thus, the existence of parietal cell antibodies does not necessarily signify the existence of pernicious anaemia, nor does it seem to presage its development. Pernicious anaemia is associated with an increased incidence of autoimmune thyroid disease, rheumatoid arthritis and gastric carcinoma.

A rare juvenile form of pernicious anaemia exists which is associated with congenital deficiency of intrinsic factor or the synthesis of a dysfunctional variant of intrinsic factor.

Gastrointestinal Disease

Of this group of causes of vitamin B_{12} deficiency, the most obvious follows surgical removal of the source of intrinsic factor or the site of absorption of the vitamin.

Total gastrectomy is associated with depletion of the body stores of vitamin B_{12} and, in the absence of supplementation, the development of megaloblastic anaemia within 5 years of surgery. The anaemia frequently is complicated by the presence of iron deficiency which also commonly follows gastrectomy.

Partial gastrectomy involves removal of part of the stomach and refashioning the junction with the gut. In one variant of this operation, an anastomosis of the stomach remnant and the jejunum is fashioned, leaving the duodenum as an afferent blind loop. The normal duodenum is not colonised by bacteria but in these conditions of stasis, bacterial growth is favoured and the loop becomes heavily colonised. These bacteria utilise considerable quantities of vitamin B_{12} which they derive from the gut, effectively leading to reduced availability of the vitamin in the terminal ileum. This malabsorptive state is known as the **stagnant** or **blind loop syndrome**. Bacterial overgrowth also occurs in ileal diverticulae, with similar results.

Pernicious anaemia was described first by Thomas Addison in 1855 as a severe anaemia of unknown cause but uniformly fatal outcome.

The first real progress in the treatment of pernicious anaemia was made by George Minot 70 years later. Minot discovered that the inclusion of about 300 g of lightly cooked liver in the daily diet elicited a reticulocyte response and a partial recovery of the haemoglobin concentration.

We now know that eating large amounts of liver provides massive doses of vitamin B_{12} which are absorbed from the gut by passive diffusion. Modern therapy consists of regular injections of hydroxocobalamin.

Because of advances in the pharmacological treatment of gastric, peptic and duodenal ulcers, total and partial gastrectomy is performed much less often than in the past.

Ileal resection or **ileostomy** involving removal or bypass of the terminal ileum predisposes strongly to the development of vitamin B_{12} deficiency.

Generalised malabsorption of nutrients from the diet is a feature of intestinal disorders such as **Crohn's disease** (regional ileitis). Crohn's disease is a granulomatous disease which, most commonly, affects the terminal ileum and ascending colon. It is a disease of early adulthood and largely is confined to developed countries. Haematological complications of Crohn's disease include malabsorption of iron, folic acid and vitamin B_{12} leading to iron deficiency and megaloblastic anaemia. The anaemia frequently is exacerbated by chronic bleeding of the inflamed ileal mucosae. In rare cases, malabsorption of vitamin K can lead to functional deficiency of the vitamin K-dependent coagulation factors which aggravates the haemorrhagic problems.

In contrast to the generalised malabsorptive states, the **Imerslund-Gräsbeck syndrome** is characterised by selective malabsorption of the intrinsic factor:vitamin B_{12} complex by the ileal mucosae. The condition is inherited as an autosomal recessive trait and is associated with the development of megaloblastic anaemia due to vitamin B_{12} deficiency once the body stores accumulated *in utero* are exhausted.

Infestation of the gut with the fish tapeworm *Diphyllobothrium latum* is relatively common in Finland where it is acquired by eating raw fish which are infected with the larval forms of this cestode. Sporadic reports of infestation are beginning to appear in other countries because of the current fashion for eating raw fish. If the parasite lodges in the upper gastrointestinal tract, it is capable of extracting substantial quantities of vitamin B_{12} both complexed with intrinsic factor and as free vitamin from ingested food, thereby reducing the amount available for absorption in the terminal ileum. Infestation typically is associated with a reduction in the body stores of vitamin B_{12} but the development of megaloblastic anaemia is unusual.

Drug-induced Malabsorption

A number of drugs have been reported to impair absorption of vitamin B_{12}, including the anticonvulsant phenytoin, the aminoglycoside antimicrobial agent neomycin, colchicine which is used in high doses in the treatment of gout and, most commonly, alcohol. Withdrawal of the drug reverses the malabsorption.

Increased Requirements

The requirement for vitamin B_{12} is increased during pregnancy because of the expansion of the blood volume and the foetal requirement. The increase is not sufficient to cause deficiency of vitamin B_{12} in a woman with normal stores prior to conception. It can, however, precipitate deficiency in a woman with previously borderline body stores of the vitamin. If a woman is severely vitamin B_{12} deficient throughout pregnancy, her baby is likely to have deficiency of the vitamin at birth. This situation is encountered most commonly in the Third World.

> **SAQ 1**
>
> Why is vitamin B_{12} deficiency in pregnancy uncommon in the UK even when the daily requirement exceeds supply?

Failure of Vitamin B_{12} Transport

Congenital deficiency of transcobalamin II, the primary transport protein of vitamin B_{12} is characterised by the development of severe megaloblastic anaemia in the first weeks of life despite the presence of a normal serum concentration of vitamin B_{12} and normal body stores of the vitamin. Early diagnosis is vital if severe neurological damage is to be avoided. Treatment involves the administration of very large doses of vitamin B_{12} by intramuscular injection.

Failure of Vitamin B_{12} Metabolism

A small number of examples of congenital failure to convert absorbed vitamin B_{12} to its active coenzyme forms have been described, resulting in excretion of methylmalonic acid and homocysteine in the urine. The affected individuals presented because of failure to thrive and mental retardation. Interestingly, only a minority of such cases developed megaloblastic anaemia. The reasons for this remain obscure.

Prolonged exposure to the anaesthetic nitrous oxide can induce megaloblastic change by inactivating vitamin B_{12} coenzymes. Inac-

Interpretation of the results of assays for vitamin B_{12} and folic acid require a knowledge of the results expected in a healthy individual. The reference intervals are shown below:

Serum vitamin B_{12}

170-1000 pg/ml

Serum folate

3-25 ng/ml

Red cell folate

145-600 ng/ml packed RBC

tivation occurs as a result of oxidation of the central cobalt ion to the Co(II) state. Chronic exposure to small amounts of nitrous oxide has been suggested as the cause of a mild neuropathy which has been described in dental surgeons.

Folic Acid Deficiency

Causes of Folic Acid Deficiency

Deficiency of folic acid can result from an inadequate diet, intestinal malabsorption, increased requirements or failure of utilisation of absorbed vitamin.

Inadequate Dietary Intake

Nutritional deficiency of folic acid is relatively common for three main reasons:

- the ideal UK diet contains about 700 µg of folate of which about half is absorbed. The daily requirement for folate is about 100 µg.

- folate is very labile to heat. Cooking can destroy up to 90% of the folate present in food.

- body stores of folate are only sufficient to last about 3 months in the absence of dietary intake.

Folate deficiency can develop rapidly where dietary intake is suboptimal, either because folate-rich foods are lacking from the diet or because of losses during cooking. An inadequate diet often is a contributory factor in the development of folate deficiency due to malabsorption or where the requirement for folate is increased.

SAQ 2

Why does assay of red cell folate give a better guide to folate status than assay of serum folate?

Malabsorption

Intestinal malabsorption is a common cause of folate deficiency. The most common cause of malabsorption of folate in the UK is **coeliac disease** (gluten-sensitive enteropathy or non-tropical sprue). Coeliac disease has an incidence of about 1 in 2, 000 in the

UK. It is unusual in blacks and in the Japanese. Malabsorption of iron and folate from the duodenum and jejunum is caused by villous atrophy secondary to gluten intolerance. The cause of coeliac disease is unknown but withdrawal of gluten from the diet reinstates jejunal absorption of iron and folate.

Tropical sprue is a similar condition to coeliac disease which is most common in the West Indies, the Indian subcontinent and in SE Asia. The cause of the disease is unknown but malabsorption of folate commonly is present. **Crohns disease** commonly causes folate deficiency, especially where the jejunum and upper ileum are involved. Surgical causes of folate malabsorption include ileal resection where the site of maximal absorption of folate is removed.

Increased Requirement

Deficiency of folic acid is especially common in pregnancy because dietary intake often fails to meet the increased demand for folate imposed by the growth of maternal blood volume and the developing foetus. The daily requirement for folate can rise to 500 μg in the third trimester of pregnancy. In the absence of folate supplementation, about 60% of pregnant women have subnormal plasma concentrations of folate (though not necessarily significant megaloblastic change). Folate deficiency commonly is accompanied by iron deficiency in pregnancy.

Because of the recently demonstrated association between folate deficiency in pregnancy and neural tube defects in the foetus, prophylactic folic acid therapy is widely recommended. However, folate therapy must start early, ideally several months before conception, if maximum protection is to be derived. Prophylactic iron therapy may be administered simultaneously although gastrointestinal disturbances may reduce compliance.

The anaemia of chronic haemolytic conditions such as sickle cell anaemia frequently is exacerbated by folate deficiency. It is not uncommon for the rate of haemopoiesis to be increased by a factor of 10 in severe haemolytic conditions. When the increased demand for folate that this massively increased haemopoietic activity imposes exceeds the amount available from dietary sources, the development of folate deficiency is inevitable.

Drug-induced Folate Deficiency

A number of drugs have been reported to cause folate deficiency by interfering with folate absorption or metabolism. With some drugs, the antifolate effect is desired, while in others it is an unwanted side effect. For example, long-term therapy with the anticonvulsant drug phenytoin is associated with the development of folate deficiency due to impaired intestinal absorption of folate. Alcohol is also thought to inhibit folate absorption and metabolism although the most common cause of folate deficiency in alcoholics is inadequate dietary intake.

The cytotoxic drug **methotrexate** is an example of a drug which is used specifically for its antifolate properties. It is a close structural analogue of folic acid which acts as a powerful competitive inhibitor of the enzyme dihydrofolate reductase. Ingestion of methotrexate rapidly causes intracellular deficiency of folate co-enzymes and depletion of thymidine and purine nucleotides. The toxic effects of methotrexate therapy include ulceration of the gastrointestinal tract, alopecia and megaloblastic change. In the treatment of leukaemia, normal tissue can be rescued from the toxic effects of methotrexate by the administration of N-5-formyl-tetrahydrofolate (folinic acid, citrovorum factor).

Failure of Folate Metabolism

A number of rare enzyme deficiencies have been reported which cause impairment of folate metabolism. Most of these have been associated with megaloblastic anaemia and with some degree of mental retardation.

Causes of Megaloblastic Anaemia Other than Haematinic Deficiency

Megaloblastic change is the result of impaired DNA synthesis caused by reduced availability of deoxyribonucleoside triphosphate precursors. Although the most common cause of this situation is deficiency of vitamin B_{12} or folic acid, with resultant deficiency of dTTP, any process which impairs the synthesis of one or more of the four deoxyribonucleoside triphosphates will cause megaloblastic change.

The first cytotoxic drug to be effective in the treatment of leukaemia was a folate antagonist called *Aminopterin*. In 1948, Sidney Farber reported that 10 of 16 children with acute leukaemia responded to treatment with this drug. As we would expect nowadays, these partial remissions were only temporary but an important step towards successful treatment of a hitherto intractable disease had been taken. Antimetabolites like methotrexate are still in common use in the treatment of leukaemia.

There are three main circumstances associated with megaloblastic change which is not attributable to deficiency of vitamin B_{12} or folic acid:

- treatment with cytotoxic drugs

- certain inborn errors of metabolism

- in association with other haematological disorders

Cytotoxic Chemotherapy

Many of the cytotoxic drugs which are used in the treatment of malignant disease act by interfering with cellular metabolism. Three groups of cytotoxic drugs are associated with the induction of megaloblastic change of variable severity:

- **inhibitors of pyrimidine synthesis** form the group of cytotoxic drugs which are most commonly associated with megaloblastic change. For example, **5-fluorouracil** acts by preventing the methylation of deoxyuridylate (dUMP) to deoxythymidylate (dTMP), thereby producing a deficiency of thymine for DNA synthesis and encouraging the misincorporation of uracil into DNA. Another pyrimidine inhibitor, **6-azauridine**, acts by inhibiting the enzyme orotidylate decarboxylase which catalyses the conversion of orotidine monophosphate (OMP) to uridine monophosphate (UMP). Treatment with 6-azauridine is associated with megaloblastic anaemia and orotic aciduria.

- **inhibitors of purine synthesis** such as **6-mercapto-purine** and **6-thioguanine** inhibit DNA and RNA synthesis by an as yet incompletely understood mechanism. Both drugs are known to be incorporated into DNA and RNA *in vivo* and to interfere with coenzyme synthesis and activity. Purine inhibitors typically induce mild megaloblastic change which remits rapidly on withdrawal of the drug.

- **inhibitors of cellular enzymes**. Inhibitors of the enzyme ribonucleotide reductase such as **cytosine arabinoside** and **hydroxyurea** are associated with the rapid induction of severe megaloblastic change. The action of **methotrexate** as a competitive inhibitor of dihydrofolate reductase was described above.

Megaloblastic Change Secondary to Inborn Errors of Metabolism

Deficiency of the purine salvage pathway enzyme hypoxanthine-guanine phosphoribosyltransferase (HGPRTase) causes the **Lesch-Nyhan syndrome** which is characterised by megaloblastic anaemia, hyperuricaemia, spasticity, mental retardation and self-mutilation. The disorder is very rare and shows an X-linked recessive pattern of inheritance.

Hereditary orotic aciduria results from a deficiency of either or both of the enzymes orotate phosphoribosyltransferase and orotidylate decarboxylase. This rare disorder of pyrimidine metabolism is associated with severe megaloblastic anaemia, growth retardation and excretion of large amounts of orotic acid in the urine. The anaemia is refractory to vitamin B_{12} or folic acid but responds well to the oral administration of uridine which bypasses the enzyme block.

Megaloblastic Change Secondary to Haematological Disorders

Some degree of megaloblastic change is common in a wide range of malignant haematological disorders. For example, in M6 acute leukaemia, the abnormal erythroblasts frequently show megaloblastic features in addition to the severe dysplasia which characterises this disease. The cause of this apparent megaloblastic change is unknown.

Megaloblastic features are common also in pyridoxine-responsive sideroblastic anaemia. The biochemical basis for the megaloblastic change is unknown. One possible explanation lies with the fact that both pyridoxal-5'-phosphate and tetrahydrofolate are required as coenzymes for the reversible conversion of serine to glycine. Disturbances of this reaction perhaps could induce sideroblastic change by impairment of haem synthesis and megaloblastic change by

> Lesch-Nyhan syndrome is associated with a severe deficiency of the enzyme HGPRTase. If the activity of this enzyme is less than 2% of normal, mental retardation results. In those cases where enzyme activity is less than 0.2% of normal, the most distressing manifestation of the disease, self-mutilation, is present.
>
> Why HGPRTase deficiency should cause neurological problems remains a mystery because the activity of the other purine salvage enzyme, APRTase, is normal. Some workers believe that an imbalance in the concentrations of purine nucleotides during development of the central nervous system is the most likely cause of this condition. The most common cause of death in these patients is renal failure secondary to hyperuricaemia.

impairment of folate metabolism. Interestingly, the megaloblastic changes in sideroblastic anaemia often are restricted to erythroid cells.

Biochemical Basis of Megaloblastic Change

As explained in Chapter 3, an adequate supply of vitamin B_{12} and folate coenzymes is essential for optimal DNA and RNA synthesis. The most significant effect of a deficiency of either of these vitamins is to reduce the rate of conversion of deoxyuridine-5'-monophosphate (dUMP) to deoxythymidine-5'-monophosphate (dTMP), the rate-limiting step in DNA synthesis. The resulting asynchrony between DNA and RNA synthesis explains many of the morphological and biochemical sequelae of megaloblastic anaemia.

Failure of dTTP synthesis results in an accumulation of dUTP relative to dTTP. DNA polymerases, the enzymes responsible for assembly of DNA from deoxynucleoside triphosphates, are unable to distinguish between dTTP and dUTP. The relative paucity of dTTP results in the misincorporation of uracil into DNA instead of thymine. An enzyme called **uracil-DNA-glycosylase** recognises the aberrant uracils and excises them. Normally, a series of other enzymes mediate the repair of the mutilated DNA by incorporating thymine in place of the excised uracil. However, when thymine is in short supply, suboptimal repair of DNA leads to fragmentation of the helical structure, impaired mitosis and premature cell death.

Pathophysiology

Individuals with megaloblastic anaemia typically display the physiological changes which are common to all types of anaemia viz pallor, weakness, shortness of breath on exertion, light-headedness, palpitations and congestive cardiac failure. In some cases, loss of appetite, weight loss and gastrointestinal disturbances also are present. In addition to these non-specific changes, a range of signs which are strongly suggestive of megaloblastic change may be noted. These typically affect the tissues which are most rapidly dividing and are attributable to impaired mitotic function and premature cell death. These effects will be described under three headings:

- general tissue manifestations

- neurological manifestations

- haematological manifestations

General Tissue Manifestations

Deficiency of vitamin B_{12} or folate affects all dividing cells but the effects are manifest most clearly in rapidly dividing tissues such as bone marrow and epithelial cells. The effects of deficiency of these vitamins on the blood are described later. Disturbances of epithelial cell turnover are responsible for the common sequelae of **angular stomatitis** (lesions at the corners of the mouth) and **glossitis** (inflammation and depapillation of the tongue). Disturbed epidermal growth promotes widespread melanin hyperpigmentation. Sterility is not uncommon.

Cytogenetic studies show that a variety of non-specific chromosomal changes such as random breaks are common in megaloblastic tissue. These almost certainly are secondary to uracil misincorporation.

Neurological Manifestations

Neurological manifestations such as symmetrical paraesthesiae in the feet and fingers, progressing to spastic ataxia and degeneration of the dorsal and lateral columns of the spinal cord are typical findings in severe megaloblastic anaemia due to deficiency of vitamin B_{12}. Once established, neurological damage is irreversible. The mechanism of neurological damage is not yet known. Some workers believe that the accumulation of methylmalonyl CoA which occurs in vitamin B_{12} deficiency promotes the incorporation of branched chain fatty acids into myelin and leads to disturbed neurological function.

Folate deficiency in pregnancy is associated with an increased incidence of neural tube defects such as spina bifida in the foetus. It is also believed to lead to mild dementia and impairment of intellectual function.

SAQ 3

Which of the following statements are true?

A. Dietary deficiency of vitamin B_{12} is common in the UK.
B. Folate deficiency inhibits RNA synthesis.
C. PA is an autoimmune condition.
D. Methotrexate is an inhibitor of folate absorption.

Haematological Manifestations

Typically, the megaloblastic bone marrow is hypercellular, with an increase in erythropoietic activity being especially prominent. There is a preponderance of immature forms of all cell lines, reflecting the premature death of cells in the process of development. This diad of increased production of blood cells and increased intramedullary cell death is known as **ineffective haemopoiesis**, and is responsible for the pancytopaenia which characterises this condition.

The increased cell turnover results in alterations in the biochemistry of the blood such as an increase in the concentrations of unconjugated bilirubin, lactate dehydrogenase and lysozyme. Bilirubin is one of the products of haemoglobin catabolism. The enzymes lactate dehydrogenase and lysozyme reflect ineffective erythropoiesis and ineffective leucopoiesis respectively. These biochemical disturbances are augmented by the shortened life span of circulating blood cells which invariably is present in this condition.

The distinctive changes in blood and bone marrow cell morphology which accompany megaloblastic anaemia are the result of asynchrony between nuclear and cytoplasmic development. Megaloblastic red cell precursors typically display retarded maturation of the nucleus relative to the cytoplasm. This is exemplified by the appearance of the late megaloblast which features an open, lace-like chromatin network and a fully haemoglobinised cytoplasm. Circulating red cells typically are macrocytic but there is a marked variation in size and shape of individual cells. Macrocytosis results from a decrease in the number of cell divisions prior to loss of the nucleus and release into the circulation. In contrast to the macrocytes which accompany alcoholic liver disease, megaloblastic macrocytes typically are oval. Absolute reticulocytopaenia invariably is present.

The twin eccentricities of megaloblastic leucopoiesis are the appearance of bizarre, giant metamyelocytes in the bone marrow and an increase in the average number of nuclear lobes in circulating granulocytes. Nuclear hypersegmentation probably results from structural abnormalities in the nuclear chromatin. Morphological changes in megaloblastic megakaryocytes include an increase in cell size and failure of cytoplasmic granulation. However, these changes often are indistinct.

Normally, peripheral blood neutrophils have between 1 and 5 nuclear lobes, with an average of 2.8. A right shift is present when the average number of nuclear lobes is significantly increased. In practice, a rigorous lobe count (Cooke-Arneth count) is seldom performed. The presence of more than 3% of 5-lobed neutrophils frequently is used as a sensitive and readily discernible alternative indicator.

The presence of a right shift is not a reliable indicator of megaloblastic anaemia. This change may be present in iron deficiency, uraemia, infection and even as an inherited condition (Undritz anomaly).

SAQ 4

Why does the plasma concentration of homocysteine rise in vitamin B_{12} deficiency?

Vitamin B_{12} deficiency is accompanied by specific biochemical changes in the blood. These include a rise in the plasma concentration of homocysteine and methylmalonate and a fall in the plasma concentration of vitamin B_{12}. Alterations in the plasma concentration of homocysteine occur early in vitamin B_{12} deficiency and can be used as a sensitive marker of the condition. Folate deficiency is accompanied by a fall in red cell and plasma folate.

Suggested Further Reading

Chanarin, I. (1992). *The Megaloblastic Anaemias (3rd ed.)*. Oxford: Blackwell.

Hoffbrand, A.V. (ed.) and Wickramasinghe, R.G. (1982). Megaloblastic Anemia. In *Recent Advances in Haematology 3*. Edinburgh: Churchill Livingstone.

Answers to Self-Assessment Questions

1. Normal body stores of vitamin B_{12} are sufficient to meet demands for about 3 years. Pregnancy only lasts for about 40 weeks.

2. Assay of red cell folate provides information about folate status over a period of 120 days: serum folate is more liable to short term fluctuation.

3. C.

4. In the absence of methylcobalamin, homocysteine is not converted to methionine and so accumulates in the plasma.

Disorders of Iron Metabolism

Iron Deficiency

Iron deficiency is by far the most common cause of anaemia world-wide, for reasons that will be explained later in this chapter. Most frequently, iron deficiency is observed as a secondary manifestation of another primary pathological state and may even be the presenting feature. Because iron is essential to the function of every cell of the body, iron deficiency causes a wide range of adverse physiological effects: anaemia is simply the best recognised of these.

The state of iron deficiency is defined as a reduction below normal limits of the total body iron content. Iron deficiency anaemia, the most severe manifestation of iron deficiency, develops slowly and insidiously through a series of successive stages, although progression from one stage to the next is not inevitable.

When the rate of absorption of iron from the diet is insufficient to meet the daily requirement, iron is mobilised from the body stores to meet the shortfall. If this **negative iron balance** persists the body iron stores eventually will become depleted, a state known as **latent iron deficiency**. In this state, the body is deficient in iron but erythropoiesis is still normal and no adverse physiological effects are present. Many people exist for prolonged periods in latent iron deficiency and never develop anaemia.

If the negative iron balance persists once the body iron stores are exhausted, **iron deficient erythropoiesis** ensues and the characteristic changes which accompany severe iron deficiency gradually develop. The final stage in this sequence of events is the development of **iron deficiency anaemia**. Because iron deficiency anaemia develops gradually, the body is able to adapt to the falling haemoglobin level and clinical symptoms often do not appear until the anaemia is moderately severe.

Spinach commonly is regarded as an extremely rich source of iron, calcium and vitamins A and C. In this regard, however, it is not particularly different from many leafy green vegetables. It is doubtful whether the iron content is assimilable because the leaves also contain a relatively high concentration of oxalic acid: iron oxalate is absorbed poorly.

In the 17th century, iron deficiency anaemia was known as "the green sickness" or chlorosis and was believed to be associated with being in love. One common treatment for the condition was to drink wine (sherris) in which iron filings had been steeped. The following extract is from Shakespeare's King Henry the Fourth: Part Two.

Falstaff: "...for thin drink doth so over-cool their blood, and making many fish meals, that they fall into a kind of male green-sickness...A good sherris-sack hath a two-fold operation in it; it ascends me into the brain, dries me there all the foolish, and dull, and crudy vapours which environ it, makes it apprehensive, quick, forgetive, full of nimble, fiery, and delectable shapes, which delivered o'er to the voice, the tongue, which is the birth, becomes excellent 'wit. The second property of your excellent sherris is the warming of the blood, which, before cold and settled, left the liver white and pale, which is the badge of pusillanimity and cowardice. But the sherris warms it, and makes it course from the inwards to the parts extreme. It illumineth the face, which as a beacon gives warning to all the rest of this little kingdom, man, to arm; and then the vital commoners, and inland petty spirits, muster me all to their captain, the heart; who, great and puffed up with this retinue, doth any deed of courage. And this valour comes of sherris."

Causes of Iron Deficiency

As explained above, iron deficiency arises where absorption of iron does not meet daily requirements. This can occur where the supply of iron is decreased or where the daily requirement for iron is increased.

Decreased Supply of Iron

A sustained decrease in the supply of iron to the body can be caused by two main conditions:

- inadequate diet

- malabsorption of iron from the diet

Inadequate Diet

As described in Chapter 3, the average adult mixed diet in the UK provides about 18 mg of iron per day: more than enough to meet normal demands. For this reason, inadequacy of the diet is seldom the sole cause of iron deficiency in this age group, although it commonly is a contributing factor to the more rapid onset of iron deficiency due to another primary cause.

Breast milk and its artificial substitutes are relatively deficient in iron. New born babies have significant body stores of iron which were accumulated *in utero*. Normally, these are sufficient to meet the relatively low demand for iron in the first weeks of life. However, introduction of a mixed diet which has a greater iron content is required to meet the increased demands imposed by growth. Prolonged breast or bottle feeding may precipitate iron deficiency in toddlers.

Inadequacy of the diet often is a significant contributory factor in the development of iron deficiency in the Third World, particularly when the iron demand is raised, for example in pregnancy.

Malabsorption of Dietary Iron

Iron deficiency secondary to malabsorption is a relatively common complication of diseases of the upper alimentary tract such as

coeliac disease (gluten-sensitive enteropathy). The incidence of this condition in the UK is about 1 in 2000. Malabsorption of dietary folate commonly exacerbates the anaemia in this disorder.

Partial gastrectomy predisposes strongly to the development of iron deficiency because the absence of stomach acid impairs absorption of dietary iron. The malabsorption is aggravated by the rapid gastrojejunal food transit times which result from removal of part of the stomach and by chronic antacid ingestion.

Increased Requirement for Iron

There are three main causes of an increase in daily iron requirement:

- loss of blood

- growth and pregnancy (physiological demands)

- loss of iron

Blood Loss

Chronic blood loss from the gastrointestinal and genitourinary tracts is the most common cause of iron deficiency. The effect of menstrual blood loss on iron requirements in adult females is described in Chapter 3.

The most common cause of bleeding in tropical areas is infestation of the gut with the hookworms *Ancylostoma duodenale* or *Necator americanus*. It is estimated that about 500 million people carry hookworms in their guts. Each worm consumes a tiny quantity of blood from its host but infestations can be very heavy (a female *Ancylostoma* produces 30,000 eggs each day!).

Outside of the tropics, the most common causes of pathological blood loss are carcinoma, duodenal ulcer, hiatus hernia, haemorrhoids and menorrhagia. Frank blood loss commonly is absent in such cases: a loss of only 4-5 ml of blood per day, if sustained, will eventually lead to iron deficiency. Even smaller losses can result in iron deficiency if the diet is poor or if malabsorption is present.

The association between spinach and strength and vigour was brought to life for most people when Max Fleischer invented the cartoon character Popeye. The pugnacious sailor has been a popular character with children of all ages since the 1930s.

In 1971, a Dr R. Hunter published a suggestion in *The Lancet* that, since laboratory animals fed on high concentrations of folic acid became tense and irritable, that perhaps it was the high folate content of spinach rather than its iron content that caused Popeye to become quarrelsome and engage Bluto in fights with such regularity!

Growth and Pregnancy

The increased requirement for iron during periods of accelerated growth makes iron deficiency very common in adolescence and in pregnancy. For example, in a normal, uncomplicated pregnancy, maternal total red cell volume increases by between 20 and 40%. This imposes an extra requirement for iron of up to 500 mg. The developing foetus, which always has first call on available iron, requires about 300 mg of iron. These dual excess demands for iron are greatest during the second and third trimester of pregnancy, when the daily demand for iron can rise to 6-7 mg! The delicate iron balance which this inevitably causes is compounded by maternal blood loss at delivery. A maternal blood loss at delivery of 500 ml which contains 250 mg of iron is not uncommon. Minimal amounts of iron are also lost in breast milk.

The excess requirement for iron in pregnancy is offset partially by amenorrhoea which saves about 200 mg of iron.

Loss of Iron

Chronic intravascular haemolysis can result in the loss of considerable amounts of iron as haemosiderin in the urine. In severe cases, this can contribute to the development of iron deficiency.

Pathophysiology

Severe iron deficiency anaemia is accompanied by a wide range of clinical manifestations. These can be considered under three broad headings:

- effects caused by the primary precipitating condition. These are beyond the scope of this book and will not be described.

- effects which are manifest in the blood and blood-forming tissue.

- effects which are manifest in other tissues.

Effects on the Blood and Blood-forming Tissue

Depletion of the iron stores means that there is insufficient iron available for incorporation into the haemoglobin of developing erythroblasts and iron deficient erythropoiesis ensues. This is manifest as a reduced mean cell haemoglobin concentration (MCHC) and an increased concentration of free protoporphyrin within the cell. The major determinant of the volume of a mature red cell is the number of mitotic divisions it undergoes before the nucleus is poisoned by the increasing concentration of haemoglobin. In iron deficiency, haemoglobin synthesis is retarded and an extra mitotic division occurs before the erythroblast nucleus dies. This results in a mature red cell which is smaller than normal. Thus, the anaemia which accompanies iron deficiency typically is hypochromic and microcytic.

In contrast to iron deficiency, vitamin B_{12} and folic acid deficiency cause a retardation of DNA synthesis but do not affect the rate of haemoglobin synthesis. Thus, fewer mitotic divisions occur before the megaloblast nucleus is poisoned by the increasing haemoglobin concentration, leading to the production of the macrocytic red cells which characterise megaloblastic anaemia.

The condition most likely to be confused with iron deficiency anaemia on morphological grounds is β thalassaemia. The differential diagnosis of these two conditions is described in Chapter 7. The main laboratory features of iron deficiency anaemia are shown in Table 5.1.

Blood Cell Features

      microcytosis and hypochromasia
      reticulocytopaenia
      poikilocytosis (pencil forms)
      defective neutrophil function
      reduced % T lymphocytes (in children)

Bone Marrow Features

      erythroid hypoplasia
      normoblasts have ragged cytoplasm
      decreased macrophage iron

Biochemical Features

      raised TIBC
      decreased % transferrin saturation
      impaired ability to maintain body temperature
      depressed muscle function
      abnormal thyroid hormone metabolism
      raised catecholamine levels
      reduced ferritin levels

Table 5.1 *Laboratory features of iron deficiency anaemia*

One of the biochemical hallmarks of iron deficiency is the combination of a raised total iron binding capacity (TIBC) and a reduced % transferrin saturation. The relationship between total iron binding capacity and % transferrin saturation in a range of conditions is shown in Figure 5.1.

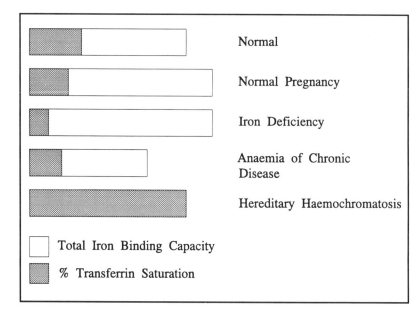

Figure 5.1 *The relationship between total iron binding capacity and % transferrin saturation in various conditions*

General Effects of Iron Deficiency Anaemia

There are three main types of generalised effect of iron deficiency:

- changes which are directly attributable to anaemia and not specific to iron deficiency.

- changes in epithelial tissue

- changes in behaviour

A reduction in circulating haemoglobin causes a reduction in oxygen carrying capacity and leads to the most widely recognised changes seen in anaemia viz pallor of skin and mucous membranes and reduced exercise tolerance. The body responds to anaemia by increasing cardiac output and increasing synthesis of red cell 2,3 DPG, thereby maintaining oxygen delivery to the tissues under basal conditions. However, there is an exaggerated response to exercise which causes shortness of breath on exertion and palpitations, the most common presenting features of iron deficiency anaemia. The response of the body to anaemia is explained in more detail in Chapter 6.

Severe iron deficiency causes deficiency of iron-containing enzymes such as cytochromes in a wide range of tissues. The effect of this is manifest most severely in epithelial cells which ordinarily are turning over relatively rapidly. Characteristic changes include:

- **koilonychia** - flattening or "spooning" of the finger nails.

- **angular stomatitis** - atrophic lesions at the corners of the mouth.

- **glossitis** - smooth, inflamed tongue.

- **atrophic gastritis** - inflammation of the lining of the stomach.

- **achlorhydria** - lack of hydrochloric acid secretion in the stomach.

- **dysphagia** - difficulty in swallowing. This is caused by the development of post-cricoid oesophageal webs which may progress to oesophageal carcinoma. This rare condition is known as the **Plummer-Vinson syndrome**.

Iron deficiency in early childhood is associated with impairment of intellectual ability and hyperactivity. Most studies have shown that these effects are at least partially reversed by suitable iron therapy.

Another characteristic but poorly understood behavioural abnormality in iron deficient subjects is manifest as a strong desire to eat unusual substances such as soil (geophagia), ice (pagophagia) or even carpet fluff. In some cases, this obsessive behaviour, known as **pica**, may exacerbate the iron deficiency. For example, ingestion of clay soil can impair intestinal absorption of dietary iron.

Iron deficiency is not a disease but, rather, it is a symptom of disease. Effective treatment of iron deficiency requires that the primary precipitating cause be removed. Excluding pregnancy and

Many workers believe that pica may be at least part of the explanation for the unusual dietary cravings experienced by some pregnant women. A number of studies have shown that the more exaggerated cases of this phenomenon correlate with depletion of the body iron stores.

menorrhagia, the most common underlying cause of iron deficiency is occult blood loss from the gastrointestinal tract.

Replacement of body iron stores is best achieved by supplementation of the diet using ferrous sulphate or, less commonly, by intramuscular injection of iron-dextran. Appropriate oral supplementation should induce a reticulocyte response within 3 or 4 days and a sustained rise in circulating haemoglobin concentration. Failure of response to an adequate dose of oral iron suggests that the underlying cause has not been removed, that patient compliance is poor or that iron deficiency is not the cause of the anaemia. It should be remembered that iron deficiency is only one of many causes of microcytic, hypochromic anaemia.

Anaemia of Chronic Disorders

Chronic inflammatory or malignant disorders frequently are accompanied by a normocytic, normochromic anaemia which is refractory to all treatment except that which causes regression of the primary condition. This form of anaemia is known by the somewhat vague descriptor, the anaemia of chronic disorders (ACD). The aetiology of this condition remains obscure although it is almost certainly multifactorial.

Disordered iron metabolism is a common finding in ACD but its relative contribution to the development of the anaemia remains a matter of debate. Chronic inflammation causes activation of tissue macrophages with a consequent upregulation of surface apotransferrin receptors. Binding of significant quantities of apotransferrin to macrophages reduces the total iron binding capacity of the plasma as shown in Figure 5.1. Inflammation also stimulates neutrophils to synthesise and release large quantities of apolactoferrin which acts as an iron-binding protein. The apolactoferrin is bound to specific surface receptors on activated tissue macrophages and acts like a magnet for circulating iron. Any iron that is bound to the apolactoferrin:receptor complex is internalised by the macrophage and stored as ferritin. Thus, tissue iron stores are increased. It is this apparent anomaly of reduced TIBC and % transferrin saturation accompanied by increased body iron stores which is the hallmark of ACD.

There is clear evidence of suppression of erythropoietic activity in ACD. There have been sporadic reports of the presence of specific inhibitors of erythropoiesis in individuals but in most cases the suppression is likely to be caused by the release of growth inhibitors such as interleukin 1, γ interferon and tumour necrosis factor in response to the primary condition. A slight reduction in red cell lifespan has also been reported in a minority of cases of ACD.

Sideroblastic Anaemias

The sideroblastic anaemias are a heterogeneous group of disorders which are characterised by disordered incorporation of iron into haem within developing erythroblasts. The resulting toxic accumulation of iron within the mitochondria of late erythroblasts leads to some degree of ineffective erythropoiesis. Demonstration of iron-laden mitochondria encircling the nuclei of late erythroblasts, the so-called "ringed sideroblast", is the *sine qua non* for a diagnosis of sideroblastic anaemia. However, ringed sideroblasts are not specific indicators of sideroblastic anaemia: they are frequently found in leukaemia, megaloblastic anaemia and alcoholism among other conditions.

The sideroblastic anaemias are classified according to their aetiology as hereditary, secondary or idiopathic (unknown aetiology).

Hereditary Sideroblastic Anaemia

Most cases of hereditary sideroblastic anaemia have shown an X-linked recessive pattern of inheritance. Affected males have hypochromic, dimorphic anaemia with mild ineffective erythropoiesis and erythroid hyperplasia. Many cases of hereditary sideroblastic anaemia have functional deficiencies of enzymes of the haem synthetic pathway, most commonly δ aminolaevulinic acid (δALA) synthetase or ferrochelatase. In some cases, however, the molecular defect remains to be determined.

The anaemia responds to the administration of vitamin B_6 (pyridoxine) in about 50% of cases of hereditary sideroblastic anaemia. Such responses are, at best, partial and usually are temporary. They do not imply correction of an underlying pyridoxine deficiency but probably are related to the presence of a variant of δALA synthetase which has an increased K_m for pyridoxal 5' phosphate.

Secondary Sideroblastic Anaemia

Drug-induced Sideroblastic Anaemia

The most common cause of secondary sideroblastic anaemia is the administration of drugs such as isoniazid, chloramphenicol or alcohol. Isoniazid and alcohol inhibit biochemical reactions which involve pyridoxal 5' phosphate, including synthesis of δALA, the first and rate-limiting step in the haem biosynthetic pathway. Chloramphenicol inhibits the synthesis of δALA synthetase and ferrochelatase. The blood picture in drug-induced or alcohol-induced sideroblastic anaemia closely resembles that of the hereditary form. All of the sideroblastic changes are reversible by cessation of therapy or withdrawal of alcohol.

Lead Poisoning

Chronic lead poisoning was a relatively common condition when most drinking water was supplied via lead pipes and lead pigments were commonly used in paints. Most cases nowadays are associated with occupational exposure.

Lead is absorbed by ingestion or inhalation: a classical route of entry in children was by sucking toys such as lead soldiers which were painted with lead-containing paint. Most absorbed lead accumulates in bone and bone marrow. In the bone marrow, lead is associated particularly with red cell precursors and, more especially, with mitochondrial membranes of developing erythroblasts. The presence of lead in the mitochondria severely disrupts haem synthesis and leads directly to sideroblastic change. Lead also causes damage to red cell membranes and inhibits glycolytic activity. These two activities result in mild haemolysis which contributes significantly to the anaemia of chronic lead poisoning.

Typically, the blood picture in chronic lead poisoning is microcytic and hypochromic with prominent basophilic stippling and a reticulocytosis. The basophilic stippling is the result of the accumulation of pyrimidine nucleotides in the cell cytoplasm and is only present in the youngest red cells. The accumulation of pyrimidine nucleotides is caused by the inhibition of the enzyme pyrimidine 5' nucleotidase by lead.

The ancient Romans made heavy use of lead. They used it in their water pipes (the name plumber is derived from the Latin for lead), their pottery drinking vessels were lead-glazed and their cooking utensils were commonly lined with lead. Archaeological evidence shows high concentrations of lead in bones found at Roman sites such as York and Cirencester. Some historians believe that the increasing sophistication of the Romans in the use of lead contributed to the fall of the Roman Empire because of a presumed high incidence of lead-induced dementia.

Idiopathic Sideroblastic Anaemia

Idiopathic sideroblastic anaemia primarily is a disease of the elderly and is the most common of the sideroblastic anaemias. It is identical to the myelodysplastic syndrome refractory anaemia with sideroblasts (RAS). Characteristic dyserythropoietic changes include macrocytosis, poikilocytosis, basophilic stippling and the appearance of ringed sideroblasts affecting all stages of erythroblast development. In the early stages of the disease platelets and leucocytes appear normal.

Cytogenetic abnormalities are demonstrable in about 50% of cases of idiopathic sideroblastic anaemia. About 10% of cases terminate as acute leukaemia, predominantly the M4 type.

Iron Overload

There are three commonly encountered forms of chronic iron overload:

- hereditary haemochromatosis

- transfusion-associated haemosiderosis

- dietary causes

Hereditary Haemochromatosis

Hereditary haemochromatosis results from an irregularity of intestinal iron absorption in which feedback control over the rate of absorption of dietary iron is lost. The inexorable accumulation of iron within the body which results damages vital organs and, if untreated, is fatal. The condition is inherited in an autosomal recessive fashion: only homozygotes express significant disease. The gene for hereditary haemochromatosis is linked closely with the HLA portion of the MHC complex on chromosome 6 and is estimated to be carried by about 1 in 16 individuals.

Absorption of dietary iron typically exceeds normal by about 2 mg per day in haemochromatosis homozygotes and is unrelated to iron requirements. Because of this, an affected adult male may have accumulated a total body iron content of over 20 g. However, in contrast to transfusion-associated haemosiderosis, bone marrow macrophages are not grossly overloaded with storage iron. Most of the excess iron is stored in the parenchymal cells of the liver and other organs.

Pathophysiology

One of the early signs of hereditary haemochromatosis is greatly increased % saturation of circulating transferrin as shown in Figure 5.1. Thus, when iron is absorbed inappropriately and released into the portal circulation some may be unable to bind to the iron transport protein transferrin because it is already fully saturated. Iron which cannot bind to transferrin circulates as hydrated complexes of ferrous and ferric ions until binding sites become available. About 30% of the circulating plasma iron exists as hydrated ionic complexes in haemochromatosis heterozygotes. These hydrated ionic complexes of iron can act as a catalyst for the formation of toxic oxygen radicals in the presence of NADPH. Oxygen radicals are short-lived and extremely reactive molecular species which are capable of causing extensive localised tissue damage. The principal villain in this regard is hydroxyl radical (OH·).

Accumulated organ damage results in the major clinical features of hereditary haemochromatosis viz hepatic cirrhosis, skin pigmentation, diabetes and progressive congestive cardiomyopathy which is the leading cause of death. In about 30% of cases, hepatic cirrhosis progresses to hepatoma.

The laboratory features of hereditary haemochromatosis include a markedly raised serum ferritin concentration (>500 mg/l), accompanied by a raised serum iron and % saturation of transferrin. If significant hepatic damage has occurred, macrocytosis and target cells may be present. Otherwise the blood picture is unremarkable.

Because the iron accumulates very slowly in hereditary haemochromatosis, tissue damage is seldom debilitating before the age of 30 years. If the diagnosis is made early, severe tissue damage can be avoided by a programme of weekly venesection involving the removal of at least 500 ml of blood on each occasion. The aim of this programme of venesection is to deplete the excess body iron stores over a 12-18 month period. Once depleted, reaccumulation can be prevented by a less energetic programme involving bimonthly venesection. Recent experience suggests that, provided that treatment is started early and controlled carefully, life expectancy and the risk of hepatoma are returned to normal.

A recent Swedish study demonstrated the potential dangers of iron fortification of food in developed countries. 350 subjects had their iron status assessed: none of the women were iron-loaded but 5% of the men had iron stores above normal limits. 2% of the men had iron stores approaching those of early haemochromatosis!

Iron fortification remains a useful public health measure in underdeveloped countries where the average diet is deficient in iron.

Transfusion-associated Haemosiderosis

As described in Chapter 7, β thalassaemia homozygotes are completely dependent on a programme of regular blood transfusion. Each transfusion of 400 ml of blood carries with it approximately 200 mg of iron which cannot be excreted. Steady accumulation of body iron results with similar consequences to those described above for hereditary haemochromatosis. The accumulation of iron in body stores is slowed appreciably by the administration of chelating agents such as desferrioxamine but, at present, these only delay the inevitable. The development of effective oral chelating agents would be a major advance in the treatment of the thalassaemia syndromes.

Dietary Causes

Iron overload due to dietary causes was reported to be a serious problem in the Bantu people of Southern Africa. The cause of this was reputed to be the local habit of cooking exclusively in iron pots coupled with enthusiastic imbibing of strong, home-brewed beer which had been brewed and illicitly stored in iron drums. For a number of reasons, **Bantu siderosis**, as this condition was called, appears to be on the wane.

Acute iron poisoning due to ingestion of a large number of iron tablets intended for therapeutic use is one of the most common causes of fatal poisoning in young children. If discovered early, gastric lavage and desferrioxamine therapy may prevent serious toxicity.

Chronic use of iron supplements in the absence of iron deficiency can lead to iron overload because the large quantities of iron present are absorbed by passive diffusion across the gut wall, regardless of the state of the body iron stores.

Suggested Further Reading

Jacobs, A. (ed.) (1986). Disorders of Iron Metabolism. *Clinics in Haematology*, **11**: 241-486.

Lee, G.R. (1983). The Anaemia of Chronic Disease. *Seminars in Haematology*, **20**: 61-80.

Bothwell, T.H. and Charlton, R.W. (1988) Historical Overview of Haemochromatosis. *Annals of the New York Academy of Sciences,* **526:** 1-10.

Marcus, R.E. and Huehns, E.R. (1985). Transfusional Iron Overload. *Clinical and Laboratory Haematology,* **7:** 195-212.

Haemoglobin Synthesis, Structure and Function

The haemoglobins are red globular proteins which have a molecular weight of about 64,500 and comprise almost one third of the weight of a red cell. Their primary function is the carriage of oxygen from the lungs to the tissues. This chapter describes the processes involved in the synthesis of normal haemoglobin, the normal structure of the haemoglobin molecule and, finally, details normal haemoglobin function. Understanding of the material in this chapter is assumed in Chapters 7 and 8 where abnormalities of haemoglobin synthesis, structure and function are described.

Over 400 different variants of haemoglobin have been described but all share the same basic structure of four **globin** polypeptide chains each with a prosthetic **haem** group. Functional haemoglobins are composed of two pairs of dissimilar globins.

Haemoglobin Synthesis

Although haem and globin synthesis occur separately within developing red cell precursors their rates of synthesis are carefully co-ordinated to ensure optimal efficiency of haemoglobin assembly.

Haem Synthesis

Haem belongs to the class of pigments known as **porphyrins**. It is composed of 4 pyrroles linked by methene bridges each bound to a central ferrous ion (Fe^{2+}) as shown in Figure 6.1. Haem is synthesised to some extent in virtually all human tissues but the most important sites are the liver (for incorporation into cytochromes) and red cell precursors.

The first step of haem synthesis involves the combination of glycine and the succinic acid derivative succinyl Co-A to produce δ **aminolaevulinic acid** (δALA). This reaction is energy dependent and so occurs within the mitochondria. It is catalysed by the enzyme δALA synthetase. This step is the rate-limiting reaction for the whole pro-

Cyclic tetrapyrroles are extremely important structures in the maintenance of life in all of its myriad forms. Three examples should suffice to demonstrate the veracity of this statement: **haem** is an essential component of the oxygen-transporting proteins of animals; **chlorophyll** is central to photosynthesis which maintains plant life and acts as an important source of atmospheric oxygen and **vitamin B_{12}** is essential for DNA synthesis.

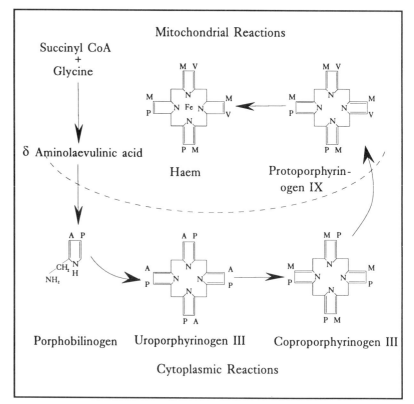

Figure 6.1 *The processes involved in haem synthesis*
P - propionyl
A - acetate
M - methyl
V - vinyl

cess of haem synthesis. It is stimulated by the presence of free globin chains and inhibited by the presence of free haem groups. This represents an important control mechanism of the rate of haem synthesis and its coordination with globin synthesis. Several cofactors are required for this first step, including the vitamin B_6 derivative pyridoxal phosphate and the presence of free ferrous and copper ions. Synthesis of the enzyme δALA synthetase is also inhibited by the presence of free haem. This represents a further feedback inhibition mechanism for haem synthesis.

Two molecules of δALA then condense asymmetrically to form a pyrrole called **porphobilinogen** (PBG) under the influence of the enzyme δALA dehydrogenase and glutathione. This and subsequent reactions occur in the cytoplasm of the cell.

The next step requires the synthesis of the porphyrin ring. The reactions involved in this process are extremely complex but can be summarised as the condensation of four PBG molecules to form the asymmetric cyclic tetra-pyrrole **uroporphyrinogen III** (UPG III). Synthesis of UPG III requires the presence of two enzymes (uroporphyrinogen I synthetase and uroporphyrinogen III cosynthetase) and involves the formation of several short-lived intermediates.

UPG III is converted to **coproporphyrinogen III** (CPG III) by decarboxylation of the acetate side chains under the influence of the enzyme uroporphyrinogen decarboxylase. CPG III enters mitochondria where it is converted to **protoporphyrinogen IX** (PPG IX) by an unknown mechanism. This reaction is catalysed by the enzyme coproporphyrinogen oxidase. PPG IX is further converted within the mitochondria to **protoporphyrin IX**. It only remains for the central ferrous ion to be inserted to complete the synthesis of haem. This reaction is catalysed by the enzyme ferrochelatase and requires the presence of reducing agents. The synthesis of haem is depicted schematically in Figure 6.1

Globin Synthesis

The various globins which combine with haem to form haemoglobins are all single chain polypeptides and, in common with all other proteins, their synthesis is under genetic control. Humans normally carry 8 functional globin genes, arranged in two duplicated gene clusters: the β-like cluster on the short arm of chromosome 11 and the α-like cluster on the short arm of chromosome 16. These genes code for 6 different types of globin chains viz α, β, γ, δ, ζ and ε globin.

Ontogeny of Globin Synthesis

Globin synthesis is first detectable in the primitive erythroid precursor of the yolk sac at about three weeks gestation. At this stage of development, the embryonic globin genes ζ and ε are synthesised, resulting in the formation of **haemoglobin Gower 1** $(\zeta\varepsilon)_2$. Activation of the α and γ genes occurs at about five weeks gestation when **haemoglobin Portland** $(\zeta\gamma)_2$ and **haemoglobin Gower 2** $(\alpha\varepsilon)_2$ are synthesised. These three embryonic haemoglobins are undetectable by routine methods after about 10 weeks gestation. This is coincident with the end of the yolk sac phase of erythropoiesis.

As the rate of synthesis of ζ and ε globins decreases, that of α and γ globins increases sharply. Thus, the predominant haemoglobin for

Key Dates

1660	Air recognised as absolute requirement for life by Boyle
1777	Oxygen identified as vital component of air by Lavoisier
1848	Guinea pig haemoglobin crystallised
1864	Name haemoglobin first coined and oxygen binding capacity demonstrated by Felix Hoppe-Seyler
1894	Hüfner demonstrated haemoglobin oxygen carrying capacity of 1.34 ml/g Hb
1913	First suggestion that haem is a cyclic tetrapyrrole
1929	First synthesis of protoporphyrin by Fischer
1946-1960	Elucidation of haem biosynthetic pathway
1960	Structure of haemoglobin elucidated by Max Perutz using X-ray crystallography
1978	β globin gene cloned
1978-Present	Rapid advances in understanding of molecular biology of globin synthesis

the remainder of foetal life is **haemoglobin F** $(\alpha\gamma)_2$. At birth, approximately 50-80% of the haemoglobin content is of this type. Maximal synthesis of γ globin coincides with the hepatic phase of foetal erythropoiesis.

Synthesis of β globin begins at about the same time as α and γ globin but it remains a minor component until just before birth. The sharp increase in synthesis of β globin coincides with the establishment of the bone marrow as the main site of erythropoiesis. After birth, β globin synthesis continues to replace γ globin synthesis until 97% of the haemoglobin present is haemoglobin A $(\alpha\beta)_2$ and haemoglobin F accounts for less than 1%. This stage is usually reached by about 6 months of age. The remaining 2-3% of haemoglobin consists of **haemoglobin A$_2$** $(\alpha\delta)_2$. δ globin synthesis begins at about 30 weeks gestation but remains a minor component throughout life. At present, the mechanism of switching from embryonic to foetal to adult globin chain synthesis is poorly understood. The relative rates of synthesis of the different globins throughout life are depicted in Figure 6.2.

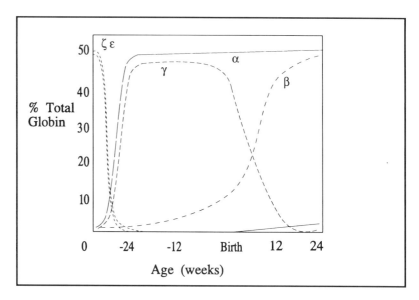

Figure 6.2 *Ontogeny of globin chain synthesis*

Structure of the Globin Gene Clusters

Mapping of the α-like and β-like globin gene clusters using recombinant DNA techniques has revealed a number of striking similarities in the structure of the individual genes:

- all globin genes contain three coding regions, or **exons**, which are interrupted by two non-coding intervening sequences, or **introns**.

- the relative positions and lengths of the exons and introns are similar in all globin genes. Homology is particularly close within clusters eg the exons of the β and δ genes show almost 90% identity.

This remarkable conservation of globin gene structure indicates that our present arrangement of two clusters of related globin genes has been arrived at by a process of gene duplication with subsequent divergence due to the gradual accumulation of mutations. Analysis of the degree of divergence between the α and β globin genes suggests that the original duplication event occurred about 500 million years ago. The degree of conservation of globin gene structure is depicted in Figure 6.3.

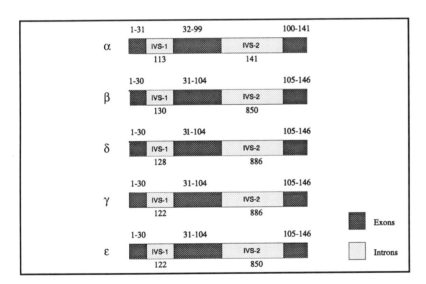

Figure 6.3 *Conservation of globin gene structure. The numbers above the exons represent the amino acid positions within the completed globin. The numbers beneath the introns represent the number of nucleotides present. The similarity in the positions and lengths of the exons and introns is obvious.*

α-like Globin Gene Cluster

The α-like globin gene cluster occupies about 30 kb at the tip of the short arm of chromosome 16. As shown in Figure 6.4 it contains three functional globin genes (ζ2, α1 and α2), three pseudogenes (ψζ1, ψα1 and ψα2) and a gene of uncertain status (θ1).

The pseudogenes are duplicates of functional genes. They show a high degree of homology with their functional counterparts but

The functional ζ gene is known as the ζ2 gene because early workers thought that both ζ globin genes were functional. Although the ζ1 gene is now known to be a pseudogene the numbered designations have been retained to avoid confusion.

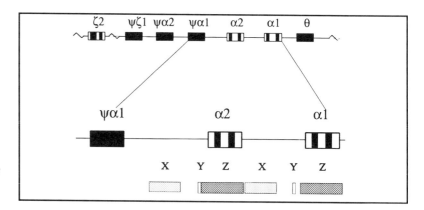

Figure 6.4 *The α-like globin gene cluster*

have acquired mutations which prevent their expression eg ψζ1 has acquired a stop (TAG) codon within exon 1.

The status of the θ1 gene in man remains uncertain. The complete gene and immediate extragenic regions have been mapped and no sequences which would prevent its expression found. Indeed, low levels of θ mRNA have been demonstrated *in utero*. However, no mature theta globin has ever been demonstrated and deletion of the gene has no apparent clinical effect.

The two functional α genes differ from each other only in the structure of IVS-2 and in the untranslated sequences downstream (3') of the stop codon. Thus, the α globin they produce is identical. Expression of the α2 gene is about three times greater than that of the α1 gene. The two functional α globin genes have been shown to lie within one of two duplicated 4 kb regions which are divided by small divergent sequences into homologous boxes labelled X, Y and Z. The two Z boxes are spaced 3.7 kb apart while the two X boxes are 4.2 kb apart. Deletions resulting from unequal crossing-over in this region result in the two most common forms of α^+ thalassaemia ($-\alpha^{3.7}$ and $-\alpha^{4.2}$). This is explained in more detail in Chapter 7. The extragenic region of the α-like gene cluster is highly polymorphic. Five hypervariable regions (HVR) have been identified:

- at the 5' end of the gene cluster.

- within IVS-1 of the ζ2 gene.

- within IVS-2 of the ζ2 gene.

- between the ζ2 and ψζ1 genes.

- at the 3′ end of the gene cluster.

These HVRs consist of a variable number of tandem repeats of short sequences of DNA eg the HVR identified within IVS-2 of the ζ2 gene consists of between 35 and 52 repeats of the sequence CGGGG. The number of repeats within each HVR usually differs for each chromosome 16 of the diploid pair. Individual HVR loci are inherited in a simple Mendelian fashion. The polymorphic nature of the α-like globin gene cluster is compounded by the presence of several restriction fragment length polymorphisms (RFLP) scattered along its length.

β-like Globin Gene Cluster

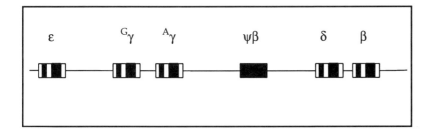

Figure 6.5 *The β–like globin gene cluster*

The β-like globin gene complex occupies about 60 kb on the short arm of chromosome 11. As shown in Figure 6.5 it contains five functional globin genes (ε, $^{G}\gamma$, $^{A}\gamma$, δ and β) and a pseudogene (ψβ).

The gene products of the $^{G}\gamma$ and $^{A}\gamma$ genes differ only in the amino acid which is inserted at position 136: glycine and alanine respectively.

The β-like globin gene cluster does not contain any hypervariable regions but does include several single base restriction fragment length polymorphisms scattered along its length. The pattern of RFLPs present within a single β-like globin gene cluster is known as its **haplotype**. A relatively small number of common haplotypes have been identified which show a close association with racial origin and also with specific β thalassaemia alleles within a population. This feature has been exploited in the antenatal diagnosis of β thalassaemia.

The δ globin gene is expressed at a much lower rate than the α or β globin genes. Many workers believe that the human δ globin gene is in the process of becoming a pseudogene.

Structure of Globin Genes

The complete nucleotide sequences of both the α-like and β-like globin gene clusters are now known. A number of features of functional significance are highly conserved in these and other structural genes. In common with other rapidly transcribed genes, the region immediately upstream (5′) of the globin genes includes three highly conserved sequences which promote effective transcription:

- the sequence ATA invariably is present 30 bp upstream of the transcription initiation site. This promotor region is known as the **ATA box**. The sequences between the ATA box and the initiation site do not appear to affect transcription significantly.

- the sequence **CCAAT** at about 70 bp upstream of the transcription initiation site.

- a **GC-rich region** of 20-50 bases just upstream of the CCAAT box.

The intervening sequences of the various globin genes, despite their similar position and length, are not highly conserved except in the region of the exon-intron junctions. The ends of both intervening sequences are constant; the dinucleotides GT and AG invariably are present at the 5′ and 3′ ends respectively. These dinucleotides appear to be an absolute requirement for splicing of the primary mRNA transcript, since any mutation abolishes this function. The adjacent sequences are moderately conserved and appear to be involved in the regulation of splicing. The region immediately downstream (3′) of the globin genes contains the sequence **AATAAA**. This is the signal for addition of the **polyadenylate (polyA) tail** to the mRNA transcript. The structure of the β globin gene is shown in Figure 6.6.

Figure 6.6 *The structure of the β globin gene*

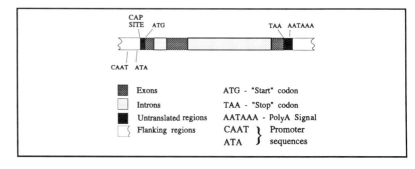

Expression of Globin Genes

Synthesis of mature globin from its gene involves a number of steps:

- transcription of the gene into mRNA.

- processing of the primary mRNA transcript.

- splicing of the introns from the transcript.

- translation of the transcript into globin.

These processes are depicted in Figure 6.7.

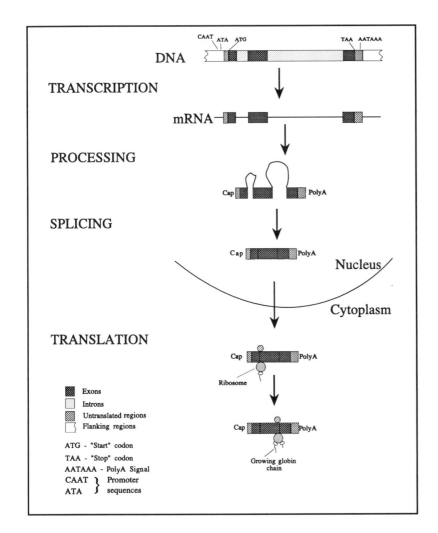

Figure 6.7 *Globin gene expression*

Transcription

Transcription involves the creation of a complementary mRNA copy of the gene and is catalysed in humans by the enzyme RNA polymerase II. Transcription of the gene begins about 30 bases downstream from the ATA box and continues well beyond the AATAAA polyA addition signal. The primary mRNA transcript thus produced is 1.5 kb in length and is a complementary copy of the complete gene, including exons, introns and untranslated leader and trailer sequences at the 5′ and 3′ ends. The primary transcript is incapable of translation.

Processing of the Primary mRNA Transcript

The primary mRNA transcript requires considerable post-transcriptional modification before its release from the nucleus as a functional mRNA molecule. The 5′ end of the primary RNA transcript is modified by the binding of a 7-methylguanylate **cap structure** in a 5′-5′ bond with the +1 nucleotide. The 5′ cap structure is required for optimal translation. The 3′ end of the transcript is cleaved about 10-30 bases downstream from the polyA addition signal. This cleavage exposes a 3′ hydroxyl group to which a string of adenylate residues are quickly bound under the influence of the enzyme polyA polymerase. This **polyadenylate tail** probably serves to stabilise the processed transcript.

Splicing

Before globin mRNA is capable of translation into functional globin the non-coding intervening sequences must be excised and the exons ligated. The exon-intron junctions of genes are identifiable by the constant presence of the dinucleotides GT at the 5′ junction and AG at the 3′ junction. In addition, the sequences adjacent to these dinucleotides are moderately conserved.

The initial step in splicing involves the cutting of the transcript at the 5′ exon-intron junction. The guanylate residue at the 5′ end of the intron then binds to the free 2′ OH group of an adenylate residue about 25 bases upstream from the 3′ exon-intron junction to form a "lariat" structure. This is followed by cleavage of the 3′ exon-intron junction and ligation of the two exons. Both intervening sequences are removed in this manner resulting in the formation of mature mRNA which is approximately 0.7 kb in length.

The naturally occurring bases found in nucleic acids are of four types:

- 6-ketopyrimidines
- 6-aminopyrimidines
- 6-ketopurines
- 6-aminopurines

In DNA, the four bases present are thymine (5-methyluracil), cytosine, guanine and adenine respectively. In RNA, the 6-ketopyrimidine is uracil, the other three bases are identical. Thus, the polyadenylation signal in DNA (AATAAA) becomes AAUAAA when transcribed into mRNA.

Translation

As will be seen in Chapter 8, the amino acid sequence of a globin chain plays a critical role in determining the structure and function of the haemoglobin molecule it forms. Substitution of a single amino acid can prove catastrophic. It is therefore essential that translation of the genetic information present on the mRNA transcript is accurate.

The nucleotide sequence of the mature mRNA transcript constitutes the genetic code from which the appropriate sequence of amino acids which constitute the globin chain is determined. The genetic code is read as a series of nucleotide triplets called **codons**. Since there are four different bases present in mRNA (cytosine (C), adenine (A), guanine (G) and uracil (U)), there are $4^3 = 64$ different codons. 61 of these code uniquely for a single amino acid as shown in Table 6.1. The remaining three codons, UAA, UAG and UGA do not code for an amino acid and therefore cause translation to stop ie they are **chain termination** or **"stop" codons**. The codon for methionine, AUG, is uniformly present as the first codon in the mRNA and acts as a signal for translation to begin, ie it acts as a **chain initiation** or **"start" codon**.

5′ Nucleotide	Central Nucleotide				3′ Nucleotide
	U	C	A	G	
U	Phenylalanine	Serine	Tyrosine	Cysteine	U
	Phenylalanine	Serine	Tyrosine	Cysteine	C
	Leucine	Serine	**STOP**	**STOP**	A
	Leucine	Serine	**STOP**	Tryptophan	G
C	Leucine	Proline	Histidine	Arginine	U
	Leucine	Proline	Histidine	Arginine	C
	Leucine	Proline	Glutamine	Arginine	A
	Leucine	Proline	Glutamine	Arginine	G
A	Isoleucine	Threonine	Asparagine	Serine	U
	Isoleucine	Threonine	Asparagine	Serine	C
	Isoleucine	Threonine	Lysine	Arginine	A
	START	Threonine	Lysine	Arginine	G
G	Valine	Alanine	Aspartic acid	Glycine	U
	Valine	Alanine	Aspartic acid	Glycine	C
	Valine	Alanine	Glutamic acid	Glycine	A
	Valine	Alanine	Glutamic acid	Glycine	G

Table 6.1 *The genetic code. Each amino acid is coded for by a nucleotide triplet eg UCA codes for serine*

Conversion of the genetic code into a sequence of amino acids is accomplished by another form of RNA, **transfer RNA** (tRNA). The tRNA molecule contains two functionally important structures:

- a **3′ terminal unpaired CCA sequence** which is the amino acid binding site. Many different tRNAs exist, each capable of binding only one specific amino acid to its CCA sequence by a process known as aminoacylation.

- an **anticodon loop** which contains a trinucleotide complementary to the codon for the amino acid which the particular tRNA can bind eg tRNA^{ala} contains an alanine anticodon. This ensures that the genetic code is accurately translated.

The process of translation is continuous but will be considered in three phases:

- initiation of translation.

- elongation of the polypeptide chain.

- termination of translation.

Initiation of Translation

The mature globin mRNA migrates from the nucleus to the cytoplasm of the erythroblast and binds, probably via the cap structure, to the 40S subunit of a ribosome. An initiator tRNA molecule then binds to the AUG initiation codon of the mRNA molecule. This initiator tRNA molecule is aminoacylated with methionine (methionyl-tRNA^{imet}) but differs structurally from the tRNA which incorporates methionine into the body of a protein chain (methionyl-tRNA^{met}). Chain initiation is aided by a number of proteins called **initiation factors**. The methionine thus introduced at the start of all globin chains is removed during the process of chain elongation. The initiator tRNA is bound to a site on the large (60S) subunit of the ribosome which is known as the P site because it binds **P**eptidyl-tRNA complexes. A second binding site exists adjacent to the P site called the A site because it binds **A**minoacyl-tRNAs. The A site is unoccupied at this stage but is close to the second codon of the mRNA transcript.

Elongation of the Polypeptide Chain

Elongation of the globin chain occurs when an aminoacylated tRNA corresponding to the second mRNA codon occupies the A site on the ribosome and a peptide bond forms between the methionine and the second amino acid. In the process of dipeptide formation, the tRNA^{imet} is dislodged from the P site and the ribosome moves along the mRNA transcript so that the dipeptidyl-tRNA occupies the P site and the unoccupied A site is adjacent to the third codon. This process is mediated by a group of proteins called **elongation factors** and continues until a chain termination codon is encountered. The process of chain elongation is shown schematically in Figure 6.8.

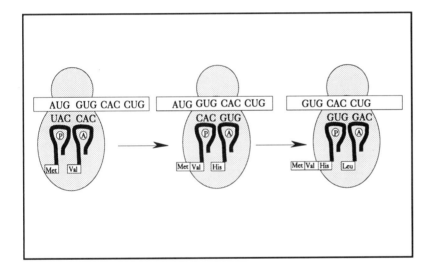

Figure 6.8 *The process of chain elongation in globin synthesis*
A - Aminoacyl binding site
P - Peptidyl binding site

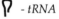 *- tRNA*

Termination of Translation

No tRNA exists which has an anticodon complementary to any of the three chain termination codons. Thus, when the A site of the ribosome lies over a chain termination codon, elongation stops. The A site is then occupied by a protein termination factor which signals the release of the completed protein chain and the dissociation of the ribosome from the mRNA.

The nascent globin chains immediately bind a haem group, fold into their secondary and tertiary configurations and associate to form tetrameric haemoglobin.

Haemoglobin Structure

Primary Structure of Globin

The primary structure of globin refers to the amino acid sequence of the various chain types. The position of individual amino acids is identified by numbering from the N-terminal end. Thus, the sixth amino acid from the N-terminal end of the β globin chain is designated β^6. However, certain amino acids perform the same essential role in all normal globin chains. The identity and position of these amino acids cannot be changed without causing gross impairment to molecular function. The positional similarities of these so-called "invariant amino acids" is not revealed by numbering according to primary sequence.

Secondary Structure of Globin

The secondary structure of all globin chain types comprises nine non-helical sections joined by eight helical sections as shown in Figure 6.9. The helical sections are identified by the letters A-H while the non-helical sections are identified by a pair of letters corresponding to the adjacent helices eg NA (N-terminal end to the start of A helix), AB (joins the A helix to the B helix) etc.

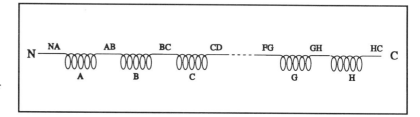

Figure 6.9 *The secondary structure of globin.*

One complete turn of the helix requires between three and four amino acid residues. The amino acid side chains point outwards from the axis of the helix. This means that the side chains of amino acids which are in closest apposition, and therefore most likely to interact with each other, are not those of sequentially adjacent amino acids but of amino acids which are one turn of the helix apart. This is an important consideration when studying amino acid substitutions in abnormal haemoglobins. Individual amino acids can be identified according to their position in the secondary structure. This is a useful notation because invariant amino acids often appear in the same positions in all types of globin chain. For example, the α^{58} and β^{63} amino acids are both histidine residues, but their position in the primary structure provides no clue that their function may be related. However, both residues occupy the position E7 in the secondary structure of their respective globin chains. This position must always be occupied by a histidine residue because it is one of the two sites to which the haem group is bound.

Tertiary Structure of Globin

The tertiary folding of each globin chain forms an approximate sphere. The intra-molecular bonds which give rise to the helical parts of the chain impart considerable structural rigidity, causing chain folding to occur in the non-helical parts. Tertiary folding gives rise to at least three functionally important characteristics of the haemoglobin molecule:

- polar or charged side chains tend to be directed to the outside surface of the subunit and, conversely, non-polar structures tend to be directed inwards. The effect of this is to make the surface of the molecule hydrophilic and the interior hydrophobic.

- an open-topped cleft in the surface of the subunit known as the **haem pocket** is created. Each globin subunit has one haem pocket in which is bound a single haem group. Within this hydrophobic cleft, the ferrous ion of the haem group is protected from the oxidative effects of water which would destroy its oxygen-binding capability.

- the amino acids which form the inter-subunit bonds responsible for maintaining the quaternary structure, and thus the function, of the haemoglobin molecule are brought into the correct spatial orientation to permit these bonds to form.

Quaternary Structure of Haemoglobin

The quaternary structure of haemoglobin has four subunits arranged tetrahedrally as shown in Figure 6.10. All functional

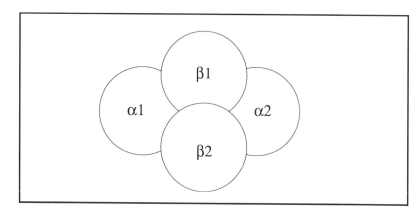

Figure 6.10 *The quaternary structure of haemoglobin*

mammalian haemoglobins are composed of two α-like and two β-like globin subunits. The structure of haemoglobin A is often written as $\alpha_2\beta_2$ but the designation $(\alpha\beta)_2$ is preferred because this implies, correctly, that the molecule is made up of two equal and identical dimers. Each dimer is held together very firmly and inflexibly by strong inter-subunit bonds involving over 30 amino acid residues, which impart stability. The area of contact is known as the $\alpha_1\beta_1$ or $\alpha_2\beta_2$ junction. Dimers have a limited ability to exist separately and a small proportion of all normal haemoglobin exists in this dissociated form.

The $\alpha_1\beta_2$ and $\alpha_2\beta_1$ contact areas which hold the tetramer together are much less tight than the $\alpha_1\beta_1$ and $\alpha_2\beta_2$ contact areas. The $\alpha_1\beta_2$ and $\alpha_2\beta_1$ contact areas involve less than 20 amino acid residues each, and it is across these junctions that the sliding molecular movements which accompany oxygen uptake and release occur.

There are two other areas of contact between globin subunits in the haemoglobin tetramer viz the $\alpha_1\alpha_2$ and the $\beta_1\beta_2$ contact areas. Bonding at these contact areas is, of necessity, considerably weaker than at the other contact areas. In deoxyhaemoglobin, the two β chains are too far apart for bonding to occur, and a functionally significant area, the β cleft, exists. On oxygenation, however, the whole molecule contracts and the β cleft disappears as the two chains move very close together. Weak interaction between the β chains is possible in this state. Strong bonding would interfere with oxygen release because deoxygenation involves the two β chains separating again. Conversely, the two α chains are some distance apart in the oxygenated state and move closer together on deoxygenation when weak interaction is possible: strong bonding between α chains would inhibit oxygenation.

Haemoglobin Function

Haemoglobin-Oxygen Binding

Oxygenation of haemoglobin is associated with considerable movement within the molecule. In the deoxygenated state, the central ferrous ions of the four haem groups are too large to fit into the plane of their porphyrin rings without causing severe distortion of the optimal ring structure. Oxygenation of the first haem group causes distortion of the electron cloud of the ferrous ion and facilitates the assumption of a truly planar configuration. Movement of the ferrous ion into the plane of the porphyrin ring pulls the attached α globin chain inwards, thereby reducing the width of the haem pocket and allowing the haem group to tilt somewhat from its upright, deoxygenated position.

Movement of the first α globin chain pulls on the other globin chains and causes a conformational change in the whole haemoglobin molecule which results in increased oxygen affinity. As each haem group is oxygenated, reduction in the size of its haem pocket induces further conformational change which further increases the oxygen affinity of the molecule. This process, whereby the sequential oxygenation of haem groups has an effect on the subsequent oxygenation of the others is known as **haem-haem interaction**, and is an important feature of normal haemoglobin function.

In the process of complete oxygenation, the diameter of the haemoglobin molecule is reduced by about 10%. Molecular compaction makes the binding of an oxygen molecule to the fourth haem group difficult despite the high oxygen affinity of this binding site. The "effort" required to oxygenate the four haem groups of a typical haemoglobin molecule is depicted graphically in Figure 6.11a. Oxygenation of the first haem group requires the greatest effort but haem-haem interaction ensures that oxygenation of the second and third haem groups is made progressively easier. Steric hindrance caused by molecular compaction makes oxygenation of the last haem group more difficult than expected.

The derivation of Figure 6.11a clearly is hypothetical and simplistic. Oxygenation is an integrated process, involving all four subunits acting in concert. It is the whole molecule that oxygenates or releases oxygen, not the individual subunits. For this reason, each haemoglobin molecule exists only in the fully oxygenated or fully

---

SAQ 1

Are the terms oxidation of haemoglobin and oxygenation of haemoglobin synonymous?

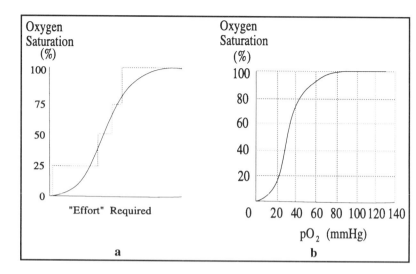

Figure 6.11a *The "effort" required to sequentially oxygenate the four haem groups of a single molecule of haemoglobin*
6.11b *The haemoglobin:oxygen dissociation curve*

SAQ 2

Myoglobin consists of a single polypeptide chain and a single haem group. Predict the shape of the myoglobin:oxygen dissociation curve.

deoxygenated states. Based on the free energy required or generated as the transition between them occurs, the fully deoxygenated and fully oxygenated conformations are known as "tense" (T) and "relaxed" (R) forms of haemoglobin respectively.

Exposure of a haemoglobin solution to increasing partial pressures of oxygen results in an increasing proportion of haemoglobin molecules which exist in the fully oxygenated (R) form. The relationship between partial pressure of oxygen and the degree of oxygen saturation it causes is shown graphically in Figure 6.11b. This curve is known as the **haemoglobin:oxygen dissociation curve** and characteristically is sigmoidal in shape. A variety of allosteric effectors, such as 2,3 DPG and H^+, can affect the position of the haemoglobin:oxygen dissociation curve by moving it left or right as described later. These do not, however, affect the shape of the curve. Maximum oxygen uptake is unaffected by the position of the curve because at normal alveolar pO_2 haemoglobin is always fully saturated. The position of the curve does, however, affect the volume of oxygen that may be donated at any given tissue partial pressure of oxygen.

The shape of the haemoglobin:oxygen dissociation curve can be represented mathematically by an equation first derived empirically by A. V. Hill in 1913:

$$Y = \frac{(pO_2)^n}{(pO_2)^n + (P_{50})^n}$$

Y   fraction of Hb saturated
pO_2 partial pressure of oxygen
P_{50} partial pressure at which 50%
      of the Hb is saturated
n   Hill coefficient
      (for normal Hb =2.8)

Alternatively, the Hill equation may be expressed:

$$\frac{Y}{1 - Y} = \left(\frac{pO_2}{P_{50}}\right)^n$$

The variables n and P_{50} are dependent on the haemoglobin under consideration and on the various factors which affect haemoglobin-oxygen binding. The oxygen affinity of haemoglobin is defined by its P_{50} value. The Hill equation is applicable in the range 10-90% oxygen saturation.

Oxygen Delivery

The haemoglobin:oxygen dissociation curve shown in Figure 6.11b is of limited value as drawn because it is difficult to interpret in terms of oxygen carriage and delivery. The Y-axis can be recalibrated to show the volume of oxygen carried per 100 ml of blood. Under physiological conditions, 100 ml of normal adult blood is capable of carrying a theoretical maximum of about 20 ml of oxygen (see sidebox).

Although the mean alveolar pO_2 of 100 mmHg is sufficient to saturate the oxygen-binding capacity of haemoglobin, not all of the alveoli are equally well ventilated. This means that some of the blood which perfuses the lungs is exposed to a lower pO_2 and so cannot saturate with oxygen. The result is that blood which enters the aorta typically carries only about 97% of the theoretical maximum quantity of oxygen ie about 19.5 ml of oxygen per 100 ml of blood. When this oxygenated blood reaches the systemic capillaries where the pO_2 typically is about 40 mmHg, it is no longer in equilibrium with its environment and so releases about 4.5 ml of oxygen per 100 ml of blood to the tissues. This reduces the oxygen saturation of the haemoglobin to 75%. The partially deoxygenated blood is then transported back to the lungs where it will, again, encounter a mean pO_2 of 100 mmHg and start the cycle all over again with 19.5 ml of oxygen per 100 ml of blood. This chain of events is shown in Figure 6.12a.

The theoretical maximum oxygen binding capacity of "normal" blood assumes a haemoglobin concentration of 14.6 g/dl. Since 1 g of haemoglobin can bind up to 1.34 ml of oxygen, it follows that 100 ml of normal blood can bind up to (1.34 x 14.6) ml of oxygen ie about 20 ml. Obviously, if the haemoglobin concentration is higher or lower, the maximum oxygen binding capacity alters proportionately.

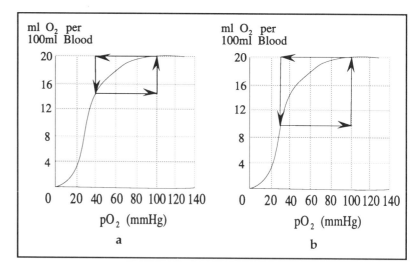

Figure 6.12a *Delivery of oxygen under normal physiological conditions* **6.12b** *Increased delivery of oxygen in response to decreased tissue pO_2*

The extra oxygen, which is apparently needlessly carried, acts as an instantly available reserve when oxygen demand increases. For example, when a muscle contracts, oxygen utilisation increases, causing a localised fall in pO_2. When blood arrives at the capillaries supplying that muscle, it encounters a pO_2 of, for example, 30 mmHg, and is forced to give up more oxygen as it equilibrates. Because of the sigmoid shape of the haemoglobin:oxygen dissociation curve, a drop in partial pressure of oxygen causes a disproportionately large increase in oxygen donation. This chain of events is shown in Figure 6.12b.

As shown in Figure 6.12, a reduced alveolar pO_2 of 70 mmHg still results in about 90% haemoglobin saturation. It is extremely unlikely that, under normal atmospheric conditions, a sufficiently low alveolar pO_2 could ever arise which would reduce significantly the oxygen saturation of blood leaving the lungs. Indeed, breathing could cease altogether for a considerable time before an alveolar pO_2 of 70 mmHg was reached and, even then, the oxygen saturation of the arterial blood would be sufficient to meet the demands of the tissues.

At rest, the typical cardiac output is about 5 litres of blood per minute. This is the minimum blood flow that meets the resting oxygen demand of the body. Since each 100 ml of blood delivers about 4.5 ml of oxygen the resting, or basal, oxygen requirement is about 225 ml of oxygen per minute. Oxygen demand increases rapidly when activity exceeds the basal level. Failure to meet this increased demand by an appropriate increase in oxygen delivery severely limits performance. The necessary increase in oxygen delivery can be achieved by increased release of oxygen per 100 ml of blood, by increasing cardiac output, or both. In normal individuals these mechanisms, along with others which are described later, interact to ensure that oxygen delivery to the tissues is adequate over a wide range of activity levels.

When severe anaemia is present, increases in oxygen demand may be difficult to meet. The value of 20 ml of oxygen carried per 100 ml of blood assumes a normal haemoglobin concentration of 14.6 g/dl. If the haemoglobin concentration falls to, for example, 7 g/dl maximal oxygen carriage falls to less than 10 ml per 100 ml of blood. Greater proportional donation of oxygen by the mechanism described above can still meet basal oxygen demands in this case, but a greatly increased cardiac output and respiration rate is required when activity levels rise. This is manifest as a normal heart rate at rest, but a greatly exaggerated cardiovascular response to exercise: the degree of exaggeration is directly related to the severity of the anaemia. This gives rise to the classical signs of shortness of breath on exertion and palpitations in anaemia.

> **SAQ 3**
>
> Why do long-distance runners often train at high altitudes before an important race?

Carbon Dioxide Transport

Carbon dioxide is excreted via the lungs in exhaled air. It is transported from the tissues to the lungs in the blood in three forms:

- approximately 78% is transported in the form of bicarbonate ions (HCO_3^-), formed by the ionisation of carbonic acid (H_2CO_3). Carbonic acid is formed by the reaction of carbon dioxide and water, a reaction catalysed by the red cell enzyme carbonic anhydrase. Haemoglobin, acting as a buffer, is an important acceptor of the H^+ ions produced along with the HCO_3^- ions.

- approximately 13% is transported bound to proteins as carbaminoproteins. About half of the total is bound to plasma proteins, principally as **carbaminoalbumin**, and the other half is bound intracellularly to globin chains as **carbaminoglobins**. The mechanism of carbon dioxide binding to globin is completely different to that of oxygen binding to haem. Carbon dioxide is acidic and therefore binds to the basic groups which are present on all proteins at physiological pH.

- approximately 9% is transported in solution in plasma and cell water.

Integration of Oxygen and Carbon Dioxide Transport

Several factors play a role in the regulation of oxygen transport by preferentially binding to and stabilising deoxyhaemoglobin, thereby promoting oxygen release. These include carbon dioxide, bicarbonate ions (HCO_3^-) and the allosteric effectors H^+ and 2,3 DPG.

The oxygen affinity of haemoglobin is affected by the presence of carbon dioxide in two ways:

- H^+ ions formed by the ionisation of carbonic acid within the red cell bind preferentially to deoxyhaemoglobin, thereby causing an equilibrium shift in favour of the deoxygenated form of haemoglobin.

- carbaminoglobins are formed by the binding of the acidic carbon dioxide to basic amino groups at the N-terminal ends of deoxygenated α and β globin chains. Carbaminoglobin formation therefore shifts the equilibrium between oxygenated and deoxygenated haemoglobin towards the deoxygenated form. However, only small amounts of carbaminoglobins are formed under physiological conditions. The effect of pH on haemoglobin oxygen affinity is much more important.

The effect of carbon dioxide on the oxygen affinity of haemoglobin is observable as a "shift to the right" of the haemoglobin:oxygen dissociation curve as shown in Figure 6.13a. Since H^+ ions are freely diffusible across the red cell membrane, a decrease in plasma pH stimulates increased oxygen donation. This is a physiologically appropriate response because acidosis results either from increased carbon dioxide tension or, under anaerobic conditions, from lactate production in the tissues where optimal oxygen delivery is

---

Animals which live only at very high altitude such as Andean llamas typically have haemoglobins which have a haemoglobin:oxygen dissociation curve which is shifted far to the left ie their haemoglobin has a high affinity for oxygen. This ensures maximal oxygen binding in the lungs at low atmospheric partial pressure of oxygen and represents an excellent example of adaptive evolution. Llamas do not develop the polycythaemia which typifies humans at high altitude.

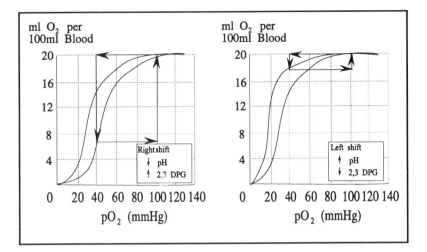

Figure 6.13a *The "shift to the right" of the haemoglobin:oxygen dissociation curve which accompanies a drop in pH or an increase in 2,3 DPG concentration*

6.13b *The "shift to the left" of the haemoglobin:oxygen dissociation curve which accompanies a rise in pH or a decrease in 2,3 DPG concentration*

demanded. The combined effect of reduced pO_2 and right shift which results can stimulate the release of up to 75% of the bound oxygen. This equates to about 15 ml of oxygen released per 100 ml of blood, or three times normal, being donated. The effect of pH on the oxygen affinity of haemoglobin is known as the **Bohr effect**. This subject is considered in more detail in Chapter 8.

Conversely, an increase in plasma bicarbonate concentration (alkalosis) leads to a shift to the left of the haemoglobin:oxygen dissociation curve ie to an increased oxygen affinity as shown in Figure 6.13b.

The transportation of carbon dioxide with respect to pCO_2 can be represented graphically as shown in Figure 6.14. There is a maximum amount of carbon dioxide that can be dissolved in a given volume of blood. The total carbon dioxide carried can be increased, however, by increasing the proportion carried as bicarbonate ions. Bicarbonate formation is favoured by haemoglobin deoxygenation and H^+ uptake. Thus, there is no absolute value for the amount of carbon dioxide that can be carried in a given blood volume at a given pCO_2. Rather, there is a range of values which is influenced by the amount of oxyhaemoglobin present as shown in Figure 6.14.

2,3 DPG and Haemoglobin Oxygen Affinity

As described in Chapter 10, one of the products of glycolysis within red cells is 2,3 diphosphoglyceric acid (2,3 DPG). This substance binds to the β globin chains of deoxygenated haemoglobin A $(\alpha\beta)_2$

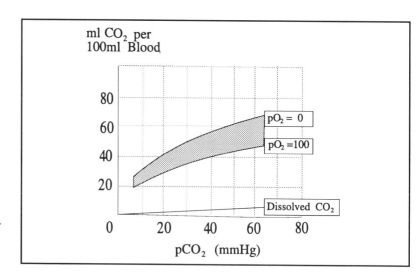

Figure 6.14 *The transportation of carbon dioxide in the blood*

in such a way that it occupies the cleft between the β chains. Since oxygenation involves contraction of the β cleft it would also require expulsion of the avidly bound 2,3 DPG. Thus, the relatively high concentration of 2,3 DPG found in red cells favours the deoxygenated form of haemoglobin A and therefore decreases its oxygen affinity.

Synthesis of 2,3 DPG is inhibited by acid conditions and potentiated by alkaline conditions. pH therefore has an indirect as well as a direct effect on haemoglobin oxygen affinity. However, unlike the Bohr effect which is immediate, the indirect effect of pH on haemoglobin oxygen affinity via 2,3 DPG synthesis is not manifest for several hours. Thus, a long-term shift of pH will affect 2,3 DPG levels, but a short-term shift will not. For example, the respiratory alkalosis which commonly accompanies severe anaemia indirectly increases oxygen delivery to the tissues by stimulating 2,3 DPG synthesis. This is a physiologically appropriate response.

Rapid correction of acute anaemia by blood transfusion increases the oxygen carrying capacity of the blood but, because of the relative deficiency of 2,3 DPG in stored blood, does not similarly increase delivery of oxygen to the tissues for up to 24 hours thereafter. In such a case, a normal haemoglobin concentration does not preclude the existence of acute tissue hypoxia.

2,3 DPG binds avidly to β globin, but not to other non-α globins. This means that haemoglobins which lack β globin chains, such as

> **SAQ 4**
>
> The concentration of 2,3 DPG rises in normal, uncomplicated pregnancy. Explain why this is physiologically appropriate.

haemoglobin F $(\alpha\gamma)_2$ and haemoglobin A_2 $(\alpha\delta)_2$, have a higher oxygen affinity than haemoglobin A in the presence of 2,3 DPG. The increased oxygen affinity of haemoglobin F confers its ability to extract oxygen from maternal haemoglobin A at the placental barrier. However, the high oxygen affinity also means oxygen is released to the tissues somewhat less readily than in the adult. This does not present a problem because foetal activity levels necessarily are restricted and the excess oxygen demand which accompanies strenuous physical exercise does not arise.

Suggested Further Reading

Bunn, H.F. and Forget, B.G. (1985). *Haemoglobin: Molecular, Genetic and Clinical Aspects.* Philadelphia: W.B. Saunders.

Darnell, J., Lodish, H. and Baltimore, D. (1990) *Molecular Cell Biology* (2nd ed). New York: Scientific American Books.

Devlin, T.M. (1992). *Textbook of Biochemistry with Clinical Correlations.* New York: Wiley-Liss.

Perutz, M.F. (1978). Haemoglobin Structure and Respiratory Transport. *Scientific American*, **205(6)**: 96-111.

Answers to Self-Assessment Questions

1. No. Oxidation of haemoglobin implies that the ferrous ions in haem are converted to ferric ions. The methaemoglobin thus produced is incapable of binding oxygen. Oxygenation, on the other hand, implies that the haemoglobin molecule has bound oxygen for delivery to the tissues but is chemically unaltered.

2. The myoglobin molecule has no haem-haem interaction. The myoglobin:oxygen dissociation curve is hyperbolic.

3. Training at altitude causes an increase in the circulating red cell count and a rise in 2,3 DPG concentration. Both increase the efficiency of oxygen donation to the tissues and therefore favour the prolonged effort required of long distance runners, particularly when they return to lower altitudes.

4. An increased concentration of 2,3 DPG reduces the oxygen affinity of the maternal haemoglobin and therefore facilitates oxygen exchange with the foetal circulation which carries a high proportion of the high oxygen affinity haemoglobin HbF.

The Thalassaemia Syndromes

The thalassaemias are a heterogeneous group of inherited disorders which are characterised by reduced or absent synthesis of one or more globin chain type. The imbalance of globin chain synthesis which results leads to ineffective erythropoiesis and a shortened red cell lifespan. In contrast to the structural haemoglobinopathies, the affected globin chain is structurally normal; it is only the *rate* at which it is synthesised which is affected.

The division of the haemoglobinopathies into structural and thalassaemia types is not always straightforward, however. Many structurally abnormal globins are synthesised at a greatly reduced rate and so do not fit clearly into either category. Several examples of such "thalassaemic haemoglobinopathies" are described in this chapter.

The name thalassaemia was coined by the eminent haematologist George Whipple in 1932 as an alternative to the eponymous "Cooley's anaemia". He wanted a name which would convey the sense of an anaemia which is prevalent in the region of the Mediterranean Sea, since most of the early cases originated there. Thalassaemia is derived by contraction of thalassic anaemia (from the Greek *thalassa* - sea, *an* - none and *haima* - blood).

Incidence and Distribution

The thalassaemias are among the most common single gene disorders in the world. They are most common in parts of the world where malaria is, or was recently, endemic: the result of positive selection for a gene which affords some protection against malaria. The incidence of thalassaemia is also high in immigrant populations which originate in these parts of the world. The areas of highest incidence of thalassaemia are shown in Figure 7.1.

The distribution of the different forms of thalassaemia is not uniform: each is most commonly found only in certain populations.

β thalassaemia is most common in people from the Mediterranean, Africa, India, SE Asia and Indonesia. The incidence of mutations which lead to β thalassaemia reaches almost 10% in some parts of Greece. The disorder is relatively rare in Northern and Western Europeans and in native Americans.

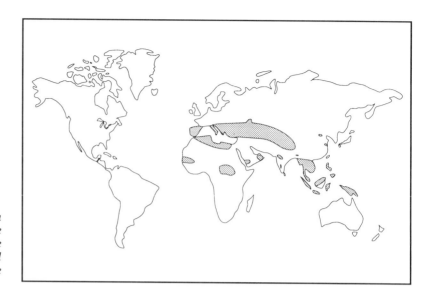

Figure 7.1 *The worldwide distribution of the thalassaemia syndromes. The shaded areas represent areas where the disease is most common, but it is found in virtually all populations of the world*

The clinically mild forms of α thalassaemia (α^+ thalassaemia) are most common in American blacks and in people from Indonesia, SE Asia, the Middle East, India, the Mediterranean and the S Pacific islands. 30% of American blacks are "silent" carriers of α thalassaemia (α^+ heterozygotes), while about 3% are homozygous. Homozygotes express minimal symptoms of disease.

The clinically severe α thalassaemias (α° thalassaemia) are most common in people from the Philippines, SE Asia and S China. The population incidence of deletions which lead to this form of α thalassaemia reaches 25% in some parts of Thailand.

Classification

The thalassaemias are classified according to three criteria:

- the affected globin gene(s) eg α, β, $\delta\beta$, etc

- whether the reduction in the rate of synthesis of the affected globin is partial eg β^+ or absolute eg β°

- the genotype eg homozygous β°

SAQ 1

Do you think that homozygous δ° thalassaemia would be a severe disease?

α Thalassaemia

More than 95% of α thalassaemias result from the deletion of one or both of the tandem α globin genes located on chromosome 16. This gives rise to five possible genotypes:

Type	Genotype	
Normal	$\alpha\alpha/\alpha\alpha$	
α^+ heterozygote	$\alpha-/\alpha\alpha$	
α^+ homozygote	$\alpha-/\alpha-$	
α^0 heterozygote	$--/\alpha\alpha$	
α^0 homozygote	$--/--$	(Barts hydrops foetalis)
$\alpha^0\alpha^+$ double heterozygote	$--/\alpha-$	(haemoglobin H disease)

Individual patients are assigned to one of the above groups according to the results of simple laboratory tests. The tests are performed on as many family members as possible and a pedigree chart constructed. The pedigree chart shown in Figure 7.2 illustrates a typical example of a Thai family with α thalassaemia. The investigation was prompted by the stillbirth of baby (III4).

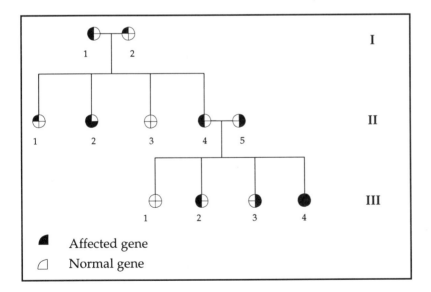

■ Affected gene
◻ Normal gene

Figure 7.2 *Pedigree chart of a typical Thai family with α thalassaemia*

Patient II2 has inherited haemoglobin H disease ($\alpha^+\alpha^0$ compound heterozygote). The dead baby (III4) had inherited haemoglobin Barts hydrops foetalis (homozygous α^0 thalassaemia).

SAQ 2

How would heterozygous γ^0 thalassaemia be manifest in an affected new-born? How would you expect the disease to change as the child grows?

SAQ 3

What type of α thalassaemia do patients I1 and I2 have?

The frequencies of the different deletions which give rise to α thalassaemia vary widely in different races. Deletion of both α globin genes on one chromosome 16 is relatively common in SE Asia and the Philippines, leading to a high incidence of haemoglobin H disease and haemoglobin Barts hydrops foetalis. Conversely, the most common deletion in American blacks is of only one α globin gene. Haemoglobin H disease is rare in the latter population and haemoglobin Barts hydrops foetalis exceedingly so.

β Thalassaemia

Most β thalassaemias result from a point mutation within or close to the β globin gene complex. Each mutation can result in a reduction or abolition of β globin gene function and so to $β^+$ or $β^\circ$ thalassaemia. Therefore, the classification of β thalassaemia is similar to that for α thalassaemia:

Type	Genotype
Normal	$β /β$
$β^+$ heterozygote	$β^+/β$
$β^+$ homozygote	$β^+/β^+$
$β^\circ$ heterozygote	$β^\circ/β$
$β^\circ$ homozygote	$β^\circ/β^\circ$

Molecular Basis

The classification scheme outlined above, although useful, greatly underestimates the complex nature of the relationship between genotype and phenotype in the thalassaemia syndromes. Greater understanding of this fascinating group of disorders can only be achieved by a detailed consideration of their molecular basis.

More than 100 different gene defects which cause thalassaemia have been described. No attempt is made in this section to provide an exhaustive list of these defects. Instead, examples have been selected which illustrate the types of defect which result in thalassaemia.

In theory, thalassaemia can arise from one of two causes: a gross deletion of one or more globin genes, or a mutation which causes defective gene expression.

Gene Deletion Forms

α Thalassaemia

Most α thalassaemias result from gross deletions within the α gene complex. At least nine deletions which result in complete abolition of α globin synthesis have been described. Each deletion is associated with a particular population, and is denoted as such. For example, almost 20% of the population in SE Asia carry the $--^{SEA}$ deletion: the $--^{FIL}$ deletion accounts for almost one third of α thalassaemia genes in the Philippines and the $--^{MED}$ deletion is most common in the Mediterranean region. The sizes and positions of these deletions are shown in Figure 7.3.

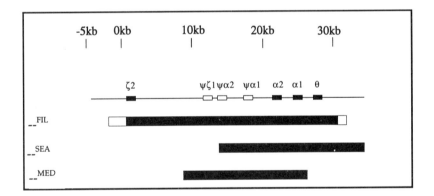

Figure 7.3 *Deletions which result in α⁰ thalassaemia. The shaded regions denote regions known to be deleted. The unfilled regions denote uncertainty over the extent of the deletion*

All three deletions remove both α globin genes on one chromosome and so result in an α⁰ haplotype. Haemoglobin Barts hydrops foetalis is most common in those parts of the world where such deletions are prevalent. The $--^{SEA}$ and the $--^{MED}$ deletions leave the ζ gene intact, allowing synthesis of haemoglobin Portland ($\zeta_2\gamma_2$) *in utero*.

Deletions which cause the removal of only one α globin gene have been described in many populations. These are the most common deletions which produce an α thalassaemia phenotype. Such deletions are denoted according to their size as shown in Figure 7.4.

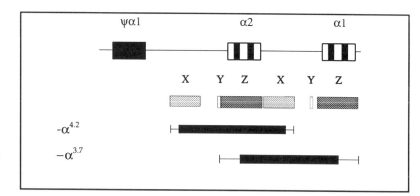

Figure 7.4 *Deletions which result in* α+ *thalassaemia*

These deletions arise from unequal crossing-over of two chromosomes 16 within the homologous X and Z regions of the α globin gene complex. Crossing-over within the X region homology blocks results in the -α$^{4.2}$ deletion while crossing-over within the Z region homology blocks results in the −α$^{3.7}$ deletion. Figure 7.5 depicts the unequal crossing-over which results in the −α$^{4.2}$ deletion. Chromosomes with three α genes are relatively common in the populations in which these deletions are found. These represent the reciprocal ααα$^{anti3.7}$ and the ααα$^{anti4.2}$ formed during the process of unequal crossing-over. Interestingly, the extra α globin gene in these cases usually is functional.

β Thalassaemia

Five different deletions which affect only the β globin gene and result in β thalassaemia have been described but all except one are extremely rare. About one third of β thalassaemias from the Indian subcontinent result from a deletion of 619 bp from the 3′ end of the β globin gene which removes part of IVS-2, exon 3 and extends beyond the gene but leaves the 5′ end intact. This mutation is most common in the Gujurati and Sind peoples.

Three further deletions have been observed which do not affect the β globin gene directly, yet disrupt its expression. All three deletions

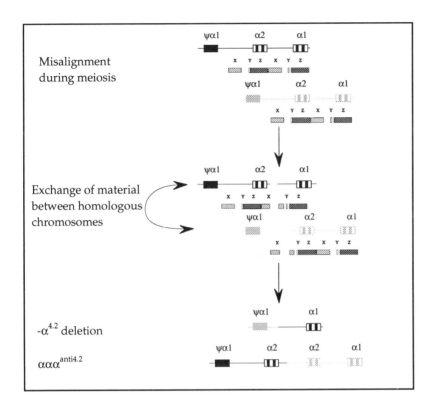

Figure 7.5 *The process of unequal crossing-over which results in the -$\alpha^{4.2}$ deletion*

include a region 5' to the ε globin gene which has been shown to be involved in activation of the β gene complex.

Non-deletion Forms

Point mutations which result in thalassaemia are classified according to the stage of globin gene expression at which the defect becomes manifest. The following effects are recognised:

- inefficient transcription of the gene into mRNA

- defective processing of the primary mRNA transcript

- defective splicing of the mRNA transcript

- improper translation into protein

- post-translational instability

If you are not completely familiar with these processes, review the appropriate section in Chapter 6 before you read the next section.

Transcription Mutants

A number of mutations which lead to inefficient transcription of the β globin gene have been described. All have been located in promoter regions such as the TATA box at -30bp and the CACACCC sequences at -90 and -105 bp upstream of the gene. Such mutations generally result in a clinically mild β^+ thalassaemia phenotype.

For example, substitution of G for A at position -29 is a common cause of β^+ thalassaemia in American blacks. This mutation results in a relatively mild condition, even in homozygotes. Interestingly, an identical mutation has been observed in Chinese populations, but associated with severe disease. The apparently anomalous difference in phenotype appears to be caused by the presence of a second substitution of C $\longrightarrow$ T at -158 to the $^G\gamma$ gene in American blacks which acts as an upregulator of γ globin gene expression. The increased synthesis of γ globin which results partially compensates for the decrease in β globin synthesis.

mRNA Modification Mutants

The substitution of C for A at the +1 nucleotide, or "cap" site of the β globin gene, results in a very mild β^+ thalassaemia. This mutation has only been described in Indians.

Point mutations of the 3' polyadenylation signal sequence (AATAAA) result in failure of cleavage and polyadenylation of the mRNA transcript. For example, the substitution AATAAG for AATAAA has been demonstrated to be the cause of impaired recognition of the polyadenylation signal in a Saudi Arabian with haemoglobin H disease.

A number of similar mutations within the 3' AATAAA sequence of the β globin gene have been described. For example, the substitution of AACAAA for AATAAA is a common cause of β^+ thalassaemia in American blacks. These substitutions do not destroy the polyadenylation signal, they merely render it less effective. Variable amounts of normal mRNA transcripts are also produced in these individuals.

mRNA Splicing Mutants

More than one third of point mutations which result in thalassaemia affect splicing of the processed mRNA transcript.

Mutations of the invariant 5' GT and 3' AG dinucleotides result in the abolition of splicing. For example, deletion of five bases from the 5' donor splice site which removes the T of the required GT dinucleotide (GGTGAGGCT —> GGCT) is a known cause of α^o thalassaemia. The removal of five bases is small enough to be considered a mutation rather than a deletion.

Mutations within the consensus sequences which surround the exon-intron junctions generally result in a less harmful phenotype caused by a variable reduction in the efficiency of splicing. Typically, such mutations reduce gene expression but do not destroy it. For example, substitution of C for G at +5 from the 5' splice site of intron 1 of the β globin gene has been shown to be the cause of about one third of β^+ thalassaemia in Indians.

A third mechanism which can impair the efficiency of the splicing mechanism arises when a point mutation creates a new splice site or causes the activation of a cryptic splice site. Cryptic splice sites contain sequences which are similar to their active counterparts but they are not normally recognised in the process of splicing.

The substitution of A for G at +110 from the 5' splice site of intron 1 of the β globin gene creates a new 3' AG dinucleotide which acts in competition with the true splice site. Thus two types of β globin mRNA can be transcribed from the defective gene. However, the mRNA which is spliced at the mutant site cannot be correctly translated. The net result is reduced synthesis of functional β globin. This mutation accounts for about one third of cases of β^+ thalassaemia in the Mediterranean region.

However, not all such mutations lie within non-coding sequences. The substitution of A for G at position +26 of exon 1 of the β globin chain (GGTGAG —> GGTAAG) causes the insertion of lysine instead of glutamic acid at this position and results in the formation of haemoglobin E. This structurally abnormal haemoglobin is synthesised at a reduced rate because the mutation activates a cryptic 5' splice site at position +25. Haemoglobin E is most common in SE Asia, where it affects about 13% of the population.

The abnormal splicing which results from the creation of a new splice site or from the activation of a cryptic splice site is depicted in Figure 7.6. The example used as illustration accounts for about one in twenty cases of β thalassaemia from the Mediterranean region. Substitution of G for C at position +745 of the second intron of the β globin gene creates a new 5′ splice site (CAGCTACCA —> CAGGTACCA). This substitution causes the cryptic 3′ splice site at position +579 to become active. Splicing at the two new sites produces a mutant mRNA with four "exons". Because the new splice sites are recognised with high efficiency, this mutation causes a relatively severe β⁺ thalassaemia.

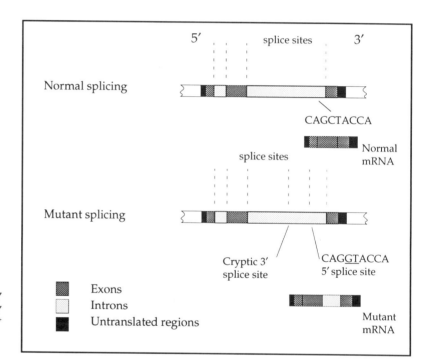

Figure 7.6 *Creation of an alternate 5′ splice site and activation of a cryptic 3′ splice site resulting in a severe β⁺ thalassaemia*

Translation Mutants

Any mutation which reduces the rate of translation of mRNA into globin will result in a thalassaemic phenotype. Some translation mutations also result in structurally abnormal globins.

Mutations within the initiation (ATG) codon or the upstream ribosomal binding site reduce the efficiency of translation of the globin mRNA. For example, deletion of two nucleotides from the ribosomal binding site of an α globin gene (CCACCATG —> CC__CATG) has been found to interfere with α globin mRNA translation in an Algerian patient with haemoglobin H disease.

Point mutations of the termination codon can result in the insertion of an amino acid where mRNA translation would normally end. In such cases, translation proceeds until the next functional termination codon is met, and an elongated globin chain results. Several abnormal haemoglobins have been described which include elongated globin chains (Table 7.1). The most common example, **haemoglobin Constant Spring,** arises from a mutation of the α2 globin gene and contains α globin chains which are 172 amino acids long, 31 longer than normal.

Affected gene	Name	Mutation	Population
α	Constant Spring	TAA—>CAA (glu)	Chinese
α	Koya Dora	TAA—>TCA (ser)	Indian
α	Icaria	TAA—>AAA (lys)	Mediterranean
α	Seal Rock	TAA—>GAA (gla)	Black
β	Tak	TAA—>ins 2nt (thr)	Thai

Table 7.1 *Variant haemoglobins caused by mutation of the chain termination codon resulting in elongation of globin chains (ins 2nt - insertion of two nucleotides)*

Point mutations within the coding regions of globin genes can generate a new termination codon, and result in premature termination of translation. For example, deletion of a single nucleotide in codon 41 of the β globin gene results in a shift in the reading frame and the generation of a termination codon (TGA) from codons 60-61, as shown in Figure 7.7. This form of β⁰ thalassaemia accounts for about 7% of β thalassaemia in the Indian subcontinent.

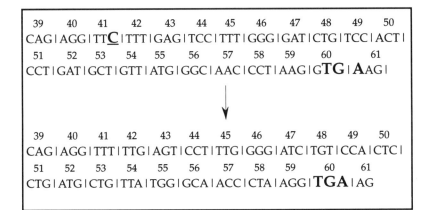

Figure 7.7 *Frame shift mutation causing early chain termination resulting in β⁰ thalassaemia*

Post-Translational Instability

As noted in the previous chapter, alterations in the amino acid sequence of globin chains can impair their stability, or that of the haemoglobin molecules which include them. In extreme cases, the resultant molecules are degraded almost as quickly as they are synthesised, leading to a severe deficiency of the affected globin chain. The resulting condition is clinically indistinguishable from thalassaemia. The most common member of this group of abnormal haemoglobins, which are known as the **hyper-unstable variants**, is **haemoglobin Quong Sze** which results from the substitution of proline for leucine at position 125 (H8) of the α globin chain. The insertion of proline at this point causes disruption of the helical structure and leads to severe instability of the globin chain.

Pathophysiology

The thalassaemia syndromes encompass a wide spectrum of clinical severity. This heterogeneity is hardly surprising, given the large number of genetic abnormalities which cause thalassaemia and their high frequency in affected populations. The heterogeneity is further increased by the relatively high frequency of coincident inheritance of a structural haemoglobinopathy such as haemoglobin S.

The myriad manifestations of this complex group of disorders can all be traced to a single cause viz the imbalanced synthesis of α-like and non-α-like globin chains. As described in Chapter 6, all normal mammalian haemoglobins are composed of two α-like and two non-α-like globin chains. Under normal circumstances, therefore, the rate of synthesis of α globin must be more or less matched by the total synthesis of β, δ and γ globin chains. Impaired synthesis of α globin results in the accumulation of unpaired non-α globins within the developing erythroblast and vice versa. Unpaired globin chains are unstable: they form aggregates and precipitate within the cell, causing decreased deformability, membrane damage and selective removal of the damaged cell by the reticuloendothelial system. Unpaired α globin chains are extremely insoluble and cause severe damage to developing erythroblasts. Unpaired β globin chains, on the other hand, form haemoglobin H which is relatively stable and only precipitates as the red cell ages. Thus moderate impairment of β globin synthesis is associated with a greater degree of ineffective erythropoiesis and haemolysis than an equivalent impairment of α globin synthesis.

α Thalassaemia

Although α thalassaemia encompasses the complete spectrum of disease severity it is convenient to consider affected individuals as belonging to one of four groups according to the increasing severity of their symptoms:

- "silent" carriers

- α thalassaemia trait

- haemoglobin H disease

- haemoglobin Barts hydrops foetalis

The groups correspond approximately to the *functional equivalent* of the deletion of 1, 2, 3 or 4 α globin genes respectively. Thus, if a point mutation completely prevents expression of an α globin gene, the result is equivalent to deletion of that gene. Similarly, the presence of two point mutations which reduce the output of their respective genes to about 50% of normal approximates to deletion of a single gene.

"Silent" Carriers

Deletion of a single α globin gene has no significant effect on the well-being of the affected individual. Such individuals are said to be heterozygous for α^+ thalassaemia. Typically, one parent of a child with haemoglobin H disease will have this genotype. As adults, no haematological abnormality can be demonstrated using standard laboratory techniques (ie excluding DNA analysis). Blood drawn from the umbilical cord of newborns may contain 1% of haemoglobin Barts (γ_4), but this determination is imprecise and an unreliable marker of the disease. Such individuals most often are identified by deduction from a pedigree chart in the course of a family study. They can only be defined with complete reliability by DNA analysis.

α Thalassaemia Trait

Individuals with the equivalent of two α globin genes deleted may be α^+ homozygotes ($\alpha-/\alpha-$) or α^0 heterozygotes ($--/\alpha\alpha$). It is important to know to which group a given individual belongs so that accurate genetic counselling may be offered. Unfortunately, the two groups are clinically indistinguishable and present identical laboratory profiles using standard laboratory techniques.

Affected individuals typically show a mild microcytic, hypochromic anaemia but exhibit no significant symptoms of disease. Precipitated haemoglobin H (β_4) can be demonstrated by supravital staining in a small minority of red cells. Blood drawn from the umbilical cord can be shown to contain up to 10% of haemoglobin Barts.

Careful consideration of a pedigree chart is often useful in such cases eg, barring spontaneous mutation, both parents of a foetus with haemoglobin Barts hydrops foetalis are obligatory carriers of α^0 thalassaemia.

Haemoglobin H Disease

Haemoglobin H disease arises from the deletion of three α globin genes or the equivalent. It is most commonly seen in SE Asian populations. The most common genotype is that of a compound heterozygote for α^+ and α^0 thalassaemia ($\alpha-/--$). Compound heterozygotes for α^0 thalassaemia and haemoglobin Constant Spring also fall into this group. Less common examples of genotypes which result in haemoglobin H disease have been described earlier in the section on the molecular basis of the thalassaemia syndromes.

The severity of haemoglobin H disease is highly variable. It is characterised by a moderately severe anaemia and hepatosplenomegaly. Typically, the haemoglobin level is maintained at around 8 g/dl and transfusion support is unnecessary. Extramedullary haemopoiesis and skeletal abnormalities are uncommon.

Characteristic findings on the peripheral blood film include microcytosis, hypochromasia, fragmented red cells, poikilocytosis, polychromasia and target cells. Multiple haemoglobin H inclusions are demonstrable in most of the red cells by supravital staining with a redox dye such as brilliant cresyl blue. These inclusions are the main cause of the haemolytic anaemia which characterises the

---

SAQ 4

Why is haemoglobin Barts hydrops foetalis extremely rare in Black Americans?

condition. Haemolysis is exacerbated by the administration of oxidant drugs such as sulphonamides. Adult blood contains between 5 and 35% of haemoglobin H and traces of haemoglobin Barts. Umbilical cord blood contains up to 40% haemoglobin Barts. The α:β globin chain synthesis ratio typically is reduced to between 0.2 and 0.4.

Haemoglobin molecules which are composed of four identical globin chains such as haemoglobin H and haemoglobin Barts do not exhibit haem:haem interaction or the Bohr effect and have a high oxygen affinity. They are therefore useless as respiratory pigments.

A rare acquired form of haemoglobin H disease is sometimes seen in a small number of cases of myelodysplasia.

Haemoglobin Barts Hydrops Foetalis

The most severe form of α thalassaemia results from the deletion of all four α globin genes and so is associated with a complete absence of α globin synthesis. It is most commonly seen in SE Asia and the Mediterranean region, in association with the --^{SEA} and --^{MED} deletions respectively.

Because of the absence of α globin synthesis, no functionally normal haemoglobins are formed after the cessation of ζ globin synthesis at about 10 weeks gestation. Instead, functionally useless tetrameric molecules such as haemoglobin Barts (γ_4) and haemoglobin H (β_4) are synthesised. Thus, although the haemoglobin concentration at delivery typically is about 6 g/dl, the *functional* anaemia is much more severe. The severity of the anaemia causes gross oedema secondary to congestive cardiac failure and massive hepatosplenomegaly. Pregnancy usually terminates in a third trimester stillbirth, often after a difficult delivery. There is a greatly increased incidence of toxaemia of pregnancy in the mothers of babies affected by haemoglobin Barts hydrops foetalis.

Intra-uterine blood transfusion can be used to combat the severe anaemia in affected foetuses. If the programme of transfusion is started early enough the changes described above can be minimised. Using this technique, a small number of cases have survived, but they remain completely transfusion dependent. The long-term health of such cases remains to be determined.

An abnormal haemoglobin which travelled faster than haemoglobin A on electrophoresis was identified in the blood of a baby with haemoglobin H disease in 1958 by Ager and Lehmann. Since the letters of the alphabet had been exhausted by then, the new variant was called after the hospital where the baby was a patient - St. Bartholomew's Hospital in London. Haemoglobin Barts was subsequently shown to be a γ globin tetramer.

Because of the characteristic changes described above laboratory investigation is seldom required to establish a diagnosis. The peripheral blood smear shows marked microcytosis, hypochromasia, poikilocytosis, fragmentation and numerous nucleated red cells. Haemoglobin electrophoresis confirms the abnormal composition described above.

β Thalassaemia

Because β thalassaemia usually results from point mutations within the β globin gene cluster, the relationship between genotype and phenotype is less straightforward than for α thalassaemia. It is still convenient, however, to group affected individuals according to the severity of their symptoms. Three groups are recognised:

- β thalassaemia minor (or trait)

- β thalassaemia major

- β thalassaemia intermedia

β thalassaemia minor

The mildest form of β thalassaemia arises from the inheritance of a single abnormal β globin gene. Typically, affected individuals exhibit no significant signs of disease, and may be unaware of their condition. A minority of heterozygotes exhibit more severe disease.

Laboratory analysis reveals a mild microcytic, hypochromic anaemia, with target cells a prominent feature on the peripheral blood film. In most cases, the red cell count appears to be inappropriately high given the degree of anaemia which is present. Bone marrow sampling is unnecessary to establish the diagnosis but, where performed, generally shows some degree of erythroid hyperplasia and mild ineffective erythropoiesis. Most cases can be demonstrated to have raised levels of one or both of the minor haemoglobins A_2 and F.

It is important to differentiate β thalassaemia minor from iron deficiency anaemia which, superficially, produces similar results. The pattern of laboratory results in these two disorders is shown in Table 7.2. A further potential source of confusion arises because iron deficiency causes a relatively greater decrease in the level of Hb A_2

Condition	Hb (g/dl)	MCV (fl)	HbA$_2$ (%)	HbF (%)	Serum ferritin (µg/l)
Normal (M)	15.5 ± 2.0	89 ± 6	<3.5	<1.0	125 ± 100
(F)	14.0 ± 2.5	87 ± 6	<3.5	<1.0	110 ± 75
β thal. minor	↓	↓	↑	↑	N or ↑
Iron defic.	↓	↓	N	N	↓

Key

N	Normal
↓	Decreased
↑	Increased

Table 7.2 *Laboratory results in β thalassaemia minor and iron deficiency*

than Hb A. This may obscure the diagnosis of β thalassaemia minor when iron deficiency is also present.

β Thalassaemia Major

β thalassaemia major results from the inheritance of two β thalassaemia genes. Affected individuals are thus either homozygous for a particular gene defect or doubly heterozygous for two distinct mutations. The original cases of thalassaemia described by Cooley in 1925 almost certainly were suffering from β thalassaemia major.

In the absence of treatment, the condition is characterised by severe anaemia, gross hepatosplenomegaly, failure to thrive and skeletal deformities such as bossing of the skull and maxillary prominence. The skeletal deformities are the result of marked erythroid hyperplasia with consequent expansion of the bone marrow volume which causes outward pressure and marked thinning of the bones.

The massive expansion of erythropoietic tissue still fails to meet demand and extramedullary haemopoiesis ensues, resulting in hepatosplenomegaly. These changes are progressive and lead to death in childhood from congestive cardiac failure or complications secondary to repeated pathological fractures of the weakened bones. Post-mortem examination reveals increased deposition of storage iron in the major organs of the body.

The peripheral blood film shows marked microcytosis, hypochromasia, numerous target cells and nucleated red cells. The prominent haemolytic component of the anaemia is manifest as tear drop poikilocytes, fragmented red cells and microspherocytes. Analysis of the haemoglobins present reveals a marked increase in the proportion of haemoglobin F, the precise value of which is dependent on the genetic defect(s) present. In homozygous β° thalassaemia, for example, Hb F accounts for up to 98% of the total. Marked reduction in the synthesis of β globin is reflected in an $\alpha{:}\beta$ globin synthetic ratio of greater than 2.5.

Bone marrow examination reveals extreme erythroid hyperplasia with marked ineffective erythropoiesis. The presence of precipitated aggregates of excess α globin chains wreaks havoc upon the normal physiology of developing red cells. In particular, α globin aggregates have been shown to cause:

- arrest of mitosis

- oxidative damage of membrane lipids

- marked increases in intracellular calcium ions

- loss of potassium ions from the cell

- decreased cell deformability

These changes all promote intramedullary death of developing erythroblasts.

The lifespan of circulating red cells is decreased by the damaging effects of the α globin aggregates described above. In addition, the cells are damaged by the selective removal of the aggregates during their passage through the spleen. This process is the main source of the fragmented red cells and microspherocytes seen on the peripheral blood film.

The mainstay of current treatment is regular blood transfusion, aimed at maintaining the haemoglobin level above about 10-12 g/dl, thereby effectively suppressing erythropoiesis and preventing skeletal changes and extramedullary haemopoiesis. However, such a programme of regular, lifelong transfusion leads to the accumulation of large amounts of iron within the body which causes a range of toxic effects:

- cardiotoxicity (the leading cause of death)

- hepatomegaly secondary to iron loading

- growth retardation

- failure of sexual development

As described in Chapter 3, the body has no effective means of excreting excess iron. On the contrary, it possesses elaborate mechanisms to prevent such loss. The toxic effects of iron overloading can only be delayed by the use of iron chelating agents such as desferrioxamine. This substance, when administered by continuous subcutaneous infusion, forms a complex with iron which is excreted in the urine and faeces. If treatment is commenced early, hepatic and cardiac toxicity may be significantly reduced in severity.

β Thalassaemia Intermedia

Not all cases of homozygous or doubly heterozygous β thalassaemia have severe disease. Because of the diversity and high frequency of gene mutations which give rise to β thalassaemia, a complete spectrum of disease severity exists. Thalassaemia intermedia encompasses all cases of β thalassaemia with significant symptoms of disease which do not require regular transfusion to maintain their haemoglobin level above about 7 g/dl.

Typically, thalassaemia intermedia arises from one of three circumstances:

- inheritance of "mild" β thalassaemia mutation(s)

- co-inheritance of a gene which increases the rate of γ globin synthesis.

- co-inheritance of α thalassaemia. Reduction in α globin synthesis reduces the imbalance in the α:non-α globin synthetic ratio.

The laboratory and clinical features of thalassaemia intermedia mirror those of the more severe phenotype. Paradoxically, despite the absence of regular transfusion, chronic iron overloading remains a major cause of morbidity in such cases. Gastrointestinal absorption of dietary iron is markedly increased in anaemic patients with

---

SAQ 5

What effect would coincident inheritance of heterozygous α° thalassaemia have on the clinical severity of a moderately severe β thalassaemia (thalassaemia intermedia)?

thalassaemia, even though total body iron is increased. This apparent anomaly is probably explained by the fact that the massively increased demand for iron imposed by erythroid hyperplasia exceeds the supply capacity of the reticuloendothelial system. Thus, functional iron deficiency is present, despite raised iron stores.

Suggested Further Reading

Bunn, H.F. and Forget, B.G. (1985). *Haemoglobin: Molecular, Genetic and Clinical Aspects.* Philadelphia: W.B. Saunders.

Thein, S.L. and Weatherall, D.J. (1988). The Thalassaemias. In *Recent Advances in Haematology,* No. 5. (Hoffbrand, A.V. (ed.)) Edinburgh: Churchill Livingstone.

Weatherall, D.J. and Clegg, J.B. (1981). *The Thalassaemia Syndromes* 3rd ed. Oxford: Blackwell.

Answers to Self-Assessment Questions

1. δ globin synthesis normally comprises less than 3% of non-α globin synthesis. Even complete absence of δ globin synthesis would not cause significant disease.

2. During the last trimester of pregnancy and for the first few months after delivery, γ globin is the predominant non-α globin synthesised. A baby with heterozygous γ^0 thalassaemia would have a moderately severe clinical phenotype. The symptoms would gradually disappear, however, as β globin synthesis increased. The condition would be clinically silent by 6 months of age.

3. Patient I1 has heterozygous α^0 thalassaemia. Patient I2 has heterozygous α^+ thalassaemia.

4. Most affected American Blacks express the clinically mild α^+ thalassaemia which precludes the transmission of haemoglobin Barts hydrops foetalis (homozygous α^0 thalassaemia).

5. The severity of the clinical manifestations of thalassaemia is proportional to the degree of imbalance of α and non-α globin synthesis. Moderately severe β thalassaemia results from a *relative* excess of α globin synthesis. Thus, coincident inheritance of α^0 thalassaemia would ameliorate the condition.

Structural Haemoglobinopathies

The structural haemoglobinopathies are characterised by the synthesis of structurally abnormal globin chains. These abnormal globins can exert a wide range of effects on the behaviour of the haemoglobin molecule. As described in the previous chapter, the distinction between structural haemoglobinopathies and thalassaemias is not always clear because many structurally abnormal globins are synthesised at a greatly reduced rate. The complexity of the situation is further compounded when co-inheritance of thalassaemia with a structural haemoglobinopathy occurs. In such circumstances, the behaviour of the abnormal molecule may be significantly altered.

Incidence and Distribution

More than 500 different structurally abnormal haemoglobins have been described, but most are rare. The four most common examples are, in order of decreasing incidence, haemoglobins S, C, D and E. Haemoglobin S is by far the most common structural haemoglobinopathy and is most prevalent in Afro-Caribbeans but it also is relatively common in Central India, the Eastern Arabian peninsula and the Southern Mediterranean. About 30% of live births in Nigeria carry the abnormal gene. In common with thalassaemia, the carrier state for haemoglobin S confers selective resistance to the malarial parasite *Plasmodium falciparum*. Haemoglobin C is most common in West and central Africa, particularly in Ghana. It frequently is co-inherited with haemoglobin S. Haemoglobin D is most common in the Punjab but is seen in a wide range of populations. Haemoglobin E is most common in SE Asia as described in Chapter 7.

In 1953 a standard nomenclature for haemoglobins was proposed. It was decided that normal adult haemoglobin should be designated HbA, foetal haemoglobin as HbF and sickle haemoglobin HbS. The two abnormal haemoglobins discovered by Itano in 1950 and 1953 were designated HbC and HbD respectively. There is no haemoglobin B because this term had been used by some workers to describe sickle haemoglobin. When the term HbS was adopted HbB was permanently abandoned.

Classification

The alteration in molecular function induced by structural abnormality is dependent upon the position of the alteration and on the properties of the amino acids involved. Functionally, the haemoglobin molecule can be considered to have a number of important areas:

- the exterior surface of the molecule, which confers solubility

- the $\alpha_1\beta_1$ and $\alpha_2\beta_2$ contact areas, which confer stability on the molecule

- the $\alpha_1\beta_2$ and $\alpha_2\beta_1$ contact areas, which confer flexibility during oxygenation and deoxygenation

- the $\alpha_1\alpha_2$ and $\beta_1\beta_2$ contact areas

- the 2,3 DPG binding site, which affects the oxygen affinity of the molecule

- the hydrophobic haem pockets, which protect the haem groups from oxidation

- the β C terminal histidines, which account for 50% of the Bohr effect

Alterations to the amino acid sequence within these areas typically lead to predictable alterations in molecular behaviour. For example, changes in the $\alpha_1\beta_1$ ($\alpha_2\beta_2$) contact areas are likely to affect molecular stability, while changes in the $\alpha_1\beta_2$ ($\alpha_2\beta_1$) contact areas are likely to affect oxygen affinity.

In general terms, the phenomena resulting from the presence of an abnormal haemoglobin will fall under one or more of the following headings:

- no apparent effect (clinically silent)

- a thalassaemia-like syndrome

- methaemoglobinaemia

- molecular instability

- altered oxygen affinity

- miscellaneous atypical effects eg haemoglobin S

Clinically Silent Haemoglobinopathies

Most structurally abnormal haemoglobins have no apparent effect. Over 200 such "silent" abnormal haemoglobins have been described. Almost all are caused by alterations to amino acids on the external surface of the haemoglobin molecule, a position where change is readily tolerated; many involve the so-called "variable" amino acid residues. Most of these silent haemoglobinopathies have been discovered by chance. They are mainly of interest to population geneticists and only a few examples merit inclusion in this chapter.

The Thalassaemia-like Syndromes

Any abnormality of globin which leads to RNA instability is likely to lead to a thalassaemia-like syndrome, since the unstable RNA will be incapable of facilitating the production of a normal quantity of globin. A number of examples of this phenomenon were described in Chapter 7. Abnormalities of this type, as with many severe abnormalities of globin, are more common in β globin chains than in α chains. This is probably because synthesis of β chains commences at a later, less critical, stage of intra-uterine development and also because severe β chain abnormality is accompanied by a life-long compensatory elevation of γ chain production. Severe abnormalities of α globin synthesis are more likely to be incompatible with life.

One important group of thalassaemic haemoglobinopathies not described in Chapter 7 are the chain fusion haemoglobins. Important members of this group are **haemoglobin Lepore** and **haemoglobin anti-Lepore** which are δ-β and β-δ fusions respectively, and **haemoglobin Kenya** which is a $^A\gamma$-β fusion. These haemoglobins result from unequal crossing-over during meiosis with the formation of hybrid globin genes as shown in Figure 8.1.

Methaemoglobinaemia

Methaemoglobinaemia is the result of irreversible oxidation of the ferrous ion in haem to the ferric state. In all instances where this occurs, molecular instability also results. Similarly, in many cases where an amino acid change causes the formation of an unstable haemoglobin there is an increase in methaemoglobin formation.

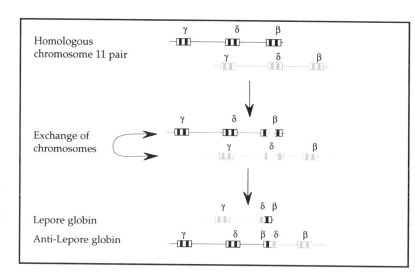

Figure 8.1 *The mechanism of unequal crossing-over which gives rise to chain fusion haemoglobins. The example shown is the fusion globin of haemoglobin Lepore*

Whether the abnormal haemoglobin is classified as an unstable or as a methaemoglobinaemia is to some extent arbitrary, but as a general rule it is classified according to which of the results predominates.

The **haemoglobin M** group are the most important of the abnormal haemoglobins which cause methaemoglobinaemia. There are four examples, and all involve the substitution of the haem-binding histidine by tyrosine. The phenolic group of the tyrosine is the cause of the oxidation.

The four members of this group and the substitutions which cause them are shown in Table 8.1.

Haemoglobin	Substitution	O_2 affinity
Hb M Saskatoon	β63 (E7) distal His —>Tyr	normal
Hb M Hyde Park	β92 (F8) proximal His —>Tyr	normal
Hb M Boston	α58 (E7) distal H is —>Tyr	reduced
Hb M Iwate	α87 (F8) proximal His —>Tyr	reduced

Table 8.1 *The M haemoglobins*

The altered oxygen affinity of the two α chain variants is due to the fact that α chains always tend to oxygenate before β chains. The oxygenation of α chains increases the oxygen affinity of β chains during the process of oxygenation through haem-haem interaction. Since oxygenation of the α chain cannot occur in Boston and Iwate, haem-haem interaction does not occur, and the subsequent oxygenation of the β chains is thus impaired.

Haemoglobin Milwaukee originally was also classified as a haemoglobin M but the substitution involved is not of a haem-binding histidine, but of β67 (E11) valine by glutamic acid. Because of the helical arrangement of this part of the β globin chain, the COO^- group of the glutamic acid is adjacent in space to the β63 histidine, being one complete turn of the helix away. The presence of this highly reactive group promotes the oxidation of the haem iron, resulting in methaemoglobin formation. Similarly, **haemoglobin Zürich**, which arises from the substitution of arginine for the β63 (E7) histidine, originally was classified as a haemoglobin M because of the methaemoglobinaemia which results. However, the predominant effect of this substitution is molecular instability and haemoglobin Zürich is now classified as an unstable haemoglobin.

It is interesting to compare the structure of haemoglobin Milwaukee with that of **haemoglobin Norfolk**, where the hydrophilic amino acid glycine at α57 (E6) is substituted by highly reactive aspartic acid. Despite the presence of the $-COO^-$ group, methaemoglobinaemia does not result because, although the substitution is numerically adjacent to the haem binding histidine at α58, the helical arrangement in this part of the chain means that the $-COO^-$ group is pointing away from the haem group, and there is no interference. Haemoglobin Norfolk is a clinically silent haemoglobinopathy.

Medical workers in Northern Japan had been puzzled for some time about the origin of a familial disease which they called *kuchikuru* or "black mouth". The mystery was solved when the abnormality was linked to a haemoglobin M. The black mouth was due to the peripheral cyanosis which accompanies methaemoglobinaemia.

Unstable Haemoglobins

More than 60 haemoglobin variants have been described where the principal defect is instability. Frequently the amino acid substitution involves the invariant amino acids. The reasons for the instability can be grouped under three main headings:

- weakened haem-globin contact

- weakened tetrameric structure

- disruption of normal or helical structure

The earliest description of an unstable haemoglobin was made in 1952. It concerned a young boy with congenital haemolytic anaemia of un-known aetiology for whom splenectomy in early child-hood had had no beneficial effect. The presence of Heinz bodies in his red cells sug-gested to the investigators that chemical poisoning was the most likely cause of the haemolysis but no culprit could be identified. It was not until 1970 that the presence of an unstable haemoglobin, Hb Bristol (β67 (E11) val—>asp), was demonstrated.

The first unstable haemo-globin to be definitively iden-tified was haemoglobin Zürich which was identified in a young girl who devel-oped acute haemolysis after ingestion of sulphonamide drugs.

Table 8.2 *Haem-contact amino acids in α and β globin chains. 16 amino acids are in identical positions in both chains, and 13, shown with an asterisk (*), are the same amino acid in both chains. This is in addition to the proxi-mal and distal histidines.*

Weakened Haem-Globin Contact

The abnormalities leading to weak haem-globin contact usually involve amino acids in the haem pocket. The 17 α chain and 19 β chain amino acids involved in haem contact in addition to the two histidine residues of each chain are shown in Table 8.2.

	α Chain		β Chain
	32 (B13)Met		31(B13)Leu
*	39(C4)Thr		38(C4)Thr
	42(C7)Tyr		41(C7)Phe
*	43(CD1)Phe		42(CD1)Phe
	45(CD3)His		44(CD3)Ser
*	46(CD4)Phe		45(CD4)Phe
	58(E7)His	Distal His	63(E7)His
			66(E10)Lys
*	62(E11)Val		67(E11)Val
			70(E14)Ala
			71(E15)Phe
*	83(F4)Leu		88(F4)Leu
*	86(F7)Leu		91(F7)Leu
	87(F8)His	Proximal His	92(F8)His
*	91(FG3)Leu		96(FG3)Leu
*	93(FG5)Val		98(FG5)Val
*	97(G4)Asn		102(G4)Asn
*	98(G5)Phe		103(G5)Phe
*	101(G8)Leu		106(G8)Leu
	129(H12)Leu		
*	132(H15)Val		137(H15)Val
*	136(H19)Leu		141(H19)Leu

In at least four unstable haemoglobins the invariant CD1 phenylala-nine is substituted, as shown in Figure 8.2. In **haemoglobin Ham-mersmith** it is the β42 (CD1) which is substituted by serine. In **haemoglobin Bucharesti**, the same amino acid is substituted, but by leucine. **Haemoglobin Hirosaki** is also a substitution of pheny-lalanine by leucine, but at α43 (CD1). **Haemoglobin Torino** involves the same amino acid (α43), but the substitution is by valine. In all cases the primary result is molecular instability, but

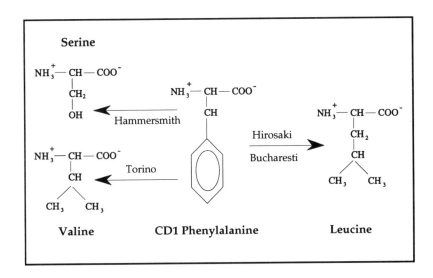

Figure 8.2 *Substitution of invariant CD1 phenylalanine leading to weakened haem-globin contact and resulting in molecular instability*

there is also an alteration in oxygen affinity as discussed later in this chapter. In the case of haemoglobin Hammersmith, the hydrophilic serine encourages water to enter the haem pocket, leading to oxidation of the haem iron and methaemoglobinaemia in addition to the molecular instability.

Another unstable haemoglobin resulting from weakened haem-globin contact is **haemoglobin Sidney** where the substitution is of β67 (E11) valine by alanine as shown in Figure 8.3. While valine is not a large molecule, its side group is somewhat larger than that of alanine and a failure of haem contact results.

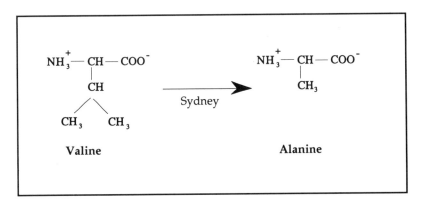

Figure 8.3 *Substitution of alanine for valine as a cause of weakened haem-globin contact in haemoglobin Sydney*

The final example of this group is **haemoglobin Gun Hill**. This is an interesting example since, unlike the others, it is not caused by a point mutation but by unequal crossing-over resulting in the deletion of several amino acids, including the β proximal histidine residue (del β91-97).

Weakened Tetrameric Structure

The $\alpha_1\beta_1$ $(\alpha_2\beta_2)$ contact areas, responsible for the stability of the molecule, involve 16 α chain and 18 β chain amino acids. Of these, 13 occupy the same position in both chains, but only 4 are the same amino acid in both chains as shown in Table 8.3.

	α Chain	β Chain
	30(B11)Glu	
*	31(B12)Arg	30(B12)Arg
	34(B15)Leu	33(B15)Val
	35(B16)Ser	34(B16)Val
	36(C1)Phe	35(C1)Tyr
		51(D2)Pro
		55(D6)Met
	103(G10)His	108(G10)Asn
	104(G11)Cys	
	106(G13)Leu	
	107(G14)Val	112(G14)Cys
		115(G17)Ala
	111(G18)Ala	116(G18)His
	114(GH2)Pro	119(GH2)Gly
*	117(GH5)Phe	122(GH5)Phe
		123(H1)Thr
*	119(H2)Pro	124(H2)Pro
		125(H3)Pro
	122(H5)His	127(H5)Gln
*	123(H6)Ala	128(H6)Ala
	126(H9)Asp	131(H9)Gln

Table 8.3 *Amino acids of the $\alpha_1\beta_1$ $(\alpha_2\beta_2)$ contact area. 13 amino acids are in identical positions in both chains, and 4, shown with an asterisk (*), are the same amino acid.*

A good example of molecular instability being caused by weakened tetrameric structure is provided by **haemoglobin Philly**, where the β35 (C1) tyrosine is substituted by phenylalanine. The lack of the polar -OH group on phenylalanine means that the $\alpha_1\beta_1$ bonding is weakened, since the bond to aspartic acid at α126 (H9) cannot be formed, leading to monomer formation and precipitation of the haemoglobin as **Heinz bodies**.

Disruption of Normal Helical Structure

A wide range of amino acid substitutions cause disruption of the structure of haemoglobin and result in molecular instability. At least six unstable haemoglobins owe their instability to a substitution of leucine by the imino acid proline. The presence of proline in the chain causes a "kink" because, unlike the amino acids, the N and α-C of this imino acid residue are constrained by the ring structure, resulting in a loss of free rotation. This kink can usually be tolerated if it occurs in a non-helical part of the chain or within the first three positions of a helical part of the chain. If a proline substitution occurs within a helical section after position three the result is disruption of the helix and molecular instability. In **haemoglobin Genova**, the leucine to proline substitution occurs in the middle of a helical section at position $\beta 28$ (B10), leading to instability and, in this case, altered oxygen affinity also.

> Proline is designated an imino acid rather than an amino acid because it contains a secondary, not a primary, α amine group.

Only one α chain variant involving a proline for leucine substitution has so far been reported. This is **haemoglobin Bibba**, and again the substitution is in a helical part of the chain at $\alpha 136$ (H19). The result in this case, in addition to the overall instability, is to cause increased dissociation of the molecule into dimers. The importance of the position of the proline substitution is exemplified by the different effects observed in **haemoglobin Duarte** and **haemoglobin Singapore** where the substitution of proline is for alanine. In haemoglobin Duarte the substitution occurs within a helical portion, at $\beta 62$ (E6), and instability and increased oxygen affinity results. In haemoglobin Singapore the substitution is at $\alpha 141$ (HC3) where distortion of the chain is tolerable: the result is a silent haemoglobinopathy.

Insertion of a polar amino acid or, even worse, a charged amino acid residue into the interior of the haemoglobin molecule is another cause of molecular instability. For example, in **haemoglobin St Louis**, the substitution is of the $\beta 28$ (B10) leucine by glutamine. The polar amino group of the glutamine induces the entry of water into the interior of the molecule, resulting in oxidation of the haem iron and instability. In **haemoglobin Wien** the substitution is of the tyrosine at $\beta 130$ (H8) by aspartic acid. The -COO⁻ of aspartic acid is strongly attractive to an adjacent positive charge, probably that of the histidine at NA2. This tends to cause the two to move closer together, thereby disrupting the alignment of the A helix and leading to molecular instability.

Finally, the importance of superficially insignificant amino acid residues is underlined by **haemoglobin Savanna**. The correct spatial configuration of each subunit is vital if they are to fit correctly together and, because of the manner in which the chains are folded, in some parts of the molecule there is a tight squeeze where two adjacent parts of the chain are in close juxtaposition. This is most likely to occur at the "corners" where one helix is joined to the next, but can occur in any area of close chain proximity. In haemoglobin Savanna, the "invariant" glycine at position $\beta25$ (B6), a "corner" position, is substituted by valine. Although the side chain of valine is not large and its properties are similar to those of glycine, the valine side chain is too big to fit into the space available in this location. Indeed molecular models suggest that the only residue that could fit here is glycine. The valine for glycine substitution in haemoglobin Savanna causes instability as a result of the disruption of the alignment of the B helix relative to the rest of the subunit.

Similar disruptive effects result from the other two reported substitutions at this position, glycine to arginine in **haemoglobin Riverdale-Bronx** and glycine to aspartic acid in **haemoglobin Moscva** as shown in Figure 8.4. The much larger side chains of the substituent are even more disruptive to the correct B helix alignment and further, being charged, will cause both compensatory

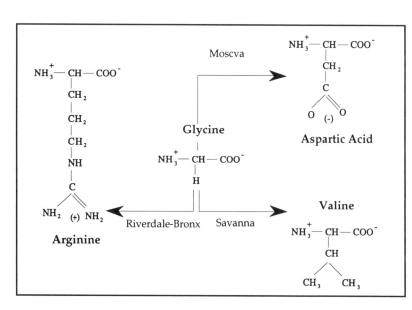

Figure 8.4 *Molecular instability resulting from substitution of invariant glycine for larger amino acids at a "corner" position*

movement of other parts of the molecule and tend to introduce water to the interior of the molecule.

Altered Oxygen Affinity

The final general type of abnormality caused by the presence of an abnormal haemoglobin is altered oxygen affinity. Changes which lead to increased oxygen affinity are about twice as common as those which lead to decreased affinity. As described above, many abnormal haemoglobins which are classified in another category exhibit altered oxygen affinity as a secondary effect.

Several mechanisms exist which result in altered oxygen affinity:

- direct interference with oxygen binding, especially of α haem

- abnormality of the $\alpha_1\beta_2$ ($\alpha_2\beta_1$) contact area

- alteration of $\alpha_1\alpha_2$ or $\beta_1\beta_2$ interaction

- changes in 2,3 DPG binding

- changes in Bohr effect H^+ binding

Interference with Oxygen Binding

Examples of direct interference with α haem oxygen binding are haemoglobins M Boston and M Iwate which were described earlier. Both of these haemoglobins exhibit decreased oxygen affinity.

The unstable haemoglobins Hammersmith, Bucharesti, Hirosaki and Torino arise by substitution of the invariant CD1 phenylalanine in either the α or β globin chain as described earlier. In addition to the molecular instability, these haemoglobins exhibit reduced oxygen affinity. The CD1 phenylalanine plays an important role in the maintenance of the correct orientation of the haem group in the haem pocket. As described in Chapter 6, the tilt of the haem on oxygenation is brought about by the CD1 phenylalanine, probably because of its size. In the absence of phenylalanine, haem tends to remain in the upright, deoxygenated position, which lowers its affinity for oxygen.

Abnormality of the $\alpha_1\beta_2$ ($\alpha_2\beta_1$) Contact

Interference with the $\alpha_1\beta_2$ ($\alpha_2\beta_1$) contact is a common cause of altered oxygen affinity. As described in Chapter 6, haemoglobin exists in equilibrium between two conformations known as "tense" (T) and "relaxed" (R). Any interference with the ability to make the salt bonds which stabilise the $\alpha_1\beta_2$ and $\alpha_2\beta_1$ interfaces will lead to reduced stability of the T form and reduced liberation of energy on transition from the T to the R form with a consequent shift in the equilibrium towards the R form. This means that the transition to the R form will occur at an earlier stage in the binding of oxygen to haem. In other words, the haemoglobin will have increased affinity for oxygen and reduced haem-haem interaction. Similarly, any substitution which led to the ability to form extra salt bonds in the R configuration would tend to stabilise that form, again shifting the equilibrium in the direction of the R form and increasing oxygen affinity.

Conversely, substitution of the amino acids involved in forming the salt bonds which stabilise the R form may inhibit salt bond formation resulting in a shift in the equilibrium towards the T form with a consequent reduction in the oxygen affinity of the molecule.

The affinity for oxygen may therefore be either increased or decreased by any factor which alters the equilibrium between the T and R forms. The amino acid residues involved in the $\alpha_1\beta_2$ ($\alpha_2\beta_1$) contact are shown in Table 8.4. Fewer amino acid residues are involved in this contact area than in the $\alpha_1\beta_1$ ($\alpha_2\beta_2$) contact area or than in haem contact, and although the amino acids are generally

Table 8.4 *Amino acids of the $\alpha_1\beta_2$ ($\alpha_2\beta_1$) contact area. Identical amino acids are shown with an asterisk (*)*

	α Chain	β Chain
		36(C2)Pro
	38(C3)Thr	37(C3)Trp
		39(C5)Gln
	41(C6)Thr	35(C6)Arg
	42(C7)Tyr	
	91(FG3)Leu	
	92(FG4)Arg	97(FG4)His
*	93(FG5)Val	98(FG5)Val
*	94(G1)Asp	99(G1)Asp
	95(G2)Pro	
	96(G3)Val	101(G3)Glu
		102(G4)Asn
	140(HC2)Tyr	

situated in similar parts of the two globin chains, there is not the close correlation between chains that exists in the other two contact areas listed earlier.

Two high affinity haemoglobins result from the substitution of the arginine at α92 (FG4). In **haemoglobin J Capetown** the substitution is by glutamine, and in **haemoglobin Chesapeake** the substitution is by leucine. The increase in oxygen affinity observed with haemoglobin Chesapeake is much greater than that of haemoglobin J Capetown. Again, the explanation for this observation lies with the nature of the amino acids involved. The α92 arginine is in Van der Waal's contact with the arginine at β35 (C2). It may also make a hydrogen bond, via its guanidinium group with another β chain amino acid. In neither substitution are these arrangements fully possible, however the polar nature of glutamine may well permit some weak interaction to take place, maintaining some of the stability of the T form, and thus reducing the severity of the effect.

One of the stabilising bonds which forms in the oxygenated (R) form is between β102 (G4) asparagine and α94 (G1) aspartic acid. Due to the sliding movement between the subunits during R to T transition, this bond is broken and a new one formed between β99 (G1) aspartic acid and β42 (C7) tyrosine, this latter serving to stabilise the T form. This important interaction between the chains in the T and R forms is shown in Figure 8.5.

Two abnormal haemoglobins, with differing effects on oxygen affinity, involve these same amino acids. In **haemoglobin Yakima**, the

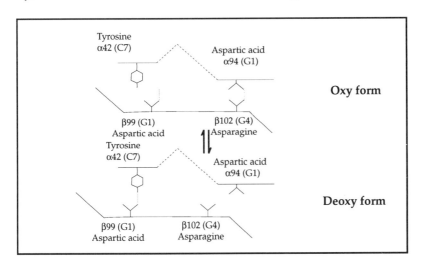

Figure 8.5 *Stabilising bonds which form between α and β globin in the oxygenated and deoxygenated states*

aspartic acid at β99 (G1) is replaced by asparagine. The asparagine is incapable of forming the stabilising bond to the tyrosine at α42 (C7). The result of this substitution is that the T form (deoxygenated) is rendered less stable than normal, favouring the R (oxygenated) form, and thus increasing the oxygen affinity. In **haemoglobin Kansas**, which has decreased oxygen affinity, the β102 (G4) asparagine is replaced by threonine. The presence of threonine precludes the formation of the stabilising bond to α94 (G1) which normally forms in the oxygenated (R) form. The absence of this stabilising bond reduces the stability of the R form, thereby favouring the formation of the T form and reducing oxygen affinity.

Alteration of α₁α₂ and β₁β₂ Interaction

Abnormalities affecting α₁α₂ and β₁β₂ interaction are very rare. Any interaction between β chains would only be possible in the oxygenated form since the chains are too far apart in the deoxygenated form. Although theoretically possible, no such amino acid changes have yet been reported.

The reverse orientation is true of α chains, in that they are too far apart to interact in the oxygenated form but move much closer together on deoxygenation. In the deoxygenated form, the terminal amino acids at both the N and C ends of the α chains form bonds with the opposite α chain as shown in Figure 8.6. These bonds serve to stabilise the T state, since they must be broken on oxygenation. An alteration in any of the three amino acids involved which led to a loss of any or all of the bonds might be expected to lead to

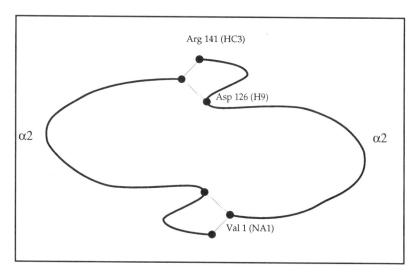

Figure 8.6 *Interaction between α globin chains which serve to stabilise the deoxygenated form.*

increased oxygen affinity because the oxygenated R state could then be adopted with a lower energy requirement. However, the bond between the NH_3^+ of the N-terminal valine and the COO^- of the C-terminal arginine is preserved by a simple amino acid substitution, irrespective of the identity of the substituent. The bond between the N-terminal valine and the α126 aspartic acid, however, involves the acid side chain of the aspartic acid. Substitution of aspartic acid by a residue lacking an acid side chain might be expected to preclude the formation of the bond.

No substitutions of α126 (H9) aspartic acid have been reported yet, only alterations at α141 (HC3) have been described. As explained above, the substitution of proline for arginine at α141 in haemoglobin Singapore, leads to no significant alteration of molecular function. However, in **haemoglobin Suresnes** the arginine is replaced by histidine, and the result is increased oxygen affinity. The most likely explanation for this apparent anomaly is that the large and rigid side chain of histidine prevents the C-terminal end of one chain coming into sufficiently close contact with the N-terminal end of the other chain for bonding to occur, despite the preservation of the COO^-. The terminal amino group of arginine is also an important CO_2 binding site. Substitution of this arginine by histidine as in haemoglobin Suresnes preserves some of this capability whereas the proline substitution of haemoglobin Singapore does not. Surprisingly, this does not appear to be significant and does not favour the deoxygenated form.

Changes in 2,3 DPG Binding

Alterations of oxygen affinity caused by changes in 2,3 DPG binding are fairly straightforward. The same three amino acid residues on each of the two β chains are responsible for the binding of 2,3 DPG as shown in Table 8.5.

The six positive charges exhibited, one from each of the six residues involved, are all required in order to fully bind the 2,3 DPG. The NA1 (β1) valine, like the α1 valine, is also capable of binding H^+

Chain Position		Amino Acid
NA1	β1	valine
EF6	β82	lysine
H21	β143	histidine

Table 8.5 *The amino acids in the β globin chain which are responsible for 2,3 DPG binding*

ions and CO_2: 2,3 DPG binding is therefore in competition with these other two alternatives. This amino acid is the last of the three to be bound to 2,3 DPG on deoxygenation, and the first to be unbound on oxygenation. Indeed, the breaking of this bond means that, as the β chains move closer together during oxygenation, the 2,3 DPG can be "popped" out of the β cleft, much like a pea from a pod. A substitution of any of these three amino acid residues on either of the two β chains which results in the loss of a positive charge must be prejudicial to 2,3 DPG binding. An obvious example occurs in normal γ chains, where the β143 (H21) histidine is replaced by serine, with the resulting loss of two of the six positive charges needed to hold the 2,3 DPG. The greatly elevated oxygen affinity of foetal haemoglobin is accounted for by this difference.

Three examples of altered oxygen affinity haemoglobin variants which result from substitution of the β82 (EF6) are shown in Figure 8.7. In **haemoglobin Rahere** the substituent is threonine, in **haemoglobin Helsinki** the substituent is methionine and in **haemoglobin Providence** the substitution is by asparagine which is partially deaminated as a post-transcriptional modification to aspartic acid. In all cases, the positive charge is lost, and in haemoglobins Helsinki and Rahere the oxygen affinity of the resulting haemoglobin is increased. In haemoglobin Providence, according to the authors who originally reported it in 1975, the oxygen affinity of the haemoglobin molecule is decreased, but that of whole blood is increased. They offer no really convincing explanation for this, and it may be that the initial observation of decreased oxygen affinity is incorrect since no independent confirmation of this unlikely phenomenon appears to have emerged.

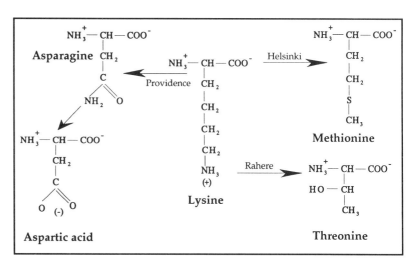

Figure 8.7 *Altered oxygen affinity haemoglobin variants which result from reduced ability to bind 2,3 DPG*

Substitutions of the histidine at β143 (H21) by arginine in **haemo-globin Abruzzo**, by glutamine in **haemoglobin Seal Rock** and by proline in **haemoglobin Syracuse** all result in loss of 2,3 DPG binding and a consequent increase in oxygen affinity. In haemoglobin Abruzzo, substitution of histidine by arginine preserves the positive charge but binding is impaired because of the greater flexibility of the arginine side chain. In haemoglobin Syracuse, the proline substitution also results in instability because of disruption of the helix.

However, not all examples of interference with 2,3 DPG binding involve substitution at these three sites. For example, **haemoglobin Shepherds Bush** results from the substitution of a charged aspartic acid for glycine at β74 (E18). The primary result of this substitution is molecular instability, but 2,3 DPG binding also is impaired.

Altered H^+ binding

As described in Chapter 6, an integral part of the oxygen association-dissociation reaction is the buffering effect of haemoglobin, whereby hydrogen ions are bound in the process of deoxygenation, but must be released for association of oxygen to occur. The shift in the position of the haemoglobin-oxygen dissociation curve which results from changes in pH is called the **Bohr effect**. A quarter of the Bohr effect is due to the N-terminal valines (NA1) of the two α chains. Half of the H^+ binding is due to the C-terminal histidines of the β chains (β146, HC3) and their links to the aspartic acid at β94 (FG1) of their own chains. The identity of the amino acid or acids responsible for the remaining 25% is as yet unknown. It cannot, however, be the N-terminal valines (NA1) of the β chains, since they are interacting with 2,3 DPG in the deoxygenated, H^+ binding state.

The complex reactions at the C-terminal end of the β chains during the processes of oxygenation and deoxygenation are shown in Figure 8.8. In the deoxygenated (T) state, the HC2 (β145) tyrosine is held in a gap between the F and H helices. On oxygenation of an α haem, this gap is reduced, forcing the tyrosine to move out. This causes the hydrogen bond from the phenolic group on tyrosine to the FG5 (β98) valine and the salt bridge and other bonds of the terminal histidine to break, with consequent loss of much of the stability of the T form. As the other α haem is oxygenated with the same breakage of stabilising bonds, the R form becomes more appropriate and the flip into this form is made. With the loss of the salt bridges, so goes the ability of the terminal histidine to bind hydrogen ions. With the movement together of the β chains so goes the

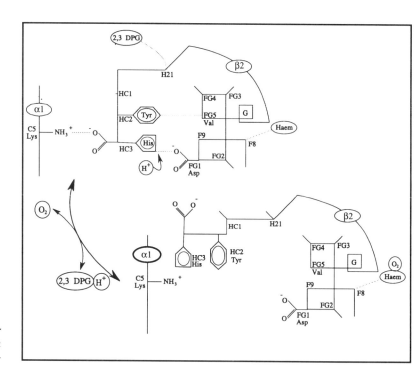

Figure 8.8 *The reactions which occur at the C-terminal end of β globin chains during the processes of oxygenation and deoxygenation*

ability to bind 2,3 DPG, as explained above. This complex series of reactions is reversed as oxygen is given up and the R form reverts to the T form again on deoxygenation.

Even if the N-terminal valines of the α chains were substituted, it would be unlikely to have an effect on the H^+ binding, since this is a phenomenon of the terminal amino group which would be preserved under such circumstances. Clearly, this is not the case with the β146 (HC3) histidines, since their role in H^+ binding involves their side chains, and the presence of the β94 (FG1) aspartic acid.

Six abnormal haemoglobins have been reported which involve β146 (HC3) histidine. In five of these cases the oxygen affinity of the resulting haemoglobin is increased. Two of these five arise by substitution: in **haemoglobin York** the substituent is proline, and in **haemoglobin Hiroshima** the substituent is aspartic acid. In **haemoglobin McKees Rock**, there is a deletion of the two terminal amino acids of the β chain (del β145,146) as a result of unequal crossing-over. The same mechanism accounts for the chain elongation variants **haemoglobin Tak** and **haemoglobin Grady** as described in Chapter 7. In the sixth and final case, **haemoglobin Cochin**, the terminal histidine is substituted by arginine which is an even more basic amino acid. The Bohr effect is therefore preserved and no change in oxygen affinity results.

Miscellaneous Effects

More than 500 haemoglobin variants have been described and the vast majority of these result in one of the five effects described above. A mere handful of abnormal haemoglobins display aberrant behaviour which is apparently unique, or at best restricted to a tiny number of variants. Some of these effects are described in this section:

- increased dissociation of the tetramer

- asymmetrical hybridisation

- polymerisation

Increased Dissociation

Several abnormal haemoglobins have been reported where there is increased dissociation of the tetramer into the dimeric $\alpha\beta$ form. In some cases increased dissociation results in altered oxygen affinity or molecular instability and these are classified accordingly. In a few cases, however, the dissociation goes no further than to dimers, and instability does not result. Such dissociation must involve substitutions in the region of the $\alpha_1\beta_2$ ($\alpha_2\beta_1$) junction. Three examples which involve substitution of the proline at $\alpha95$ (G2) are **haemoglobin G-Georgia**, where the substituent is leucine; **haemoglobin Rampa**, where the substituent is serine, and **haemoglobin St Lukes**, where the substituent is arginine. Interestingly, substitution at this point by alanine, which occurs in **haemoglobin Denmark Hill**, causes no increased dissociation but for unexplained reasons causes increased oxygen affinity.

Asymmetrical Hybridisation

Only one example has been reported of asymmetrical hybridisation. **Haemoglobin Richmond** arises by substitution of lysine for the $\beta102$ (G4) asparagine. Unlike haemoglobin Kansas, which also involves substitution at this site, haemoglobin Richmond does not have altered oxygen affinity; instead, it forms asymmetrical hybrid haemoglobins. Normally, when an aberrant globin gene is present in the heterozygous form each haemoglobin molecule formed which includes the aberrant globin will be of the same form eg $\alpha\beta^A\alpha\beta^X$, where A represents normal β globin and X represents a β globin abnormality. When the aberrant gene present is the abnormal β gene of haemoglobin Richmond, however, a mixture of molecules forms ie $(\alpha\beta^R)_2$, $\alpha\beta^A\alpha\beta^R$ and $(\alpha\beta^A)_2$. This is called asymmetrical hybridisation. Haemoglobin Richmond is clinically silent.

Polymerisation

Polymerisation of haemoglobin in oxidising conditions is observed with **haemoglobin Porto Allegro** which arises from the unusual substitution of serine by cysteine at the "variable" $\beta9$ (A6) position. The polymerisation is thought to be mediated by the formation of disulphide bonds from adjacent sulphydryl groups between haemoglobin molecules under oxidising conditions. The presence of haemoglobin Porto Allegro has no apparent clinical implications.

The most significant structural haemoglobinopathy in terms of its clinical consequences and its incidence is **haemoglobin S**. The myriad clinical consequences of the presence of this abnormal haemoglobin all stem from its tendency to polymerise, causing deformation of the red cell into elongated and poorly deformable sickle shapes. All haemoglobin molecules can be induced to polymerise *in vitro* under the appropriate conditions of concentration, salt and pH strength, and oxygen tension. Where haemoglobin S differs is that it will readily do so under physiological conditions.

The mechanism of polymer formation by haemoglobin S is poorly understood but important insights into possible interactions have been obtained by X-ray crystallographic analysis of the polymers. This provides detailed information about the relative positions of amino acids in the polymers thereby permitting analysis of possible intermolecular interactions. The behaviour of haemoglobin variants which have similar substitutions and the behaviour of mixtures of haemoglobin S and other normal and abnormal haemoglobin molecules have also proved to be important in helping to unravel the complex molecular interactions which govern this important phenomenon.

Haemoglobin S results from a substitution of the glutamic acid residue in the external and "variable" position $\beta6$ (A3) by valine. Substitution of the same amino acid by lysine gives rise to **haemo-**

globin C which is the second most common of the structural haemoglobinopathies. A third, much rarer, haemoglobin variant, **haemoglobin G-Makassar**, results from the substitution of the valine by alanine. Neither haemoglobin C nor haemoglobin G-Makassar polymerise under physiological conditions, which tends to suggest that it is the presence of valine at position β6 rather than the loss of glutamine which is an important determinant of the tendency towards polymer formation. **Haemoglobin C Harlem** is the result of a double substitution: the same substitution as haemoglobin S, but in addition it also has a substitution of aspartic acid to asparagine at β73 (E17). Haemoglobin C Harlem can be induced to sickle but not as readily as haemoglobin S. This implicates the aspartic acid at E17 as an important factor in the full manifestation of the sickling phenomenon. This implication is strengthened by the observation that mixtures of haemoglobin S with **haemoglobin Korle-Bu**, which has the same substitution of asparagine for aspartic acid at β73 as a single alteration, display the same reduced tendency to sickle as identical mixtures of haemoglobins S and C Harlem. The presence of foetal haemoglobin in a mixture with haemoglobin S has an even more marked tempering effect on sickling: an observation which has important clinical consequences.

In contrast, the presence of **haemoglobin O Arab** and **haemoglobin D Punjab** have an enhancing effect on sickling. An analysis of the alterations occurring in these haemoglobins reveals that both haemoglobin O Arab and haemoglobin D Punjab are substitutions of the glutamic acid at β121 (GH4). In haemoglobin O Arab the substitution is by lysine and in D Punjab the substitution is by glutamine. In both cases the substitution results in the loss of a negatively charged amino acid residue. In the case of D Punjab, the replacement amino acid residue is polar, but in the case of O Arab, the replacement means the substitution of a negative charge by a positive charge. The fact that haemoglobin O Arab produces a stronger interaction with haemoglobin S than do either haemoglobin D Punjab or haemoglobin S itself is strongly suggestive that the presence of the positive charge is even more important than the presence of a second β^S chain. This may well be due to the manner in which the molecules align themselves during polymerisation. The other β6 amino acid residue appears not to be in contact with another chain, whereas the β121 residue is in contact with an α globin chain, at about α114.

Another haemoglobin that can be induced to sickle is **haemoglobin Memphis.** Like haemoglobin C Harlem, haemoglobin Memphis involves a double substitution. Again one of the substitutions is the β6 glutamic acid to valine substitution of haemoglobin S. The second substitution, however, is an α chain substitution. The substitution is at α23 (B4), and is of glutamine for glutamic acid. The fact that haemoglobin Memphis sickles considerably less readily than haemoglobin S, despite possessing the same substitution, is strongly suggestive of an important role for the glutamic acid at α23 in the polymerisation process, a role which glutamine, probably because of the lack of the negative charge, cannot adequately perform.

At least two other α chain variants have been reported which, when co-inherited with haemoglobin S, exacerbate the sickling tendency. **Haemoglobin G Philadelphia** arises from the substitution of lysine for the polar asparagine at α68 (E17): **haemoglobin Stanleyville II** arises from the same substitution at α78 (EF7). The fact that both changes lead to enhanced sickling strongly suggests that these two chain positions are in close contact during polymer formation, and that the presence of the charge leads to firmer inter-chain bonding.

The study of the interactions of the globin chains during the process of polymerisation in haemoglobin S and in other haemoglobins is incomplete. Structural analysis has only been possible for a relatively few years. The application of recently developed tools such as computer-aided analysis and molecular modelling are likely to help explain the complex interactions which result in polymerisation, but for the moment we can only gather what evidence we can and wait.

Pathophysiology

The clinical manifestations of the structural haemoglobinopathies stem from the behaviour of the aberrant haemoglobin molecule and largely coincide with the classification scheme used in this chapter.

Methaemoglobinaemia

The haemoglobins M are only seen in the heterozygous state: the homozygous state is incompatible with life. Methaemoglobin is incapable of oxygen carriage because the iron in haem is in the Fe^{3+} state. Thus haemoglobin M heterozygotes display reduced arterial oxygen saturation. Capillary blood normally is rich in oxyhaemoglobin which characteristically is bright red. However, when the oxygen saturation of capillary blood is greatly reduced, as in haemoglobin M heterozygotes, it assumes the bluish-red colour normally associated with the high levels of deoxyhaemoglobin seen in venous blood. This is manifest as a bluish tinge to the complexion of affected individuals, a condition known as **peripheral cyanosis**. Apart from this cosmetic change, haemoglobin M heterozygotes typically are asymptomatic.

Unstable Haemoglobins

The unstable haemoglobins precipitate within the red cell, forming aggregates called **Heinz bodies**. These are "pitted" from the cell during passage through the spleen, resulting in a shortening of the red cell lifespan. The typical symptoms of a haemolytic state are present in affected individuals but are highly variable in their severity. Typically, α globin variants manifest symptoms from birth and, occasionally, the condition may be confused with haemolytic disease of the newborn. β globin variants seldom are manifest before 3 months of age.

Increased Oxygen Affinity Haemoglobins

The presence of a haemoglobin with an increased affinity for oxygen results in decreased delivery of oxygen to the tissues and so leads to an erythrocytosis. It is important to differentiate between this condition and other causes of erythrocytosis such as the myeloproliferative disorder, polycythaemia rubra vera.

Sickling Disorders

Sickle cell disease is associated with a variety of clinical pictures, depending on whether the affected individual is heterozygous or homozygous for haemoglobin S and on which other abnormal globin genes are present. Heterozygotes for haemoglobin S are said to have sickle cell trait, while homozygotes have sickle cell anaemia. Typically, individuals with sickle cell trait are clinically normal and may be unaware of their condition. Such cases are only reliably detectable by laboratory analysis, which will reveal the presence of about 40% HbS. Sickle cell crises are extremely rare but affected individuals should be warned of the potential dangers of severe hypothermia or hypoxia. Rare cases of sickling in, for example, unpressurised aircraft have been reported.

Sickle cell anaemia follows a highly variable clinical course; some patients die in infancy from the disabling effects of recurrent crises

> The first published description of a case of sickle cell anaemia was made in 1910 by James Herrick. The patient described was a young West Indian student who demonstrated many of the classical clinical features of this condition recognised today.
>
> *Archives of Internal Medicine*, 6: 517-521

or overwhelming infection; others may live for a normal lifespan. The precise causes of this variability are poorly understood but it is clear that the physical and social environments of the patient play a large part. Symptoms of sickle cell anaemia are seldom manifest before the age of about 6 months when the level of circulating foetal haemoglobin falls to the adult level. Between crises, the condition is characterised by a chronic haemolytic state with jaundice and a relatively constant haemoglobin level of 7-8 g/dl. The anaemia may be exacerbated by the presence of folate deficiency. This quiescent state is punctuated by crises of four main types:

- **vaso-occlusive sickling crises**. The most common manifestation of sickling in young children is the **hand and foot syndrome**. This is an extremely painful dactylitis, which is accompanied by swelling of the affected joint, pyrexia and a moderate leucocytosis. It is caused by infarction of the haemopoietic bone marrow secondary to sickling in the microcirculation of the fingers and toes. In some cases, this may result in premature fusion of the epiphyses, and a selective growth defect of the affected joint.

- **aplastic crises**. These are manifest as a sudden fall in the haemoglobin value with no compensatory reticulocytosis. Aplastic crises usually are secondary to intercurrent infection, most commonly with parvo virus.

- **acute splenic sequestration**. This is manifest as sudden weakness and dyspnoea with left abdominal pain and marked abdominal distension. The symptoms result from sequestration of a large proportion of the circulating red cell mass by the spleen. Splenic sequestration is a major cause of infant mortality in sickle cell anaemia.

- **infections**. Susceptibility to bacterial infection is a hallmark of sickle cell anaemia, and a common cause of infant mortality. The most common infections are pneumococcal septicaemia and meningitis and staphylococcal osteomyelitis.

Repeated sickling crises cause cumulative damage to a wide range of tissues but two examples deserve special mention. Repeated small infarctions within the microcirculation of the spleen ultimately result in its destruction, a condition known as **autosplenectomy**. The presence of features of severe hyposplenism in an individual who has not undergone splenectomy may indicate the presence of sickle cell disease. The most common type of sickling crisis in adults, and also potentially the most dangerous, is the **chest syndrome** which is characterised by severe pleural pain of sudden onset, fever and severe difficulty in breathing. The precise cause of this complication is obscure; it may be triggered by pulmonary infection, local infarction caused by sickling, pulmonary embolism or, in some cases, a combination of these.

Co-inheritance of other haemoglobinopathies can influence the clinical course of sickle cell trait or anaemia. For example, HbS homozygotes which also inherit a thalassaemia trait typically have higher haemoglobin levels and a less severe clinical picture. On the other hand, compound heterozygotes for HbS and β^o thalassaemia have relatively severe disease. One particularly important example of such an interaction is where sickle cell anaemia is co-inherited with the benign condition hereditary persistence of foetal haemoglobin (HPFH) in which levels of HbF do not fall. The presence of significant amounts of haemoglobin F has a protective effect against sickling and such individuals express relatively mild disease.

One of the most important measures in the effective treatment of sickle cell disease is to minimise the number of crises by educating sufferers and their families about circumstances which may trigger a sickling crisis. They should be advised to avoid sudden cold, dehydration, hypoxic conditions, and infections.

Other measures intended to reduce the incidence of sickling crises are more controversial. Hypertransfusion or even exchange transfusion with normal blood can lower the proportion of haemoglobin S sufficiently to reduce greatly the incidence of sickling crisis. This is most useful as a short-term measure, for example in pregnancy or as prophylaxis before and during major surgery. This treatment should not be maintained for longer periods because of the risks of haemosiderosis, red cell sensitisation and infection associated with transfusion. A number of different drugs have been claimed to prevent sickling *in vivo*, but none have proved to be effective without unacceptably severe side effects. The possibility of therapeutic manipulation of HbF levels with drugs such as 5-azacytidine is currently under investigation.

Suggested Further Reading

Bunn, H.F. and Forget, B.G. (1985). *Haemoglobin: Molecular, Genetic and Clinical Aspects.* Philadelphia: W.B. Saunders.

Winslow, R.M. and Anderson, W.F. (1983). The Haemoglobinopathies. In Stanbury, J.B., Wyngaarden, J.B., Fredrickson, D.S., Goldstein, J.L. and Brown, M.S. (eds.) *The Metabolic Basis of Inherited Disease* 5th ed., London: McGraw-Hill.

Embury, S.H. (1986). The Clinical Pathophysiology of Sickle Cell Disease. *Annual Review of Medicine,* **37:** 361-376.

Serjeant, G.R. (1985). *Sickle Cell Disease.* Oxford: Oxford University Press.

The Red Cell Membrane

The primary function of the mature red cell is the transport of respiratory gases to and from the tissues. The effective performance of this task requires that the cell should be capable of traversing the microvascular system without mechanical damage and that the cell should normally retain a shape which facilitates gaseous exchange. These demands require the red cell membrane to be extremely tough yet highly flexible. During its 120 day lifespan, a red cell travels about 300 miles along blood vessels with a diameter of as little as 3 μm and is subject to the extreme stresses of passage through the heart at least 5×10^5 times. The secret of the success of the red cell membrane in meeting the conflicting demands of strength and flexibility lies in the design of its **protein cytoskeleton** and the way in which the cytoskeleton interacts with the membrane **lipid bilayer**.

The main functions of the red cell membrane may be summarised as follows:

- to separate the contents of the cell from the plasma

- to maintain the characteristic shape of the red cell

- to regulate intracellular cation concentrations

- to act as the interface between the cell and its environment via membrane surface receptors

The role of the membrane in separating the contents of the cell from the plasma allows the red cell to control its own internal environment. For example, a constant supply of glucose from the plasma is required by the red cell to supply its energy needs and requirement for reducing potential. The transport of glucose into the red cell is facilitated by a specific transport protein in the membrane. Conversely, it is important that, once inside the cell, the phosphorylated intermediates of glycolysis are retained or the glycolytic pathway would fail in its purpose. Retention is assured because the red cell membrane is impermeable to phosphorylated sugars. This property of controlling which substances can cross the membrane is called **selective permeability** and is vital to the economy of the cell.

Mature red cells are biconcave discs with an average diameter of 7.2 μm, a volume of about 85 fl and a surface area of about 140 μm^2. This unusual shape maximises the surface area:volume ratio (a sphere of the same volume has a surface area of 95 μm^2) and so facilitates gaseous exchange across the membrane. Bi-concave discs also are readily deformable, assuming an "arrowhead" conformation to allow passage through narrow capillaries.

The red cell membrane contains channels which facilitate the rapid passage across the membrane of water and monovalent anions such as Cl$^-$ and HCO$_3^-$. In contrast, the passage of monovalent cations such as Na$^+$ and K$^+$ across the membrane is relatively slow. Large plasma:cell concentration gradients exist for these cations. The intracellular Na$^+$ concentration is relatively low (about 8 mmol/l) while the plasma Na$^+$ concentration is relatively high (about 140 mmol/l). This results in a slow leakage of Na$^+$ from the plasma to the cell. On the other hand, the intracellular K$^+$ concentration is relatively high (about 100 mmol/l) while the plasma concentration is relatively low (about 5 mmol/l). Thus, there is a slow leakage of K$^+$ from the cell into the plasma. In the absence of some mechanism to counter the leakage of monovalent cations, their concentrations would gradually equalise. However, the red cell membrane contains a protein which acts as a **"cation pump"** ie it actively pumps Na$^+$ from the cell into the plasma and pumps K$^+$ in the opposite direction. The energy required to drive the pump is derived from the conversion of ATP to ADP by a membrane ATPase. The ADP thus formed is utilised by the Embden Meyerhof pathway of glycolysis and so is reconverted to ATP (see Chapter 11). The activity of the pump is stimulated by extracellular K$^+$ or by a rise in the intracellular Na$^+$ concentration. The activity rate of the cation pump is controlled in such a way that it precisely balances the rate of leakage of cations across the membrane. Thus, the intracellular Na$^+$ and K$^+$ concentrations are maintained within very narrow limits.

Composition of the Red Cell Membrane

The approximate composition of the red cell membrane is shown in Table 9.1.

50% Protein
10% Carbohydrate (glycoproteins and glycolipids)
40% Lipid - 30% free unesterified cholesterol
           10% glycerides & free fatty acids
           60% phospholipid - 30% phosphatidyl choline
                             30% phosphatidyl ethanolamine
                             25% sphingomyelin
                             15% phosphatidyl serine

Table 9.1 *Composition of the red cell membrane*

Lipids

All of the lipid associated with red cells is present in the cell membrane. The mature red cell has no capacity to synthesise lipid: alterations in membrane lipid content can only occur by exchange with plasma lipids.

As shown in Table 9.1, about 60% of the red cell membrane lipid is composed of one of four different phospholipids viz **phosphatidyl choline, phosphatidyl ethanolamine, sphingomyelin** and **phosphatidyl serine**. Phospholipid molecules are characterised by a polar head group attached to a non-polar fatty acid tail. The polar head group is hydrophilic (water-loving) while the fatty acid tail is hydrophobic (water-fearing) or lipophilic (fat-loving). Thus, the phospholipid molecules in the cell membrane tend to arrange themselves in a bilayer with their hydrophilic heads pointing towards the inner and outer aqueous phases (the cytoplasm and plasma respectively) while the hydrophobic tails point towards each other as shown in Figure 9.1. Small amounts of phosphatidic acid, phosphatidyl inositol, lysophosphatidyl choline and glycolipids also are present.

The distribution of the different phospholipids between the two leaflets of the bilayer is not symmetrical. The choline phospholipids phosphatidyl choline and sphingomyelin are mainly present in the plasma layer while the amino phospholipids phosphatidyl ethanolamine, phosphatidyl serine and phosphatidyl inositol are restricted to the cytoplasmic layer.

The membrane **cholesterol** is unesterified and lies between the two layers of the lipid bilayer as shown in Figure 9.1. The concentration of cholesterol in the membrane is an important determinant of membrane surface area and fluidity: an increase in membrane

The lysophospholipids such as lysophosphatidyl choline (lysolecithin) differ from their phospholipid cousins in that they have only one fatty acid attached to their glycerol backbone instead of two. The *lyso* prefix alludes to their pronounced detergent-like properties which can induce red cell haemolysis if they accumulate within the red cell membrane.

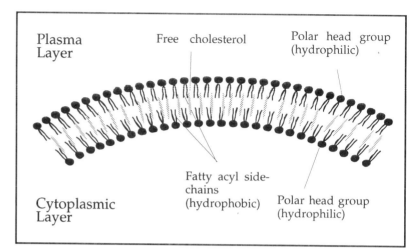

Figure 9.1 *Arrangement of phospholipids in the lipid bilayer*

cholesterol leads to an increased surface area and decreased deformability. Red cell membrane cholesterol is in rapid exchange with the unesterified cholesterol of plasma lipoproteins. Plasma lipoproteins contain cholesterol in the free and esterified states in a ratio of about 1:3. The ratio of free to esterified cholesterol is controlled by the action of the enzyme **lecithin:cholesterol acyl transferase (LCAT)**. A decrease in LCAT activity leads to an increased plasma concentration of free cholesterol and thus, indirectly, to an increased concentration of cholesterol levels in the red cell membrane. In extreme circumstances, the decreased deformability which results can lead to premature destruction of the red cell.

Red cell lysophosphatidyl choline, phosphatidyl choline and sphingomyelin also are in exchange with their plasma lipoprotein counterparts. The rate of exchange of phosphatidyl choline and sphingomyelin is slow (less than 1% is exchanged per hour). The phospholipids of the cytoplasmic layer cannot exchange with the plasma.

Proteins

Most red cell membrane proteins are tightly associated with the lipid bilayer, and require treatment with powerful detergents such as sodium dodecyl sulphate (SDS) to extract them for analysis by polyacrylamide gel electrophoresis (PAGE). This technique separates substances according to their molecular weight, the lightest travelling the furthest from the origin. Red cell membrane proteins have been named according to their relative positions on SDS-

SAQ 1

Which of the following statements are true?

A. The RBC membrane is rich in esterified cholesterol.
B. Phosphatidyl serine is concentrated in the outer leaflet of the lipid bilayer.
C. RBC membrane sphingomyelin is in rapid exchange with the plasma.
D. Lysolecithin is present at high concentration in RBC membranes.

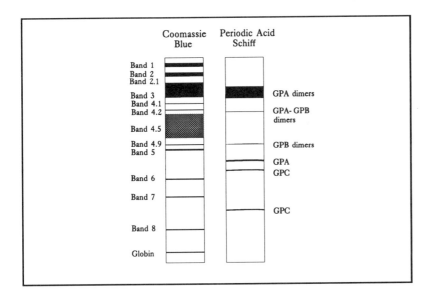

Figure 9.2 *Red cell membrane proteins separated by SDS-PAGE electrophoresis. Coomassie blue is a protein stain. Periodic acid Schiff stains carbohydrate and therefore reveals the glycophorins.*

PAGE electrophoresis, as shown in Figure 9.2. Some of the better characterised proteins also have trivial names, as shown in Table 9.2.

Protein	Trivial Name	Molec. Wt.
band 1	spectrin	240,000
band 2	spectrin	220,000
band 2.1-2.6	ankyrin	200,000
band 3	anion exchange channel	95,000
band 4.1		80,000
band 5	actin	42,000
band 6	glyceraldehyde-3-phosphate dehydrogenase	35,000
band 7		29,000
PAS-1	glycophorin A	29,000

Table 9.2 *Red cell membrane proteins.*

Red cell membrane proteins can be grouped into two types:

- **integral proteins** which penetrate the lipid bilayer and are firmly anchored within it via interactions with the hydrophobic core. Only a relatively small portion of an integral protein molecule is exposed to the inner and outer aqueous phases. About 60-80% of red cell membrane proteins are of this type.

Examples of important integral proteins include **band 3** and the **glycophorins**. Band 3 acts as the anion transport channel while the glycophorins are associated with the MNSs blood group system. Both of the named examples of integral proteins are bound tightly to the protein cytoskeleton.

- **peripheral proteins** which are in contact with the lipid bilayer but are not strongly attached to it. About 20-40% of red cell membrane proteins are peripheral proteins. Examples of important peripheral proteins include haemoglobin, the enzyme glyceraldehyde-3-phosphate dehydrogenase and the cytoskeletal proteins **spectrin** and **actin**.

Red Cell Membrane Integral Proteins

Band 3

Band 3 is a single chain molecule with a molecular weight of about 95,000. It accounts for close to 25% of the total protein content of the red cell membrane. Band 3 has two major functions within the red cell membrane, each associated with a distinct functional domain. Its primary function is to facilitate anion transport across the membrane but it also acts as an important binding site for cytoskeletal and other red cell proteins.

The central portion of the band 3 molecule consists of a series of hydrophobic helices which traverse the lipid bilayer. These helices are linked by short hydrophilic sequences which are exposed to the inner and outer aqueous phases. This arrangement forms a transmembrane channel which facilitates the rapid transport of Cl^- and HCO_3^- anions. Band 3 is not particularly selective because SO_4^{2-} and PO_4^{3-} anions also are transported, albeit much more slowly, via this channel. A large carbohydrate side chain which carries the Ii blood group antigens is attached to one of the external hydrophilic linking sequences.

The N-terminal portion of band 3 is hydrophilic and projects into the cytoplasm of the cell. This functional domain has a molecular weight of about 43,000 and contains binding sites for haemoglobin, the glycolytic enzymes glyceraldehyde-3-phosphate dehydrogenase, aldolase, and phosphoglycerate kinase and the cytoskeletal proteins ankyrin, band 4.1 and band 4.2.

Glycophorins

The three members of the red cell glycophorin family most commonly are known as glycophorins A, B and C. An alternative classification scheme exists in which glycophorin A is known as glycoprotein α, glycophorin B as glycoprotein δ and the three forms of glycophorin C are known as glycoproteins β, β$_1$ and γ.

Glycophorin A accounts for close to 2% of the mass of the red cell membrane. The glycophorin A molecule has been shown to consist of three distinct domains: a **receptor domain** which projects into the outer aqueous phase, a **transmembranous domain** which spans the lipid bilayer and an **interior domain** which projects into the cytoplasm of the cell. The receptor domain is very hydrophilic and contains large amounts of carbohydrate and sialic acid. The M, N and Wr^b blood group antigens are located on this portion of the molecule. The glycophorin A receptor domain contains receptors for a variety of lectins such as phytohaemagglutinin and wheat germ agglutinin as well as a number of viruses including influenza virus and myxovirus. The transmembranous domain is hydrophobic and therefore serves to anchor the molecule in the membrane. Red cell membrane glycophorin A is thought to exist as a dimer, coupled at the transmembranous domains. The interior domain is hydrophilic and contains an assemblage of cationic amino acid residues near to the C-terminal end. The function of this portion of the molecule remains obscure but it is known to bind to anionic phospholipids and to certain cytoskeletal proteins. The glycophorins are thought to act as transmembrane signal transducers. Glycophorins A, B and C have been shown to act as receptors for the malarial parasite *Plasmodium falciparum*.

Glycophorins B and C are similar in gross structure to glycophorin A. The N, Ss and U blood group antigens are located on the receptor domain of glycophorin B.

Na$^+$/K$^+$ ATPase

The Na$^+$/K$^+$ ATPase enzyme exists as an oligomer containing two large α subunits of molecular weight 110,000 and two smaller gly-

The haematocrit of venous blood normally is greater than that of arterial blood. This interesting phenomenon is explained by changes in anion concentrations within the red cell as it passes from the arterial to the venous system.

As explained in Chapter 6, deoxyhaemoglobin is a weaker acid than oxyhaemoglobin and so has a lower net polyvalent anionic charge. Thus, deoxygenation is accompanied by a reduction in the net negative charge within the red cell. Electrochemical neutrality is restored by the rapid uptake of Cl$^-$ ions via the band 3 anion exchange channel and water, leading to a slight swelling of the cell. Venous blood largely is deoxygenated and so the mean red cell volume and haematocrit is increased with respect to fully oxygenated arterial blood.

coprotein β subunits of molecular weight 55,000. The α subunits span the lipid bilayer while the β subunits project into the outer aqueous phase. As its name suggests, this enzyme catalyses the hydrolysis of ATP to ADP, liberating energy in the process. The action of the Na^+/K^+ ATPase is mediated by phosphorylation and dephosphorylation of a specific aspartic acid residue on the α subunit. Phosphorylation of the aspartic acid requires the presence of Na^+ and Mg^{2+} ions but not K^+ ions while dephosphorylation requires K^+ but not Na^+ or Mg^{2+} ions. Each ATP molecule hydrolysed via this system results in the ejection of three Na^+ ions from the cell and the transport of two K^+ ions into the cell. This mechanism is present in all mammalian cells and accounts for about one third of all ATP hydrolysis at rest. The action of the red cell cation pump is shown schematically in Figure 9.3.

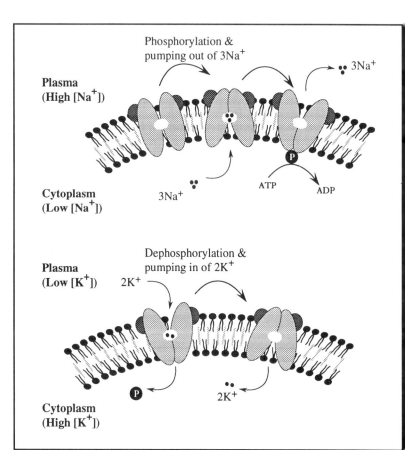

Figure 9.3 *Action of the red cell membrane cationic pump*

Glucose Transport Protein

The glucose transport protein has a molecular weight of 60,000 and shows some structural similarity to band 3, the anion transport protein. The motive force for transport of plasma glucose into the red cell is derived from the electrochemical gradient of Na^+ ions across the cell membrane. ATP hydrolysis is not required for glucose transport. Each molecule of glucose transported into the red cell is accompanied by a Na^+ ion, leading to a net reduction in the transmembrane gradient of Na^+ ions. Failure of the cation pump constantly to regenerate the Na^+ ion gradient would, therefore, result in failure of glucose transport. This, in turn, would lead to glycolytic failure and a consequent lack of ATP generation. The net result would be a rapid downward spiral leading to the death of the cell.

Surface Receptors

Physiologically, the most important surface receptor of red cells is the **transferrin receptor**. This membrane protein has a molecular weight of 85,000 and consists of a short N-terminal interior domain, a lipophilic transmembrane domain and a large C-terminal receptor domain. The receptor domain is capable of binding two transferrin molecules. Binding of plasma transferrin to its receptor causes aggregation of receptor-transferrin complexes in clathrin-coated pits on the red cell surface. The complexes are then internalised, whereupon the iron is released from the transferrin and the apo-transferrin:receptor complex is recycled to the cell surface. The transferrin receptor has a relatively low affinity for apotransferrin at plasma pH, causing the release of the binding protein into the plasma to rejoin the iron transport cycle. Transferrin receptors are present on the surface of most cells but are present at particularly high concentration on the red cell surface. The concentration of transferrin receptors is highest on intermediate normoblasts, when haemoglobin synthesis is maximal.

A large variety of other surface receptors have been demonstrated on the red cell membrane, including those for insulin, parathyroid hormone, vitamin E, the Complement components C3b and C4b, opiates and oestradiol. In most cases, the function of these receptors in the context of red cells remains obscure.

Red Cell Membrane Peripheral Proteins

The red cell membrane peripheral proteins interact to form a **cytoskeleton** which, as its name suggests, acts as a tough supporting framework for the lipid bilayer. Four proteins play a key role in the structure of the red cell cytoskeleton viz spectrin, ankyrin, band 4.1 and actin, although many others play ancillary roles in this complex structure.

Spectrin (Bands 1 and 2)

Spectrin constitutes about two thirds of the total weight of the cytoskeleton. This protein is a heterodimer composed of two subunits designated α and β which have molecular weights of 240,000 and 220,000 respectively. These subunits are bound together in an antiparallel ie "head to tail" configuration. Further, the two subunits are twisted around one another as shown in Figure 9.4. Spectrin heterodimers can associate head to head to form heterotetramers or can form higher oligomers in a branching, radial structure. *In vivo* red cell membrane spectrin is thought to be composed of a mixture of these three forms, with the heterotetrameric form predominating. Spectrin also associates with ankyrin, band 4.1, actin and anionic phospholipids.

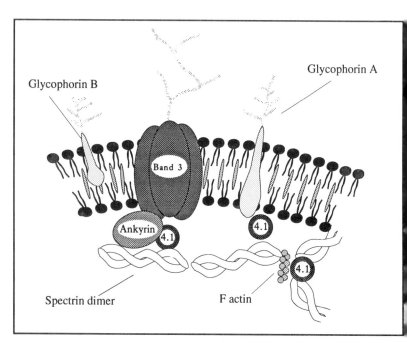

Figure 9.4 *Structure of the red cell membrane*

Ankyrin (Bands 2.1-2.3 and 2.6)

Ankyrin has a molecular weight of 210,000 and serves to anchor assembled spectrin molecules to the lipid bilayer. This is accomplished by binding simultaneously to spectrin tetramers and to the interior domain of the integral protein, band 3.

Actin

Actin is synthesised as a globular protein, a form known as **G actin**. An alternative configuration, **F actin**, is formed by the assembly of G actin molecules "head to tail" into double helical filaments. Assembly and disassembly of actin filaments is an important process in neutrophil locomotion as described in Chapter 13. Red cell membrane actin takes the form of relatively short F actin filaments. These filaments bind weakly to the tail end of both α and β spectrin. The result is a two-dimensional lattice of spectrin tetramers held together by actin filaments. The lipid bilayer is attached to this lattice via band 3.

Band 4.1

Band 4.1 is a globular protein of molecular weight 80,000 which serves two distinct functions in the red cell membrane. It binds to spectrin close to the actin binding site, thereby strengthening and stabilising the cytoskeletal lattice. It also binds directly to glycophorins A and C, band 3 and phosphatidyl serine, and therefore strengthens the links between the lipid bilayer and the protein cytoskeleton.

The currently accepted model of the structure of the red cell membrane is shown in Figure 9.4.

Red Cell Blood Group Antigens

Study of red cell blood group antigens has provided important insights into such diverse fields as population genetics, mechanisms of gene expression, blood transfusion, forensic pathology and organ transplantation. There are 19 different blood group systems and nine collections recognised in humans, encompassing well over 200 different antigens. Only the clinically most important blood

---

SAQ 2

Which of the following statements are true?

A. Spectrin is an RBC membrane integral protein.
B. Band 3 acts as an exchange channel for negatively charged ions.
C. Glycophorin A carries MN blood group antigens.
D. Ankyrin binds to both spectrin and band 3.
E. RBC membrane actin is mainly in the globular form.

group systems are described in this chapter: an exhaustive review is beyond the scope of this book.

The following conventions are used to describe blood group antigens, antibodies and genes:

- the location of a gene which encodes a blood group antigen is called its **locus**

- the various forms of the gene which encode the different antigens of the blood group system are **alleles** and are mutually exclusive

- the genes present in an individual constitute the **genotype** irrespective of expression

- the expressed blood group antigens constitute the **phenotype** of the individual

- to differentiate between genes and antigens, genes are written in italics ie A is an antigen whereas *A* refers to the gene which encodes A

The ABO Blood Group System

The ABO blood group system was the first to be discovered and is by far the most important. Transfusion of ABO-incompatible blood results in an acute haemolytic reaction which may be life-threatening.

The ABO blood group system is controlled by the allelic genes *A, B, H* and *h* which are located on chromosome 9 and are inherited in a simple Mendelian fashion. The dominant *H* allele encodes a transferase enzyme (α2-L-fucosyltransferase) which converts a precursor substance in the red cell membrane to **H substance**. In the absence of *H* (*hh*), this conversion cannot occur and the result is a complete absence of ABO antigens. This rare abnormality is known as the **Bombay phenotype.**

The *A* and *B* alleles also encode transferase enzymes which are called α3-N-acetylgalactosaminyltransferase (A-transferase) and α3-D-galactosyltransferase (B-transferase) respectively. These enzymes add specific sugar molecules to the terminal galactose of

In 1900, Karl Landsteiner performed a series of mixing experiments with the blood of 22 colleagues in which the red cells of each individual were mixed with the serum of each of the others. On the basis of the patterns of agglutination observed, Landsteiner could discern three groups of individuals which he named A, B and C. The red cells of group A individuals were agglutinated by the serum of group B and C individuals. The red cells of group B individuals were agglutinated by the serum of group A and C individuals. The red cells of group C individuals were not agglutinated by serum from any individual.

It is easy to see that Landsteiner's groups A, B and C equate with the blood groups A, B and O recognised today. The fourth ABO blood group, AB, was not recognised until two years later when the experiment was repeated with a much larger sample.

H substance, forming A or B substance on the cell surface. In the case of A-transferase, the added sugar is N-acetylgalactosamine, in the case of B-transferase the added sugar is galactose. It is these terminal sugars which determine the ABO specificity. The development of A, B and H antigens is shown schematically in Figure 9.5.

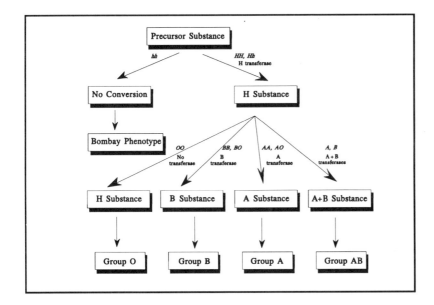

Figure 9.5 *Synthesis of ABO blood group antigens*

Because ABO-like polysaccharides are widespread in nature, exposure to A and B substance with subsequent immunisation occurs early in life. This means that neonates typically do not have ABO antibodies in their plasma but that, in the first months of life, exposure to A and B substance elicits the formation of IgM immunoglobulins with ABO specificity complementary to the host ABO type. The ABO blood group system is summarised in Table 9.3.

Blood Group	Genotype	Phenotype	Red Cell Antigens	Plasma Antibodies	Frequency
A	*AA* *AO*	A	A	β	0.44
B	*BB* *BO*	B	B	α	0.08
O	*OO*	O	H	α, β	0.45
AB	*AB*	AB	A+B	none	0.03

Table 9.3 *The ABO blood group system*

SAQ 3

A group O woman has given birth to a group O baby. Which of the following men could be the father?

A. Steve, who is group O
B. Phil, who is group A
C. Chris, who is group AB
D. Mike, who is group B

The Secretor System

In addition to carrying ABO antigens on their red cells, about 80% of Caucasians secrete ABO blood group substances in body fluids such as saliva and seminal fluid. This fact is exploited in the field of forensic pathology for typing of blood and semen stains at scenes of violent crime. Whether an individual secretes blood group substances is governed by a pair of allelic genes designated *Se* and *se*.

The dominant allele, *Se*, controls the expression of the enzyme H-transferase in body fluids and hence governs whether the precursor substance present is converted to H substance. Subsequently, the presence of A- and B-transferases governs the synthesis of A and B substance. Thus, a group O secretor secretes H substance in their body fluids while a group A secretor secretes A substance and a smaller amount of unconverted H substance. In the absence of the *Se* allele (*se/se*), blood group substances are absent from body fluids: only unaltered precursor substance is detectable.

The Lewis Blood Group System

The Lewis blood group system is governed by a complex interaction between three pairs of allelic genes *H* and *h*, *Se* and *se* which have been described above and the Lewis genes *Le* and *le*. The dominant Lewis allele, *Le*, encodes yet another transferase enzyme, α4-L-fucosyltransferase, which adds a fucose to the subterminal N-acetylglucosamine of either precursor substance or H substance in body fluids. Thus, two different Lewis antigens exist: Lewis transferase converts precursor substance into Le^a antigen while it converts H substance into Le^b antigen.

As shown in Figure 9.6, synthesis of Le^b substance requires the presence of the *H* gene to encode H-transferase, the *Se* gene to permit secretion of this enzyme into body fluids and the *Le* gene to convert the H substance which results. When either of the *H* or *Se* genes is absent, H substance cannot be synthesised in body fluids and so Le^b substance is absent. In these circumstances, the *Le* gene encodes Le^a substance. In the absence of the *Le* gene, no Lewis antigens are synthesised.

The Lewis substances Le^a and Le^b are soluble antigens which are synthesised solely in body secretions. The red cell Lewis antigens

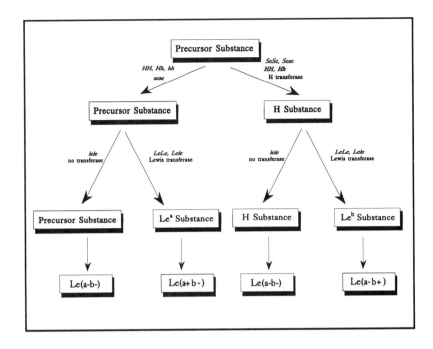

Figure 9.6 *Synthesis of Lewis blood group antigens*

are acquired by adsorption of soluble Lewis substances onto the cell membrane from plasma. The Lewis blood group system is summarised in Table 9.4.

Genotype	Blood Group Substances		Red Cell Phenotype	Frequency (Caucasians)
	Body Fluids	**Red Cells**		
hh, Le	Le^a	Le^a	Le(a+b-)	Rare
hh. lele	None	None	Le(a-b-)	Rare
H, sese, Le	Le^a	H, Le^a	Le(a+b-)	0.20
H, sese, lele	None	None	Le(a-b-)	0.04
H, Se, Le	H, Le^a, Le^b	H, Le^b	Le(a-b+)	0.75
H, Se, lele	H	H	Le(a-b-)	0.01

Table 9.4 *The Lewis blood group system*

Antibodies against Lewis antigens are present as naturally occurring IgM immunoglobulins in about 1% of Caucasians. Typically, these antibodies are of low titre and react best below 30°C and so create minimal problems in the selection of blood suitable for transfusion. Rarely, a high-titre anti-Le^a antibody with a high thermal amplitude is encountered. Such an antibody is capable of causing a haemolytic transfusion reaction if Le(a+b-) blood is transfused and so Le(a-b+) or Le(a-b-) blood is required.

Lewis antibodies do not cause haemolytic disease of the newborn as they cannot cross the placental barrier and, even if they could, foetal red cells type as Le(a-b-). The red cell Lewis phenotype typically is not expressed until after 1 year of age.

The Ii Antigens

The I and i antigens are located on the oligosaccharide chains which carry the ABO and Lewis antigens. The I antigen is present on the red cells of virtually all adults but is expressed only weakly on cord red blood cells. Conversely, the i antigen is expressed most strongly on cord red cells but diminishes with increasing age as I antigen activity increases. Naturally occurring, cold-reactive anti-I and anti-i antibodies are present at low titre in the plasma of most individuals, regardless of age. In normal circumstances, these antibodies are insignificant but, as described in the next chapter, a range of pathological conditions can affect the expression of the Ii antigens and can alter the titre and thermal range of the anti-I and anti-i antibodies resulting in haemolysis.

The Rh Blood Group System

The Rhesus or Rh blood group system is clinically the most important after the ABO system because Rh antigens are highly immunogenic and frequently are associated with haemolytic transfusion reactions and severe haemolytic disease of the newborn. The Rh system is highly polymorphic with more than 40 different antigens described although, in practice, only 5 antigens (C, c, D, E and e) are clinically important.

The genetics of the Rh system are complex and still not fully understood. For all practical purposes, however, the system can be considered to be the product of three closely linked alleles, C and c, D and d and E and e which are inherited *en bloc*. This arrangement gives rise to 8 possible haplotype combinations viz *CDE, CDe, CdE, Cde, cDE, cDe, cdE*, and *cde*. The d allele is thought to be amorphic: no red cell antigen with d specificity has ever been described. For this reason, the "d antigen" can be thought of as an absence of D

In 1940, Landsteiner and Wiener were immunising rabbits with the blood of rhesus monkeys. The antibody obtained was named anti-rhesus and was shown to agglutinate the red cells of 85% of caucasians. These individuals were said to possess the rhesus factor or to be rhesus positive. Rhesus negative individuals were assumed to lack the rhesus factor on their red cells.

Although this discovery formed the basis of the Rh blood group system, it was subsequently discovered that the antigen involved did not belong to the Rh system and so was renamed the LW antigen in honour of its discoverers. The genes for the Rh system are located on chromosome 1 while the *LW* gene is located on chromosome 19.

antigen and homozygotes are said to be Rh negative. Conversely, individuals who possess at least one *D* gene are said to be Rh positive. The frequency of the different haplotypes and the most common genotypes in UK whites are shown in Tables 9.5 and 9.6.

Haplotype	Designation	Frequency
CDE	R^z	Rare
CDe	R^1	0.41
CdE	r^y	Rare
Cde	r'	0.01
cDE	R^2	0.14
cDe	R^0	0.03
cdE	r''	0.01
cde	r	0.39

Table 9.5 *Frequency of Rh haplotypes in UK whites*

The Rh antigens are found in association with red cell membrane proteins of unknown function. The U, LW and Duffy blood group antigens are thought to be associated with the same protein. In contrast to the ABO and Lewis antigens, Rh antigens do not contain sugars.

Genotype	Designation	Phenotype	Frequency
CDe/cde	R^1r	CcDe	0.31
CDe/CDe	R^1R^1	CDe	0.16
cde/cde	rr	ce	0.15
CDe/cDE	R^1R^2	CcDEe	0.13
cDE/cde	R^2r	cDEe	0.13
cDE/cDE	R^2R^2	cDE	0.03

Table 9.6 *Frequency of most common Rh genotypes in UK whites*

Most Rh antibodies are IgG immunoglobulins which are produced in response to contact with foreign Rh antigens as a result of blood transfusion or pregnancy. Because the most immunogenic of the Rh antigens is the D antigen, antibodies with anti-D specificity are particularly common. Antibodies with anti-C, anti-E or anti-c specificity are also relatively commonly encountered in clinical practice.

The Kell Blood Group System

The Kell blood group system, in common with the Rh system, is under the control of three closely linked alleles K and k, Kp^a and Kp^b and Js^a and Js^b. The synthesis of the Kell antigens is incompletely understood but most workers currently believe that a gene on the X chromosome encodes a Kell precursor antigen, K_x, which is subsequently converted to the final Kell antigens. The location of the genes which control this conversion process is unknown. The frequency of the Kell antigens is shown in Table 9.7.

| | Frequency | |
Antigen	Caucasians	Blacks
K	0.090	0.035
k	0.998	>0.999
Kp^a	0.02	<0.001
Kp^b	0.999	>0.999
Js^a	<0.001	0.195
Js^b	>0.999	0.989

Table 9.7 *Frequency of Kell blood group antigens*

The Kell blood group system is clinically important because Kell antigens are highly immunogenic and antibodies with Kell system specificity have been implicated in haemolytic transfusion reactions and haemolytic disease of the newborn. The most commonly encountered immune antibody outside of the Rh system is anti-K. The K antigen is lacking (ie the K-k+ phenotype) in 91.1% of individuals in the UK. Anti-k is a rare immune antibody which reacts with 99.8% of blood in the UK (the frequency of the K+k+ phenotype is 8.7%).

SAQ 4

A sample of red cells has the phenotype CcDe. What is the most likely genotype?

The Duffy Blood Group System

The Duffy blood group system is encoded by a number of alleles located on chromosome 1. As shown in Table 9.7, almost all caucasians possess one or both of the two major Duffy antigens (Fy^a and Fy^b) while in blacks, the most common phenotype is Fy(a-b-). Interestingly, the Duffy phenotype plays an important role in determining susceptibility to certain forms of malaria. The Duffy antigens are associated with the surface receptor which facilitates

Genotype	Phenotype	Frequency
Fy^a, Fy^b	Fy(a+b+)	0.46
Fy^a	Fy(a+b-)	0.20
Fy^b	Fy(a-b+)	0.34
Fy	Fy(a-b-)	Rare

Table 9.7 *The frequency of the Duffy blood group antigens in Caucasians*

invasion of the red cell by the malarial parasite *Plasmodium vivax*. Individuals with the Fy(a-b-) phenotype are highly resistant to *Plasmodium vivax* infection. Invasion of the red cell by *Plasmodium falciparum* is independent of Duffy phenotype. This parasite binds to sialic acid residues on red cell membrane glycophorins. Accordingly, individuals who lack the S, s and U blood group antigens are resistant to attack by this parasite.

The Fy[a] antigen is moderately immunogenic and IgG anti-Fy[a] antibodies are not uncommon following transfusion of Fy(a+) red cells to Fy(a-) individuals. The Fy[b] antigen is much less immunogenic; anti-Fy[b] is a relatively uncommon antibody.

Suggested Further Reading

Surgenor, D.M. (ed.) (1974). *The Red Blood Cell* (2nd ed.). New York: Academic Press.

Schrier, S.L. (1985). Red Cell Membrane Biology - an Introduction. *Clinics in Haematology*, **175:** 1-12.

Mollison, P.L., Engelfriet, C.P. et al. (1987). *Blood Transfusion in Clinical Medicine* (8th ed.). Oxford: Blackwell Scientific Publications.

Answers to Self-Assessment Questions

1. A. False, RBC cholesterol is unesterified.
   B. False, phosphatidyl serine is restricted to the inner layer.
   C. False, sphingomyelin is exchanged slowly.
   D. False, accumulation of lysophosphatidyl choline would cause haemolysis.

2. A. False, spectrin is a peripheral protein.
    B. True.
    C. True.
    D. True.
    E. False, RBC membrane actin is in the filamentous form.

3. A. Yes.
    B. Yes, if Phil has the genotype AO.
    C. No, except in the extremely rare instance of a compound AB
       gene when Chris could have the genotype ABO.
    D. Yes, if Mike has the genotype BO.

4. R^1r.

Disorders of Red Cell Survival

A normal, mature red cell survives in the circulation for about 120 days. The ageing process within red cells is associated with a reduction in glycolytic activity, reduced concentrations of 2,3 DPG and ATP, accumulation of Na^+ and Ca^{2+} ions and increased rigidity due to loss of membrane lipid and changes in the cytoskeleton. These changes promote the sequestration and destruction of senescent cells in the reticuloendothelial system. Normally, the rate of destruction of senescent cells is balanced by the rate of synthesis and release of juvenile cells from the bone marrow.

Any condition which leads to a reduction in the mean lifespan of the red cell is designated as a **haemolytic disorder**. Any reduction in red cell lifespan requires a balancing increase in the rate of erythropoiesis if anaemia is to be avoided. The reserve erythropoietic capacity of normal bone marrow usually is sufficient to prevent the development of anaemia until the mean red cell lifespan falls to about 15 days, when **haemolytic anaemia** ensues. The onset of anaemia is often accelerated by the presence of a haematinic deficiency or by another complicating pathological condition. Such conditions are said to have a **haemolytic component** in their pathogenesis but typically are not considered to be haemolytic disorders.

The haemolytic disorders can be classified in several different ways:

- **site of haemolysis**. Most haemolytic disorders result from the premature destruction of red cells by the macrophages of the reticuloendothelial system. These are known as the **extravascular haemolytic disorders**. Conversely, where haemolysis occurs mainly within the circulatory system, an **intravascular haemolytic disorder** is said to exist. This scheme groups together some highly disparate disorders and says little about the pathogenesis of particular disorders.

The earliest reliable determination of red cell lifespan was performed by Hawkins and Whipple in 1938. They created an opening in the bile ducts of dogs to enable the measurement of the amount of bile excreted daily. A number of experimental animals were rendered acutely anaemic by the administration of acetylphenylhydrazine, thereby eliciting a marked reticulocytosis. About 120 days after the reticulocyte response was noted, a peak of bile pigment production was observed. This was interpreted to be due to the destruction of the reticulocyte response cohort, suggesting that newly-released red cells survive in the circulation for 120 days.

SAQ 1

What is the main site of extravascular destruction of red cells?

- **site of the defect**. Haemolytic disorders can be divided into those caused by a structural or functional defect within the red cell (ie an **intrinsic defect**) and those caused by an abnormality in the red cell environment (ie an **extrinsic defect**). Knowledge of the site of the defect is useful in that transfused blood survives normally where the defect is intrinsic but may be rapidly destroyed in the presence of an extrinsic defect.

- **nature of the defect**. Grouping haemolytic disorders according to the pathogenetic mechanism involved can aid understanding of underlying processes but can lead to confusion between hereditary and acquired types and unnecessary investigation of blood relations.

- **inherited or acquired**. Typically, inherited haemolytic disorders are caused by an intrinsic defect whereas acquired haemolytic disorders are caused by an extrinsic defect. However, there are several exceptions to this rule. For example, paroxysmal nocturnal haemoglobinuria (PNH) is an acquired intrinsic defect and severe hereditary G-6-PD deficiency typically requires the presence of an extrinsic trigger such as an antimalarial drug for this intrinsic defect to be manifest. Recognition that a disorder is hereditary can facilitate diagnosis in blood relations.

None of these classification schemes is universally applicable and, in practice, an amalgam of all four schemes is used.

Inherited Haemolytic Disorders

The inherited haemolytic disorders can be subclassified into three main groups, according to the nature of the defect:

- disorders of globin synthesis and/or structure

- enzyme disorders

- primary membrane disorders

The disorders of globin synthesis and/or structure are the thalassaemia syndromes and structural haemoglobinopathies which are described in Chapters 7 and 8 respectively. Disorders of red cell metabolism are described in Chapter 12. The remaining group of inherited haemolytic disorders, the membrane defects, are described in detail below.

Primary Membrane Disorders

Primary disorders of the red cell membrane are associated with alterations of cell shape. Many of these disorders are classified according to the shape of the abnormal red cells. Although this scheme says little about the pathogenesis of these disorders and in some cases is misleading in this regard, it remains by far the most commonly employed, and so will be used in this book.

Hereditary Spherocytosis

Hereditary spherocytosis (HS) is the most common of the inherited primary red cell membrane abnormalities, having an incidence of at least 1 in 5000 in North European populations. The condition typically is transmitted as an autosomal dominant characteristic although a less common autosomal recessive variant exists. To date, no homozygotes for the autosomal dominant form have been described, suggesting that this state is incompatible with life.

The principal features of HS include congenital haemolytic anaemia with a variable degree of spherocytosis, increased red cell osmotic fragility, episodic jaundice and variable splenomegaly. The severity of haemolysis in HS is episodic and highly variable. It is not uncommon for the diagnosis to be missed until adulthood. Less common manifestations of HS include pigment gallstones (cholelithiasis), often at an unusually young age and aplastic crisis in which erythropoiesis is almost completely suppressed for up to 72 hours, leading to severe but self-limiting anaemia. Aplastic crises commonly follow infection with type B19 human parvovirus.

In most cases of HS, the exact nature of the red cell defect is unknown. A variety of cytoskeletal defects have been described in affected families but whether these are primary or secondary manifestations of the disorder remains uncertain.

> The earliest description of a case of HS was published in 1871 by two Belgian physicians, Vanlair and Masius. The index case presented with the classical symptoms of an aplastic crisis, jaundice, splenomegaly, abdominal pain and collapse. Microscopic evaluation of the blood of this patient revealed numerous microspherocytes which remained after the apparent remission of the crisis. Similar symptoms were noted in her sister and mother.
>
> Vanlair and Masius, who named this hitherto unknown condition *microcythemie* thought it was caused by an overproduction of the spherocytes by the spleen coupled with a deficiency in their removal by the liver.

Primary red cell membrane disorders caused by deficiency of a known cytoskeletal protein deficiency are denoted by the abbreviation for the disease state followed by the name of the affected protein in brackets. A complete deficiency is denoted by a ° superscript while a partial deficiency is denoted by a + superscript eg HE[4.1°] denotes hereditary elliptocytosis caused by a complete lack of band 4.1 in the red cell membrane.

Where a primary membrane disorder is caused by a defect in a cytoskeletal protein, the affected protein is underlined eg HS[Sp-4.1] denotes hereditary spherocytosis caused by a defective spectrin molecule which cannot bind band 4.1.

Structural abnormalities of α spectrin are denoted by the abbreviation Spα followed by the affected domain and the size of the peptide obtained by tryptic digestion eg HE[Spα$^{I/74}$] denotes hereditary elliptocytosis in which maps of tryptic digests reveal a decrease in the normal 80kDa αI domain and its replacement by an abnormal 74kDa αI domain. Two truncated forms of β spectrin have been described in HE. These are denoted by the abbreviation Spβ followed by the molecular weights of the normal and the truncated form eg Spβ$^{220/216}$.

- **deficiency of spectrin (HS[Sp+]).** Severe deficiency of the red cell cytoskeletal protein spectrin has been described in a number of cases of HS. All have shown an autosomal recessive mode of inheritance and are presumed to be homozygous for an as yet undetermined defect of α spectrin synthesis. In these families, the severity of the haemolysis mirrors the degree of spectrin deficiency.

- **defective binding of band 4.1 (HS[Sp-4.1]).** A number of families have been described in which about 40% of their red cell membrane spectrin cannot bind to band 4.1, resulting in a severe weakening of the cytoskeletal framework. Most cases are associated with a structural defect of the tail end of β spectrin. The red cell membrane spectrin content in these cases is about 80% of normal, presumably as a result of proteolysis of the abnormal β spectrin.

- **deficiency of band 4.2 (HS[4.2°]).** Complete deficiency of band 4.2 has been described in a small number of Japanese families with HS. How this might contribute to the development of HS is unknown.

Typical autosomal dominant HS has been linked to deletions or translocations involving the short arm of chromosome 8. The gene which encodes ankyrin is located in this region. Since ankyrin is responsible for binding spectrin to the lipid bilayer, defective ankyrin function is a plausible, if not likely, cause of HS. However, definitive proof that such a relationship exists is lacking. The genes which encode α spectrin and band 4.1 are located on chromosome 1 while the β spectrin gene is located on chromosome 14. Mild deficiency of red cell membrane spectrin is present in most cases of typical HS, but this is thought to be a secondary phenomenon.

The major site of haemolysis in HS is the spleen. As described in Chapter 2, there are two routes through the spleen; the faster, open circulation and the slower and more challenging closed circulation. Red cells which take the closed route face an inhospitable environment which tests to the limit the deformability and metabolic competence of the cell. The defective red cells in HS have an increased flux of Na$^+$ ions into the cell leading to greatly increased activity of the cation pump and necessitating an increased rate of glycolysis.

Because of this, HS red cells find passage through the spleen particularly hazardous. Detention in the glucose-poor environment of the splenic cords rapidly leads to metabolic exhaustion in HS red cells, thereby promoting the loss of intact portions of membrane. The cell which results has a reduced surface area:volume ratio and so is less readily deformable. Reduced deformability of the cell leads to increased splenic transit times thereby increasing the time of exposure to the hazards of the splenic circulation. HS reticulocytes have a normal biconcave discoid shape and normal deformability but, with each passage through the spleen, they become progressively spherocytic and rigid. This vicious circle leads inevitably to the early demise of the spherocyte within the splenic circulation. It is estimated that HS red cells survive an average of 30 passages through the spleen before they succumb.

The damage inflicted upon HS red cells by passage through the spleen is augmented by splenic macrophages. Oxygen radicals derived from activated macrophages directly damage spectrin in the red cell membrane and weaken its capacity to bind membrane lipid, thereby promoting membrane loss. The acidic pH of the spleen also promotes metabolic exhaustion of the cell by inhibiting the activity of hexokinase and phosphofructokinase, the rate-determining enzymes of glycolysis.

> **SAQ 2**
>
> Why does chronic haemolysis predispose to folate deficiency but not vitamin B_{12} deficiency?

The clinical severity of HS is highly variable. In mild cases, increased erythropoiesis compensates for the shortened red cell lifespan and the haemoglobin concentration remains within normal limits. A common consequence of chronic erythroid hyperplasia such as this is depletion of body folate stores. Oral folate supplementation may be required to prevent the development of megaloblastic anaemia. Where haemolysis is troublesome, the only effective treatment is splenectomy. Although this procedure does not affect the red cell defect, removal of the main site of haemolysis effectively "cures" the condition and returns the mean red cell lifespan to normal.

> **SAQ 3**
>
> Where in the body is the major site of folate storage?

Hereditary Elliptocytosis

The term hereditary elliptocytosis (HE) encompasses a disparate group of primary red cell membrane disorders which are characterised by the presence of a large proportion of oval or elliptical red cells.

The frequency of HE is difficult to estimate because most forms are clinically silent but may be as high as 1 in 1000. The condition typically is transmitted as an autosomal dominant characteristic. In contrast to HS, homozygous HE is well recognised as a severe, transfusion-dependent haemolytic anaemia. An unusual autosomal recessive variant of HE exists but appears to be restricted to Melanesian aborigines and Philippinos.

The clinical severity of HE ranges from clinical silence to severe, life-threatening haemolysis. Broadly, HE can be divided into four major forms which share many clinical and laboratory features but show no correlation with cytoskeletal defect:

- **Common HE** has been described in virtually all races of the world. In most cases, despite the presence of moderate numbers of elliptocytes, a mild haemolytic process exists which is fully compensated by an increased rate of erythropoiesis: anaemia and splenomegaly are absent. However, in a minority of cases, compensation is only partial and mild anaemia and splenomegaly are present. Cholelithiasis, chronic leg ulcers and aplastic crises are more common in association with incompletely compensated haemolysis. Homozygotes have a severe, transfusion-dependent haemolytic anaemia which is characterised by the presence of marked poikilocytosis, microelliptocytosis and red cell fragmentation. The major site of red cell destruction in these cases is the spleen and splenectomy provides an effective "cure".

- **HE with infantile poikilocytosis** is almost restricted to blacks and presents as a moderately severe congenital haemolytic disorder with neonatal jaundice. It is characterised by elliptocytosis, marked poikilocytosis, red cell fragmentation and susceptibility of the red cells to heat damage. In this regard, it is clinically and morphologically indistinguishable from hereditary pyropoikilocytosis (HPP). However, in contrast to HPP, this condition progressively moderates until, by the age of one year, it is clinically and morphologically indistinguishable from common HE.

- **HE with spherocytosis** has mainly been described in Caucasians and is characterised by the presence of rounded elliptocytes, microspherocytes, micro-elliptocytes and a mild, incompletely compensated haemolytic state. About one in five cases of HE in Caucasians is of this type.

- **HE with stomatocytosis** is characterised by the presence of elliptocytes which show one or more slit-like areas of pallor, or stomas, an autosomal recessive mode of inheritance and mild or absent haemolysis. The condition is most common in Melanesian aborigines but has also been described in Philippinos. The high incidence of HE with stomatocytosis in such a geographically restricted area is probably explained by the fact that the red cells in this condition are highly resistant to invasion by malarial parasites, and therefore confer a selective survival advantage to those affected.

A wide range of cytoskeletal defects have been described in association with HE as shown in Table 10.1. The most common cytoskeletal defects are structural abnormalities of domain I of α spectrin, the region responsible for dimer-dimer self-association in the cytoskeleton. Heterozygotes for these abnormalities synthesise an abnormal α spectrin which forms heterodimers but cannot self-associate to form tetramers and higher oligomers as well as an equal amount of structurally and functionally normal α spectrin. This results in a clinically mild form of HE. As a group, α spectrin variants are responsible for about one third of common HE.

Three rare abnormalities of β spectrin have been described in association with HE. Two involve the synthesis of truncated β spectrin chains (HE[$\underline{Sp}\beta^{220/216}$-Sp] and HE[$\underline{Sp}\beta^{220/214}$-Sp]) which cannot self-associate to form tetramers and higher oligomers. In many of these patients, $Sp\alpha^{I/74}$ is present as a secondary phenomenon. The third defect (HE[$\underline{Sp}\beta$-Ank]) involves the synthesis of a structurally abnormal β spectrin which has defective ankyrin binding properties. This abnormality appears to be transmitted as an autosomal recessive characteristic.

Deficiency of band 4.1 is a common cause of HE in Southern France and Northern Africa, accounting for more than one third of cases in this area. Heterozygotes have a partial deficiency of band 4.1 and

---

SAQ 4

Which of the following statements are true?

A spectrin accounts for 70% of the weight of the red cell cytoskeleton
B α spectrin has a molecular weight of 10,000
C spectrin associates with ankyrin in the red cell cytoskeleton
D spectrin associates with band 4.1 in the red cell cytoskeleton

Molecular Defect	Frequency	Affected Groups	Severity
Defective self-association of α chains			
Sp$\alpha^{I/74}$-Sp	Common	Worldwide	Mild HE
Sp$\alpha^{I/65}$-Sp	Common	N Africa blacks	Mild HE
Sp$\alpha^{I/46}$-Sp	Common	USA blacks	Mild HE
Sp$\alpha^{I/43}$-Sp	Rare	S Africa blacks	HE with Poik
Defective self-association of β chains			
Sp$\beta^{220/216}$-Sp	Rare	UK, France	Severe HE
Sp$\beta^{220/214}$-Sp	Rare	UK, France	Mild HE (+)
Defective binding of ankyrin			
Spβ-Ank	Rare	S Africa white	Mild HE (+)
Deficiency of band 4.1			
4.1^+, 4.1°	Uncommon	France, N Africa	HE with Sphero
Defect of band 4.1			
Sp-4.1	Rare	USA whites	HE with Sphero
Defect of band 3			
Ank-3	Uncommon	N America	HE (+)

Table 10.1 *Molecular defects observed in association with various forms of HE. HE (+) denotes HE with clinically significant haemolysis*

mild HE with spherocytosis whereas homozygotes have a complete absence of this protein and a severe haemolytic anaemia. Deficiency of band 4.1 appears to be rare in other parts of the world. Various functional defects of band 4.1 have also been described, at least some of which are associated with the spherocytic variant of HE.

Finally, abnormal binding of the integral protein band 3 to ankyrin has been described in association with HE with moderately severe haemolysis. The molecular basis for this abnormality remains obscure.

The mechanisms involved in elliptocyte formation are poorly understood at present. HE reticulocytes are normal in shape but

---

SAQ 5

What are the two main functions of the cytoskeletal protein band 3?

become progressively elliptocytic with age. Normal red cells are highly deformable, a property which permits passage through the tiniest capillaries of the microvasculature which have a diameter of less than half that of the red cell. Normal red cells rapidly regain their normal biconcave disc shape when deformed for short periods but, when deformation is prolonged, the shape change becomes irreversible due to realignment of the cytoskeletal proteins. Most workers currently believe that, because of the weakened forces holding the cytoskeleton together in HE red cells, realignment of the cytoskeletal proteins occurs more readily and that repeated passage through the microvasculature causes the progressive elliptocytic transformation of the cell. In severe cases of HE with prominent haemolysis, the cytoskeleton is thought to be so weakened that it cannot stand the stresses imposed by passage through the microvasculature, resulting in red cell fragmentation, poikilocytosis and microelliptocytosis.

Elliptocytes are poorly deformable and so are sequestered in the spleen. In most cases of HE, haemolysis is so mild that clinical intervention is unnecessary. Where haemolysis is troublesome, splenectomy typically provides a functional cure.

Hereditary Pyropoikilocytosis

Hereditary pyropoikilocytosis (HPP) is characterised by moderately severe haemolysis, microspherocytosis, micropoikilocytosis and an unusual susceptibility of the red cells to heat damage. The condition is inherited as an autosomal recessive characteristic and is most common in blacks.

Virtually all cases of HPP examined so far have had one of the defects of α spectrin self-association described above in association with HE. About 80% of cases of HPP have the $Sp\alpha^{I/74}$ defect while most of the rest have the $Sp\alpha^{I/46}$ defect. In common HE where these defects are present, the red cell membrane spectrin content is normal and the level of spectrin heterodimers is relatively low whereas in HPP membrane spectrin content is reduced to 70% of normal and the level of spectrin heterodimers is high. That HPP is closely related to HE is further suggested by the fact that common HE usually is demonstrable in one parent and one or more siblings of affected neonates. In most cases, the other parent is haematologically normal. This is consistent with the hypothesis that HPP represents a double heterozygous state for a defect of α spectrin

The earliest published description of hereditary elliptocytosis is attributed to M Dresbach, a physiology lecturer at Ohio State University. The abnormality first came to the his attention during a student practical class in which students were examining their own blood. Unfortunately, the index case died soon thereafter, raising doubts about the veracity of Dresbach's observation.

The hereditary nature of the condition was not established until 1929 when W C Hunter demonstrated transmission of HE through three generations of a white US family.

self-association and a defect of α spectrin synthesis. The latter defect would be clinically silent in isolation because α spectrin synthesis normally exceeds β spectrin synthesis by at least 50%.

Splenectomy ameliorates the haemolysis in most cases of HPP but does not provide the "cure" seen in HS or HE with haemolysis.

Hereditary Stomatocytosis

Hereditary stomatocytosis (HSt) is characterised by the presence of bowl-shaped red cells which on dried films have a slit-like area of central pallor. These stomatocytes result from an increased sodium transport into the cell which cannot adequately be compensated for by increased activity of the cation pump, resulting in the ingress of water and the deformation of the cell. Hereditary stomatocytosis is inherited in an autosomal dominant fashion and presents as a congenital haemolytic anaemia of variable severity which is incompletely resolved by splenectomy. The molecular defect responsible for this disorder remains obscure. Stomatocytes are sometimes known as hydrocytes because of their increased water content.

> Hereditary stomatocytosis was first described in 1961 by S P Lock, R Sephton-Smith and R M Hardisty. The index cases were a mother and daughter with chronic haemolytic anaemia which had failed to respond to splenectomy. The name is derived from the Greek στομα (stoma), meaning mouth and refers to the slit-like area of central pallor which characterises this condition.

Hereditary Xerocytosis

In contrast to hereditary stomatocytosis, the red cells of hereditary xerocytosis (HX) are characterised by an excessive leakage of K^+ from the cell, leading to progressive water depletion. Xerocytes are thus dehydrated cells which are irregularly contracted and have an abnormally high MCHC. The degree of haemolysis usually is mild and compensated by erythroid hyperplasia. Splenectomy has no clinical effect. Hereditary xerocytosis is inherited as an autosomal dominant characteristic. The molecular defect which causes this condition remains obscure.

Hereditary Acanthocytosis

In contrast to the other disorders described in this section, hereditary acanthocytosis (HAc) is caused by an extracellular defect. Abetalipoproteinaemia is an autosomal recessive trait which is characterised by an absence of low and very low density lipoproteins from the plasma because of defective synthesis of apoprotein B, and by steatorrhoea, failure to thrive, retinitis pigmentosa and neurological abnormalities. How the plasma lipid abnormalities cause the red cell defect is uncertain. The total red cell membrane lipid content in the acanthocytes is normal but the distribution of phosphatidyl choline and sphingomyelin within the bilayer is disturbed. These changes are not reversed by incubation of affected red cells in normal plasma. Typically haemolysis in HAc is mild. Treatment consists of dietary control and supplements of vitamins A, K and E; there is no cure for this condition.

Rh Null Disease

The red cells in Rh null disease are completely devoid of Rh antigens, including the LW antigen. This rare condition is characterised by a moderately severe haemolytic anaemia with stomatocytosis and spherocytosis. In contrast to the stomatocytes of hereditary stomatocytosis, however, these cells have a decreased water content. Rh null disease is caused by deletion of the Rh genes or by deletion of the Rh regulator gene. A milder variant of Rh null disease, designated Rh mod disease, is caused by the action of a suppressor gene which leads to partial expression of the Rh antigens.

McLeod Phenotype

The McLeod phenotype denotes a deficiency of the Kell precursor substance K_x on the red cell surface and is associated with a mild, fully compensated haemolytic state with acanthocytosis, poikilocytosis and reticulocytosis. This disorder is transmitted in an X-linked recessive fashion and has been described in association with chronic granulomatous disease. Individuals with the McLeod phenotype are highly susceptible to immunisation by Kell blood group antigens.

Familial LCAT Deficiency

The enzyme lecithin:cholesterol acyl transferase (LCAT) controls the level of free cholesterol in plasma lipoproteins and plasma cell membranes by transferring a fatty acid group from phosphatidyl choline to the cholesterol, forming cholesterol ester and lysophosphatidylcholine. Deficiency of this enzyme causes a marked accumulation of free cholesterol and phosphatidyl choline in the red cell membrane, although total membrane lipid content is normal

SAQ 6

Sort the following Rh haplotypes into order of increasing frequency in the UK white population

A   CDE
B   cde
C   CDe
D   cDE

because sphingomyelin and phosphatidyl ethanolamine content is correspondingly low. LCAT deficiency is clinically silent in childhood but in adults is manifest as renal disease, corneal opacities and a mild, incompletely compensated haemolytic state.

Acquired Haemolytic Disorders

The acquired haemolytic disorders can be subclassified into five groups, according to the nature of the defect:

- haemolysis secondary to immune mechanisms

- haemolysis secondary to the action of chemicals, drugs or toxins

- haemolysis secondary to infection

- haemolysis secondary to physical damage

- miscellaneous disorders

Haemolysis Secondary to Immune Mechanisms

Immune haemolysis can be defined as a shortening of red cell lifespan caused by the binding of antibodies to the red cell surface with consequent Complement activation. The antibodies concerned may be synthesised by the host immune system and be directed against host red cell antigens leading to **autoimmune haemolysis** or they may be derived from exogenous sources or be directed against foreign antigens leading to **alloimmune haemolysis**. Therapy with certain drugs can also stimulate immune haemolysis.

Autoimmune Haemolysis

The autoimmune haemolytic anaemias (AIHA) can be divided into three types:

- **warm-reactive antibody AIHA** where the offending autoantibody reacts most strongly above 32°C

- **cold-reactive antibody AIHA** where the offending autoantibody reacts most strongly below 32°C

- **drug-induced AIHA** where immune haemolysis is triggered by the presence of a drug

Warm-reactive Antibody AIHA

Warm-reactive antibody AIHA is a relatively common condition affecting all ages and races. Some reports suggest that women are affected more commonly than men and that the incidence is higher after the age of 45 years. Most cases appear to be associated with viral infections, lymphoproliferative disorders such as infectious mononucleosis or chronic lymphocytic leukaemia, immunodeficiency states or autoimmune disorders such as systemic lupus erythematosus (SLE). The underlying causes of autoimmunity are incompletely understood at present.

The severity of the clinical manifestations in warm-reactive antibody AIHA is highly variable. At one extreme, haemolysis may be so mild that the diagnosis is missed. This is especially likely in conditions such as CLL and SLE where other causes of anaemia may be suspected. At the other extreme, severe acute haemolysis can be immediately life-threatening. When AIHA is associated with an underlying lymphoproliferative or autoimmune condition, the intensity of the haemolysis often mirrors the clinical course of the condition, abating during remission and accelerating during relapse.

Typically, the offending autoantibody in warm-reactive antibody AIHA is a polyclonal IgG immunoglobulin which binds to antigenic determinants common to most red cells. In some cases, specificity against Rh, Wr^b, LW, U, N and En^a blood group antigens has been demonstrated. The most common IgG subtype involved is IgG_1 which is capable of activating Complement via the classical pathway. The presence of IgG antibody and C3b fragments on the red cell surface promotes attachment of the cell to Fc and C3 receptors on the macrophages of the reticuloendothelial system, leading to increased extravascular haemolysis.

Treatment of warm-reactive antibody AIHA involves the use of adrenocorticosteroids such as prednisone to suppress antibody production or immunosuppressive cytotoxic drugs such as

6-mercaptopurine or cyclophosphamide. If this strategy fails, splenectomy to remove the major site of red cell destruction may be required.

Cold-reactive Antibody AIHA

Autoimmune haemolysis caused by antibodies which bind to red cell antigens most strongly at temperatures less than 32°C can be divided into two main types: **cold agglutinin syndrome** and **paroxysmal cold haemoglobinuria (PCH)**.

Cold Agglutinin Syndrome

Cold agglutinin syndrome typically is a disease of old age with a peak incidence over the age of 70 years. It is associated with *Mycoplasma pneumoniae*, Epstein-Barr virus and cytomegalovirus infection, where the offending autoantibody is polyclonal and also with lymphoproliferative disorders such as Waldenström's macroglobulinaemia, CLL, multiple myeloma and lymphoma where monoclonal antibodies are produced.

The temperature of capillary blood in the body extremities can be as low as 25°C, allowing the cold-reactive antibody to agglutinate the red cells and activate Complement, leading to intravascular and, more importantly, extravascular haemolysis and obstruction of capillary blood flow. Capillary obstruction is manifest as a purplish discolouration of the tips of the fingers, ear lobes or the tip of the nose, called **acrocyanosis**. Although these changes are reversible on warming, over a period of time necrotic tissue damage and even gangrene can result.

The earliest clear description of a cold-reactive antibody AIHA was published in 1873 by R Druitt. In this paper, he described two cases of haematinuria, one of which was a fellow doctor who had suffered from acrocyanosis with haematinuria and loss of sensation in the hands and feet for several years. Apparently miraculously, these distressing symptoms disappeared completely when the patient moved to the warmer climate of India.

Typically, the autoantibody is an IgM immunoglobulin with anti-I, anti-i or anti-Pr specificity. The most important determinant of the severity of haemolysis in individuals with cold agglutinin syndrome is the thermal amplitude of the autoantibody. Complement-mediated haemolysis does not occur below about 15°C and accelerates with increasing temperature. Conversely, cold-agglutinins are most active at very low temperatures and their avidity decreases with increasing temperature. Clinically significant cold agglutinins, therefore, are those which have a large thermal amplitude and thus are capable of binding to red cells at higher temperatures when Complement activity is greater.

Ii antigens are not restricted to red cells: T and B lymphocytes, neutrophils, monocytes, macrophages and platelets all carry Ii-like antigens. Cold agglutinins have been shown to induce lymphocytolysis, to impair neutrophil function and to aggregate platelets, causing their removal from the circulation.

The most important measure in the treatment of cold agglutinin syndrome is the avoidance of cold. In contrast to the treatment of warm-reactive antibody AIHA, attempts to suppress autoantibody production with adrenocorticosteroids such as prednisone or immunosuppressive cytotoxic drugs such as the thiopurines or cyclophosphamide have met with limited success. Plasmapheresis may prove useful in the management of acute haemolytic episodes.

Paroxysmal Cold Haemoglobinuria

Classically, PCH is a chronic haemolytic condition which is characterised by intravascular haemolysis following exposure to cold, and is found in association with tertiary or congenital syphilis, and viral illnesses such as measles or mumps. It is caused by a unique haemolytic IgG antibody called the **Donath-Landsteiner antibody** which has anti-P blood group specificity.

Haemolysis in PCH is biphasic, requiring both exposure to cold and subsequent warming. Because the Donath-Landsteiner antibody binds to red cells most strongly at temperatures below 15°C, exposure to cold promotes red cell sensitisation and the early stages of Complement activation. At this low temperature Complement activation is restricted to C1q, C1r and C1s binding. However, following warming, the Complement cascade is completed and rapid intravascular haemolysis ensues.

The classical form of PCH is now a rare condition. However, a variant form which is associated with viral illnesses also exists. This acute form is seen most commonly in young children where it usually is an isolated, self-limiting event which recovers without clinical intervention.

Alloimmune Haemolysis

Alloimmune haemolysis results from the immunisation of the host to transplanted foreign antigen or the action of foreign antibody to normal host antigen. Broadly, there are three circumstances where this can occur:

PCH has been well recognised for over a century. The first description of this condition was published in 1854 and involved a young boy who probably had congenital syphilis. In the years that followed, several reports appeared of an association between inclement weather and haemoglobinuria.

The relationship between cold and haemolysis in affected individuals was clearly demonstrated by Ehrlich 27 years later. His experiment involved the isolation of blood flow in a single finger of an affected individual by tying tightly a cord around its base. The finger was then held in iced water for some time. Serum obtained from the chilled finger was tinged red due to haemolysis whereas serum from a similarly isolated but unchilled finger remained unchanged.

- haemolytic transfusion reactions

- haemolytic disease of the newborn

- allograft versus host reactions

Haemolytic Transfusion Reactions

Transfusion of blood from one individual to another is fraught with dangers. Chief among these is the risk of antibody-mediated haemolysis of donor or recipient red cells, a condition which can be life-threatening. The most severe haemolytic transfusion reactions are seen when ABO-incompatible blood is transfused. For example, if group A blood is transfused into a group O individual the IgM anti-A in the recipient plasma will immediately bind to the donor cells and activate the Complement cascade. The resultant acute intravascular destruction of the donor cells can cause renal failure, hypotension and disseminated intravascular coagulation and may be fatal.

SAQ 7

What genotypes are denoted by R^1R^1 and rr?

Transfusion of red cells which carry an antigen to which the recipient has previously been sensitised also causes an immediate haemolytic transfusion reaction. For example, transfusion of ABO-compatible R^1R^1 blood into a rr recipient with a circulating antibody which has anti-D specificity results in immediate binding of the IgG antibody to the donor red cells. However, the concentration of the antibody on the red cell surface typically is not high enough to activate Complement efficiently so intravascular haemolysis does not occur. Instead, the donor cells are destroyed via Fc receptor-mediated phagocytosis, primarily in the liver and spleen. Phagocytosis of antibody-coated red cells is accelerated by the presence of small amounts of the Complement component C3b.

Less commonly, haemolytic transfusion reactions can be delayed, often for several days following transfusion. In these cases, the recipient usually has previously been sensitised to donor red cell antigen, but the titre of the immune antibody is very low. Transfusion of red cells which carry the offending antigen stimulates a vigorous synthesis of antibody and, after a variable delay of up to several days, haemolysis ensues.

Haemolytic Disease of the Newborn

During pregnancy, the mother supplies nutrients to the developing foetus via the placenta and umbilical cord. Nutrient-rich maternal arterial blood drains into large placental sinuses which are punctuated by a huge number of placental villi. Foetal blood flows from the umbilical arteries into the capillaries of the placental villi and then drains into the umbilical vein which feeds the foetal liver directly. A proportion of the oxygen and nutrients in the maternal blood diffuse across the chorionic epithelium that covers the placental villi and into the foetal circulation. Foetal waste products are transported in the opposite direction and excreted by the mother.

Given this close association between foetal and maternal circulations, it is inevitable that minor bleeds occur, even in normal pregnancy, allowing small amounts of foetal blood to enter the maternal circulation. At delivery, compression of the placenta can result in the injection of much larger amounts of foetal blood into the maternal circulation. If these foetal red cells carry paternal antigens which are foreign to the mother, she may respond by producing antibody directed against the offending antigen. For example, an Rh negative mother (rr) carrying an Rh positive foetus (eg R^1r) is likely to respond to the presence of foetal red cells in her circulation by synthesising an antibody with anti-D specificity. In subsequent pregnancies, further stimulation by foetal R^1r red cells can provoke the synthesis of a high-titre IgG anti-D which can cross the placental barrier and trigger the premature destruction of foetal red cells.

Although Dr P Levine is credited with the first unequivocal demonstration that most cases of erythroblastosis foetalis, or HDN, could be attributed to maternal immunisation against a shared foetopaternal Rh factor, a much less well known figure deserves much of the credit for this discovery. In 1938, three years before Levine's seminal observation, Dr Ruth Darrow published a theoretical account of the pathogenesis of HDN in which she speculated that the most likely cause was maternal immunisation against a hitherto unrecognised foetal antigen. Sadly, her remarkable prescience is all too often forgotten.

In severe cases, acute haemolysis in the foetus results in profound anaemia, hepatosplenomegaly, gross oedema secondary to cardiac failure and portal hypertension. This full-blown manifestation of HDN is known as **hydrops foetalis**, and was a relatively common cause of stillbirth in the first half of this century. In less severe cases, the baby is born alive, and the cord haemoglobin level may be normal. However, haemolysis continues after birth, causing progressive anaemia and hyperbilirubinaemia as a result of haemoglobin catabolism. Unless treated by exchange transfusion, the hyperbilirubinaemia may cause severe neurological damage leading to spasticity, deafness and mental retardation. This condition is known as **bilirubin encephalopathy** or **kernicterus** and is irreversible once established.

Prior to 1970, the most common cause of severe HDN was maternal antibodies with anti-D specificity. The incidence of this form of

HDN has been greatly reduced by the routine injection of IgG anti-D into all Rh negative mothers immediately following delivery. This procedure elicits the rapid destruction of any Rh positive foetal red cells which may be present, thereby minimising the risk of maternal sensitisation.

The most common cause of HDN today is ABO incompatibility of maternal and foetal blood. This form of HDN is almost always associated with group O mothers and group A or B babies. It is caused by the presence of naturally-occurring IgG antibodies with anti-A or anti-B specificity in maternal plasma crossing the placental barrier and eliciting the destruction of foetal red cells which carry the A or B antigen. Typically, ABO-incompatibility produces a mild, self-limiting HDN: kernicterus and hydrops foetalis are rarely observed.

Allograft versus Host Reactions

Occasionally, mild immunohaemolysis has been detected in the recipients of a renal, cardiac or hepatic transplant. The offending antibody in these cases is derived from activated lymphocytes transplanted along with the new organ.

Drug-induced Immune Haemolysis

Treatment with a wide range of drugs can stimulate immune haemolysis by one of three mechanisms:

- **penicillin-type immune haemolysis** in which the drug binds non-specifically to the red cell surface where it acts like a foreign antigen stimulating the production of IgG anti-drug antibodies. These antibodies bind to the surface-bound drug, leading to the selective removal of affected cells by the macrophages of the reticuloendothelial system. This type of immune haemolysis most commonly is associated with high dose intravenous penicillin therapy, although cephalosporins and, rarely, tetracyclines have also been implicated.

- **α-methyldopa-type immune haemolysis**. A minority of patients on long-term treatment with this anti-hypertensive drug produce a warm-reactive autoantibody which, in most cases, has anti-Rh specificity. Less than 1% of treated individuals respond in this way and the time taken for auto-antibody synthesis varies from only a few months to more than 4 years. It is unknown why α-methyldopa therapy elicits autoantibody synthesis but the drug has been shown to inhibit T suppressor cell function *in vitro*. There is a strong association between the HLA antigen B7 and autoantibody production. Other drugs implicated in this form of immune haemolysis include levodopa and mefenamic acid.

- **rifampicin-type immune haemolysis** in which the drug forms a stable complex with plasma protein and induces the synthesis of IgG and IgM anti-drug antibodies. Subsequent reaction between the drug-protein complex and the anti-drug antibody forms a relatively large immune complex which is adsorbed onto the surface of red cells, platelets and neutrophils, resulting in Complement activation and brisk intravascular haemolysis. This form of immune haemolysis has been observed with a wide range of drugs, and is not restricted to high dose treatment. Because the red cells are not directly the subject of the antibody attack, this mechanism is sometimes known as **"innocent bystander" immune haemolysis**. Withdrawal of the offending drug typically results in rapid resolution of the haemolysis.

Haemolysis Secondary to the Action of Chemicals, Drugs or Toxins

Immune-mediated haemolysis is not the only mechanism whereby drug therapy can promote premature destruction of red cells. Free oxygen radicals and peroxides generated by the action or metabolism of a wide range of drugs can inflict severe oxidative damage to haemoglobin and red cell membrane components and lead to the early demise of the cell. For example, the precipitation of denatured haemoglobin within the red cell results in the formation of particulate inclusion bodies called **Heinz bodies** which are bound to the cytoplasmic aspect of the membrane cytoskeleton via disulphide bonds. These inclusion bodies are removed selectively from the cell by phagocytosis, or "pitting" during passage through the spleen, a process which inflicts considerable collateral damage on the cell. Similarly, peroxidation of membrane lipids and cytoskeletal proteins causes a loss of deformability, thereby favouring sequestration of the cell in the spleen.

Alternatively, some drugs are powerful oxidising agents in their own right, and directly inflict oxidative damage to the red cell. The drugs which most commonly are associated with haemolysis are shown in Table 10.2. Haemolysis is favoured when the activity of the red cell glutathione cycle is impaired such as occurs in G-6-PD deficient individuals. This aspect of oxidative haemolysis is described in more detail in the following chapters.

Substance	Comment
Sulphonamides and Sulphones Sulphadiazine Sulphanilamide Sulphapyridine	Antimicrobial drugs less used nowadays because of bacterial resistance and side effects
Antimalarials Chloroquine Primaquine Quinine Maloprim	Used in the treatment and prevention of malaria
Nitrofurans Nitrofurantoin	Antimicrobial used in urinary tract infection
Others Salazopyrin Para-amino salicylic acid Vitamin K derivatives	
Chemicals Potassium chlorate Naphthalene Arsine	Widely used as a weedkiller Used in moth balls AsH_3 encountered in extraction and refining of metal ores.

Table 10.2 *Drugs commonly associated with non-immune haemolysis*

The bite of a number of venomous spiders and snakes has been reported to cause acute intravascular haemolysis. For example, the bite of the brown recluse spider *Loxosceles reclusa* is associated with the development of painful necrotic lesions which heal slowly and, after a variable delay of up to several days, with acute intravascular haemolysis which may be life-threatening. The bite of the king cobra *Ophiophagus hannah*, the Indian cobra *Naja naja* and the Egyptian cobra *Naja haje* have also been reported to cause acute intravascular haemolysis. In all cases, the severity of the haemolysis is related to the venom concentration: symptoms typically are worse in children or following multiple bites. In extreme cases, even multiple honeybee *Apis mellifera* stings have caused acute haemolysis in children.

Haemolysis Secondary to Infection

A wide range of infections are associated with secondary haemolysis, and only a few illustrative examples are given here. By far the most prevalent of these are the parasitic infestations such as malaria, trypanosomiasis, leishmaniasis, toxoplasmosis and babesiosis. The most common parasitic disease which is associated with a haemolytic component is malaria. Malaria in humans is caused by four species of *Plasmodium*: *P vivax*, *P falciparum*, *P malariae* and *P ovale*. The malarial parasites are present in the saliva of infected female *Anopheles* mosquitoes and are injected into the bloodstream of the human host during feeding. Once in the bloodstream, the parasites invade red cells and begin to grow and undergo asexual division. Interestingly, the different species have a preference for particular stages of red cell maturity: *P vivax* and *P ovale* invade only reticulocytes, *P malariae* invades only mature red cells and the malignant form *P falciparum* invades red cells of any age. This partly explains why *P falciparum* parasitaemia often is higher than *P vivax*.

Asexual division of the intracellular parasite produces up to 32 merozoites and prompts lysis of the red cell. The newly released merozoites quickly invade further red cells, thereby propagating the infection. The intravascular haemolysis caused by the rupturing of infected red cells is supplemented by preferential splenic sequestration and pitting of parasitised red cells and also by Complement-mediated haemolysis.

Oroya fever is caused by infection with the flagellated bacillus *Bartonella bacilliformis*. The infection is transmitted by the bite of the *Phlebotomus* sandfly and is found most commonly in Peru and surrounding countries. The acute phase of the disease frequently is accompanied by severe, acute extravascular haemolysis.

Infections with the anaerobic bacterium *Clostridium perfringens*, the causative organism of gas gangrene, are most commonly seen in poorly treated or contaminated wounds but are also seen in association with malignant disease and necrotising enterocolitis. This organism secretes a number of different toxins at least one of which, phospholipase C, is associated with severe, acute intravascular haemolysis which commonly results in death. Several case reports exist which describe affected patients as having no circulating red cells at all!

Haemolysis Secondary to Physical Damage

Haemolysis secondary to physical damage to red cells is characterised by the presence of fragmented red cells, or **schistocytes**, in the peripheral blood. Physical damage may be inflicted by abnormalities within the circulatory system or by external changes such as thermal injury or repeated physical trauma.

The classical cause of haemolysis secondary to physical damage to red cells occurs in a minority of patients who have undergone surgery to replace diseased aortic or mitral valves. In most cases, haemolysis is associated with extreme turbulence due to regurgitation of blood around an improperly fitted or faulty prosthesis. Local shear stresses in such circumstances may be sufficient to tear the red cell apart, resulting in intravascular haemolysis. The presence of non-physiological material in the prosthesis almost certainly is an important contributor to the promotion of red cell fragmentation. Recent improvements in surgical technique and the design of implants have made this form of haemolysis much less common.

Disorders of the microvasculature frequently are associated with intravascular deposition of fibrin, thrombocytopaenia and intravascular haemolysis secondary to physical trauma. This clinical syndrome is termed **microangiopathic haemolytic anaemia** and encompasses a number of important disease states including **haemolytic-uraemic syndrome (HUS), thrombotic thrombocytopaenic purpura (TTP), disseminated intravascular coagulation (DIC)** and **eclampsia of pregnancy**. The haemostatic component of these disorders is described in detail in Chapter 23. All are characterised by the deposition of fibrin within the microvasculature which acts like a cheese-wire, "slicing" passing red cells to form schistocytes.

Prolonged and repeated physical trauma, especially to the hands and feet can cause transient intravascular haemolysis with haemoglobinuria. This condition was first described in 1881 in a soldier following prolonged marching and was termed **march haemoglobinuria**. The haemolysis is thought to result from the crushing action on red cells in surface capillaries caused by repeatedly striking a hard surface. March haemoglobinuria has also been described in long-distance runners, in bongo drum players and in karateka following prolonged training on a makiwara. The full-blown condition is uncommon but subclinical haemolysis may be present in most individuals following prolonged strenuous physical exercise.

Severe and extensive burns frequently are accompanied by intravascular haemolysis induced by thermal injury to the red cells. Subjecting red cells to temperatures above 49°C, even for relatively short periods, causes irreversible denaturation of the cytoskeletal protein spectrin with consequent membrane disruption. In most cases, the haemolysis is acute and self-limiting, resolving within 48 hours of the initial injury. The intravascular haemolysis is augmented by the sequestration of minimally heat-damaged red cells in the spleen.

Miscellaneous Disorders

Paroxysmal Nocturnal Haemoglobinuria

Paroxysmal nocturnal haemoglobinuria (PNH) is an acquired clonal disorder which arises following a somatic mutation in a multipotential stem cell. It is characterised by the presence of red cells which are unusually susceptible to the lytic action of Complement, leading to chronic but episodic intravascular haemolysis. In the classical form of the disorder, intravascular haemolysis occurs mainly during sleep, leading to the passage of haemoglobin in the early morning urine. However, this pattern of haemolysis is noted only in a minority of cases: most patients have no discernible pattern of haemolysis. In addition to intravascular haemolysis, moderately severe panhypoplasia, neutrophil dysfunction, renal insufficiency, dysphagia and a tendency to venous thrombosis frequently are present in PNH.

Broadly, the red cells in cases of PNH can be divided into three groups: PNH I red cells are normal with regard to their sensitivity

The earliest description of PNH was published in 1866 by Gull. In his report, he describes an anaemic patient whose early morning urine contained "haematin". Urine passed later in the day appeared normal. As is so often the case, Gull failed to recognise that this was a hitherto unrecognised condition, blaming instead the cold and damp living conditions that his patient had to endure as the trigger for the haemolysis. A further 16 years passed before the connection between sleep and haemolysis in this condition was noted. The name PNH does not appear to have been used until 1928.

to Complement-mediated lysis; PNH II red cells show a moderately increased sensitivity and PNH III red cells show a markedly increased sensitivity. Most cases of PNH carry a mixture of PNH I and PNH III red cells, although mixtures of PNH II and PNH III red cells and mixtures of all three cell types are not uncommon. The major determinant of the severity of haemolysis is the size of the PNH III red cell population. Where more than 50% of the circulating red cells are PNH III cells haemolysis is severe and relatively constant. Typical episodic or sleep-related haemolysis is seen when between 20 and 50% of the circulating red cells are PNH III cells.

Deficiency of several red cell membrane proteins has been noted in PNH, at least some of which contribute to the pathogenesis of the haemolysis.

- **Acetylcholinesterase** deficiency is a relatively constant finding in PNH red cells and was originally thought to be implicated in the pathogenesis of the condition. However, this is now known to be untrue because artificially-induced inhibition of this enzyme has no apparent effect on red cell life-span either *in vitro* or *in vivo*. PNH II and III red cells typically have a complete absence of acetylcholinesterase.

- **Decay Accelerating Factor (DAF)** is a red cell membrane integral protein which binds to the Complement components C3b and C4b on the membrane surface, thereby inhibiting the construction of the C3 convertases. DAF therefore protects normal red cells from Complement-mediated haemolysis. Deficiency of DAF causes a relatively mild increase in susceptibility to Complement-mediated haemolysis similar to that observed in PNH II cells.

- **Membrane Inhibitor of Reactive Lysis (MIRL)** is a red cell membrane protein which protects normal red cells from Complement-mediated haemolysis by inhibiting the assembly of the Complement membrane attack complex, C5b-9. Experimentally induced inhibition of MIRL in normal red cells produces cells with a sensitivity to Complement-mediated lysis equivalent to that seen in PNH III red cells.

- **Homologous Restriction Factor (HRF)** is a red cell membrane integral protein which, in normal red cells, limits the assembly of the Complement membrane attack complex by binding C8. HRF has been shown to be absent in PNH III cells.

These membrane protein deficiencies are not restricted to red cells in PNH. Similar deficiencies are present in granulocytes, monocytes, platelets and in some lymphocyte subsets but not in T lymphocytes. In addition, PNH neutrophils are deficient in the enzyme alkaline phosphatase. In contrast to normal membrane proteins, which are anchored to the membrane lipid bilayer via hydrophobic amino acid residues, these proteins bind specifically to glycophospholipids containing phosphatidyl inositol. It seems likely, therefore, that the primary defect in PNH involves the mechanisms which mediate this attachment.

The clinical course of PNH is punctuated by episodes of acute intravascular haemolysis with haemoglobinuria, haemorrhage, infection and thrombotic complications. In some cases, haemolysis can be related to events such as infection, vaccination, blood transfusion or the menstrual cycle but in most cases the trigger for haemolysis is unknown. Nocturnal haemolysis was once thought to be associated with the slight drop in plasma pH during sleep, but this is now known to be untrue. The excess of bacterial and fungal infection in PNH is secondary to leucopaenia and neutrophil dysfunction and is a common cause of death. The leading cause of death in PNH, however, is venous thrombosis, particularly repeated and progressive cerebrovascular and hepatic vein thromboses. The pronounced thrombotic tendency in PNH is explained in part by the release of thromboplastin-like material from lysed red cells and in part by the induction of platelet aggregation in response to the binding of C3b to the cell surface.

In a minority of patients with PNH, the abnormal clone regresses spontaneously and a complete or partial remission of the disease occurs. Progression of PNH to ANLL or other haematological malignancy has also been reported.

Pathophysiology of Haemolytic Disorders

The specific pathophysiology of individual haemolytic disorders has already been described. This section describes those features which the various haemolytic disorders have in common. Perhaps surprisingly, given the diversity of the mechanisms of haemolysis, the signs and symptoms produced by the various haemolytic disorders are very similar.

A haemolytic state is defined by the presence of a shortened red cell lifespan and a compensatory increase in the rate of erythropoiesis. These two features are responsible for the characteristic physiological changes which permit the recognition of haemolytic disorders on clinical grounds:

- **anaemia** frequently is absent because of the compensatory increase in the rate of erythropoiesis. Severe, decompensated haemolysis can lead to moderate or severe anaemia, particularly where folate deficiency is also present.

- **acholuric jaundice.** Haemolysis is accompanied by a concomitant increase in the rate of haem catabolism and accumulation of haem breakdown products. The primary breakdown product, **bilirubin**, is a bright yellow pigment. An increased plasma bilirubin is responsible for the characteristic yellow discolouration of jaundice. The form of bilirubin which predominates in haemolytic jaundice is unconjugated and circulates tightly bound to albumin. Because unconjugated bilirubin is not excreted into the urine, an increase in this form of bilirubin leads to jaundice, but no increase in bilirubin excretion in urine ie acholuric jaundice.

- **cholelithiasis.** The most common cause of an inflamed gall bladder, or **cholecystitis**, is the development of gall stones which are composed of a mixture of cholesterol crystals and calcium salts. This form of cholelithiasis is associated with middle age. The increased concentration of bilirubin which accompanies chronic haemolysis can lead to the formation of gall stones which are composed of a mixture of bilirubin crystals and various phosphates and carbonates. These **pigment stones** are associated with much younger people.

- **splenomegaly** is a common feature of haemolysis but typically is slight. Marked splenomegaly may indicate the presence of an underlying condition such as lymphoma as the cause of the haemolysis.

- **haemoglobinuria**. The passage of dark red or even black urine is strongly indicative of intravascular haemolysis.

- **intractable leg ulcers** are relatively common in chronic haemolytic states such as HS and sickle cell disease.

- **aplastic crisis**. Acute arrest of erythropoiesis accompanied by a dramatic fall in circulating red cell count following parvovirus infection is associated with chronic haemolytic disorders such as HS.

- **growth retardation and delayed puberty** are seen in association with severe congenital haemolytic disorders such as homozygous β thalassaemia as described in Chapter 7.

- **hypertrophic skeletal changes** due to expansion of erythropoietic marrow is only seen in severe congenital haemolytic disorders.

Once a haemolytic disorder is suspected on clinical grounds, further enquiry may provide useful indicators of the mechanism or cause of the haemolysis:

- **family history**. If the putative disorder is present in other family members, especially if several generations are involved, a hereditary condition may be suspected. Construction of a pedigree chart can sometimes provide information about the possible mode of inheritance of the putative disorder.

- **ethnic origin**. Some inherited haemolytic disorders are associated with particular ethnic groups. For example, G-6-PD deficiency is most common in Mediterranean and Chinese populations. However, such associations cannot be used to *exclude* any possible cause of haemolysis.

- **patient history**. Neonatal jaundice may be indicative of congenital conditions such as HS or G-6-PD deficiency whereas a late age of onset suggests an acquired condition. Again, this information must be interpreted with caution because diagnosis of a mild congenital disorder may be missed until adulthood.

- **triggering events**. A history of drug ingestion, infection, exposure to cold, surgery or other event which appears to be associated with the onset of haemolysis may provide strong evidence of a cause of an acquired condition.

Clinical findings are seldom sufficient to enable a definitive diagnosis of a particular haemolytic condition to be made; laboratory investigation plays a central role in the accurate diagnosis of haemolysis. The various laboratory features of the different haemolytic disorders can all be grouped under two headings: signs of increased haemolysis and signs of an increased rate of erythropoiesis.

As described earlier, haemolysis is accompanied by an increased rate of haem catabolism and clearance and, typically, a compensatory increase in the rate of erythropoiesis. Recognition of a haemolytic state is dependent, therefore, upon recognition of these changes.

An increased rate of haem catabolism is indicated by an increased concentration of unconjugated bilirubin in the serum, urobilinogen in the urine and stercobilin in the faeces. The iron released from haem is bound by transferrin, leading to an increase in plasma transferrin saturation.

About 7 g or so of haemoglobin is released from effete red cells every day. Almost all of this haemoglobin is recycled; the body possesses a variety of mechanisms designed to prevent the loss of this valuable substance. Pathological increases in the rate of red cell destruction cause easily recognisable disturbances in these mechanisms.

Haemoglobin released from lysed red cells is bound rapidly by a plasma glycoprotein of molecular weight 85,000 known as **haptoglobin (Hp)**. The HbHp complexes thus formed are rapidly cleared by the hepatic parenchymal cells. When the rate of release of haemoglobin increases suddenly, the rate of clearance of Hp from the plasma is similarly increased and the plasma Hp concentration falls. Thus, a decreased plasma concentration of Hp is indicative of an increased rate of haemolysis. However, since Hp is an acute phase protein, the presence of a normal or raised plasma concentration of Hp cannot be taken as evidence that haemolysis is not present.

Depletion of plasma haptoglobin permits the circulation of free haemoglobin in the plasma. This free haemoglobin rapidly dissociates to form αβ dimers which are small enough to be absorbed and degraded by the renal proximal tubular cells, thereby preventing loss of haemoglobin in the urine. This process results in the gradual accumulation of iron within the renal proximal tubular cells. Thus, the presence of exfoliated iron-laden renal proximal tubular cells in the urine is indicative of chronic intravascular haemolysis. Acute intravascular haemolysis may cause the release of sufficient haemoglobin into the plasma to saturate these protective mechanisms resulting in the presence of haemoglobin in the urine.

Oxidation of free plasma haemoglobin results in the formation of methaemoglobin and methaemalbumin which cause a brownish discolouration of the plasma.

An increased rate of erythropoiesis is indicated by marrow erythroid hyperplasia and peripheral blood reticulocytosis which is manifest as the appearance of polychromasia on blood films stained with Romanowsky dyes. In severe cases, nucleated red cells may be present in the peripheral blood. These changes may be absent, however, for example when folate deficiency is also present.

In cases of doubt, the red cell lifespan can be measured directly by labelling the cells with radioactive ^{51}Cr. This technique permits an accurate assessment of the severity of haemolysis and also provides information about the site of haemolysis.

Recognition that a haemolytic state exists requires that further investigations are made to determine the nature and mechanism of the haemolysis. A detailed consideration of this process is beyond the scope of this book, but a summary of a typical schema is shown in Figure 10.1.

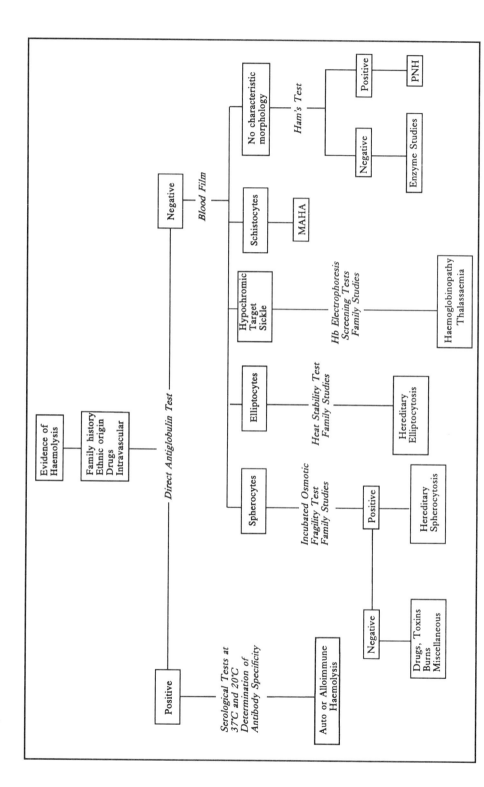

Figure   10.1   *Simplified schema for the investigation of a haemolytic disorder*

Suggested Further Reading

Surgenor, D.M. (ed.) (1974). *The Red Blood Cell* (2nd ed.). New York: Academic Press.

Mollison, P.L., Engelfriet, C.P. et al. (1987). *Blood Transfusion in Clinical Medicine* (8th ed.). Oxford: Blackwell Scientific Publications.

Dacie, J. (1985). *The Haemolytic Anaemias* (3rd ed.). Edinburgh: Churchill Livingstone.

Beutler, E. (1978) *Haemolytic Anaemia in Disorders of Red Cell Metabolism.* New York: Plenum.

Petz, L.D. and Garratty, G. (1980) *Acquired Immune Haemolytic Anaemias.* Edinburgh: Churchill Livingstone.

Williams, W.J., Beutler, E. et al. (eds.) *Hematology*, 4th ed. New York: McGraw-Hill

Answers to Self Assessment Questions

1. The spleen.

2. The total body store of folate is about 10 mg and is sufficient to last for about three months. The total body store of vitamin B12 store is about 3-4 mg and is sufficient to last for about three years. Thus, the excess erythropoietic demands imposed by chronic haemolysis tend to exhaust folate stores relatively quickly.

3. Folate is stored mainly in the liver.

4. A. True.
   B. False, a spectrin has a molecular weight of 240,000
   C. True.
   D. True.

5. Band 3 functions as an anion transport channel and serves to stabilise the membrane by binding to several cytoskeletal proteins.

6. **Genotype**   **Frequency**

   CDE   Rare
   cDe   0.03
   cDE   0.14
   cde   0.39
   CDe   0.41

7. R^1R^1 - CDe/CDe
   rr - cde/cde

Red Cell Metabolism

In the process of maturation, red cells lose their nucleus, mitochondria and ribosomes. Loss of its nucleus and ribosomes renders the mature red cell incapable of protein synthesis. Loss of its mitochondria deprives the red cell of the most efficient means of energy production, oxidative phosphorylation. The cell is thus entirely dependent upon the relatively inefficient mechanism of anaerobic glycolysis via the **Embden Meyerhof pathway** (shown in Figure 11.1) for the fulfilment of its considerable energy requirement. Protection of the red cell against the oxidative stresses imposed by its environment and metabolic processes is provided primarily via the **hexose monophosphate pathway** (also shown in Figure 11.1). Because of the utter dependence of the red cell upon the proper functioning of these two pathways, defects in the enzymes which catalyse them can be catastrophic. Enzyme defects and their effects on the economy of red cells is the subject of the next chapter.

The glucose which is used by the red cell in the two glycolytic pathways is derived from plasma. It enters the cell via a specific transport protein in the red cell membrane. Normally, about 95% of red cell glucose is metabolised via the Embden Meyerhof pathway while the remainder enters the hexose monophosphate pathway. The accumulation within the red cell of the main products of glycolyis, lactate and pyruvate is minimised by excretion via specific transport proteins.

The Embden Meyerhof Pathway

As described above, the primary role of the Embden Meyerhof pathway in the economy of the mature red cell is the generation of ATP. Large quantities of energy are released from ATP during its conversion to ADP. Thus, ATP can be thought of as an energy store for use by the cell. The Embden Meyerhof pathway is also a source of nicotinamide adenine dinucleotide (NADH) which acts as a cofactor for the enzyme methaemoglobin reductase in the conversion of methaemoglobin to functional haemoglobin. The physiologically vital intermediate 2,3-diphosphoglycerate (2,3-DPG) is formed via a diversion from the main pathway known as the **Rap-**

The ability of cells to extract energy from glucose in the form of ATP in the absence of oxygen (anaerobic glycolysis) represents an extremely important survival mechanism. Anaerobic glycolysis can provide a short-term energy reserve for vital organs when oxygen supply is cut off and aerobic glycolysis ceases. For example, at parturition, changes in the foetal blood circulation temporarily starve all of the major organs except the brain of oxygenated blood. During this period, the energy demand of the foetal organs are met via anaerobic glycolysis until normal blood circulation resumes. In other words, if anaerobic glycolysis did not exist, nor could we!

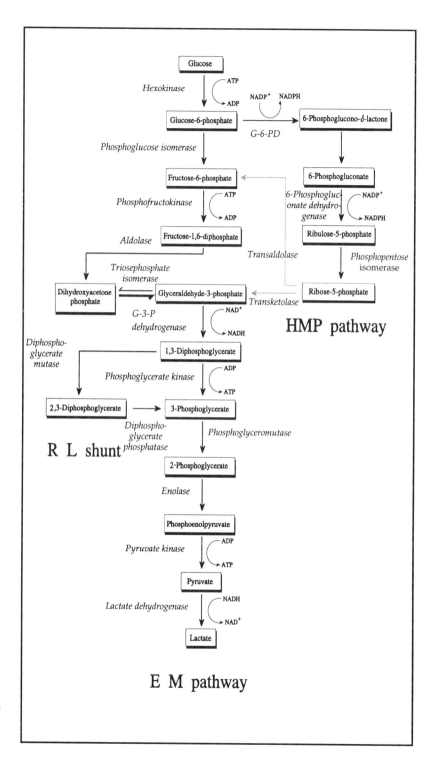

Figure 11.1 *Glycolytic pathways within the mature red cell*

paport Luebering shunt (also shown in Figure 11.1). This molecule functions to increase oxygen delivery to the tissues by altering the oxygen affinity of haemoglobin as described in Chapter 6.

There are three main requirements for energy within normal red cells:

- **maintenance of intracellular cation balance.** The intracellular concentrations of Na^+ and K^+ differ markedly from those of the surrounding plasma. This difference is maintained by the active pumping out of Na^+ from the cell and pumping-in of K^+ from the plasma. The energy required to drive this process is provided via the dephosphorylation of ATP by a membrane-bound ATPase. Failure of the cation pump results in rapid loss of K^+ and water, leading to desiccation and the premature death of the red cell.

- **maintenance of cell shape.** Maintenance of the characteristic biconcave shape and deformability of the red cell is an energy-consuming process. The precise mechanism involved remains obscure although plausible theories abound. Whatever the mechanism, failure results in loss of deformability and shape changes which shorten the lifespan of the affected cell.

- **phosphorylation of glucose and fructose-6-phosphate.** In the early stages of the Embden Meyerhof pathway, the phosphorylation of glucose to glucose-6-phosphate and, later, of fructose-6-phosphate to fructose-1,6-diphosphate are achieved at the expense of ATP. Failure of these steps results in failure of the pathway and a consequent reduction in ATP synthesis. Low levels of ATP lead to failure of these phosphorylation steps, thus establishing a vicious circle which can only culminate in the death of the cell.

> Strictly, phosphorylated intermediates such as fructose-1,6-diphosphate (F-1,6-DP) and 2,3-diphosphoglycerate (2,3-DPG) should be called fructose-1,6-bisphosphate and 2,3-bisphosphoglycerate because the two phosphate groups are located on separate carbon atoms. However, the abbreviations F-1,6-DP and, more especially, 2,3-DPG have been used so extensively that to replace them with the correct forms viz F-1,6-BP and 2,3-BPG would be likely to lead to confusion. I hope that this decision doesn't offend any readers who are biochemical purists!

The Reaction Steps of the Embden Meyerhof Pathway

The first reaction of the Embden Meyerhof pathway involves the **phosphorylation** of glucose to form glucose-6-phosphate (G-6-P).

Enzymes are classified into six major classes, each with several subclasses:

Class 1 Oxidoreductases catalyse redox reactions and include **dehydrogenases, oxidases** and **peroxidases**

Class 2 Transferases catalyse the transfer of functional groups and include **aminotransferases** (amino groups), **kinases** (phosphoryl groups) and **glucosyltransferases** (activated glucosyl residues)

Class 3 Hydrolases catalyse the transfer of functional groups to water and include the **peptidases, esterases** and **deaminases**

Class 4 Lyases catalyse the addition or removal of the elements of water, ammonia or carbon dioxide and include the **decarboxylases** and the **dehydratases**

Class 5 Isomerases catalyse isomerisation reactions and include the **epimerases**, the **racemases** and the **mutases**

Class 6 Ligases catalyse synthetic reactions where two molecules are joined together and include the **synthetases** and **carboxylases**

This reaction consumes a mole of ATP for every mole of glucose phosphorylated and is catalysed by the enzyme hexokinase in the presence of divalent metal ions such as Mg^{2+}. The catalytic action of hexokinase is inhibited by the product of the reaction, G-6-P, thus providing an important control mechanism on the rate of glycolysis. An important effect of this reaction is to "lock" the intermediates of glycolysis within the red cell: the red cell membrane is impermeable to phosphorylated sugars.

G-6-P is subsequently converted to fructose-6-phosphate (F-6-P) in a reaction called an **isomerisation**. This reaction is catalysed by the enzyme phosphoglucose isomerase.

F-6-P is further phosphorylated, again at the expense of ATP, to form fructose-1,6-diphosphate (F-1,6-DP), a reaction catalysed by the enzyme phosphofructokinase. The catalytic function of phosphofructokinase is inhibited by high levels of ATP. Thus, in the presence of adequate levels of ATP, glycolysis is inhibited and, conversely, when the supply of energy falls glycolysis is stimulated. This mechanism provides the most important regulator of the rate of glycolysis. The metabolic strategy in the conversion of G-6-P into F-1,6-DP is to form a six-carbon molecule which is easily cleaved into two phosphorylated three-carbon molecules.

The **cleavage** of F-1,6-DP into dihydroxyacetone phosphate and glyceraldehyde-3-phosphate (G-3-P) is catalysed by the enzyme aldolase. These two products are isomers and are interconvertible under the influence of the enzyme triose phosphate isomerase. Because G-3-P is constantly consumed in the next step of the pathway, the dynamic equilibrium which exists between dihydroxyacetone phosphate and G-3-P is shifted to the right. Thus, in effect, one mole of F-1,6-DP is cleaved to form two moles of G-3-P.

The next reaction involves the conversion of G-3-P to 1,3-diphosphoglycerate (1,3-DPG). This reaction is catalysed by the enzyme glyceraldehyde-3-phosphate dehydrogenase and also results in the formation of NADH.

At this stage of the Embden Meyerhof pathway, no ATP has been generated. On the contrary, two moles of ATP have been sacrificed to reach this stage. However, everything is now in place to commence production of ATP. 1,3-DPG has a high potential to donate one of its phosphoryl groups to ADP thus forming 3-phosphoglycerate (3-PG) and ATP. This reaction is catalysed by the enzyme phosphoglycerate kinase. However, remember that one mole of glucose has been converted into two moles of 1,3-DPG. Thus, for each mole of glucose which enters the Embden Meyerhof pathway, two moles of ATP are generated by this reaction. This balances the energy equation of the pathway: two moles of ATP have been expended and two moles have been generated.

The final stages of the Embden Meyerhof pathway are designed to generate two further moles of ATP in the conversion of 3-PG to lactate. This outcome requires the synthesis of a molecule which, like 1,3-DPG, has a high phosphoryl group transfer potential. The first step towards achieving this goal occurs under the influence of the enzyme phosphoglyceromutase and involves the rearrangement of 3-PG to form 2-phosphoglycerate (2-PG). 2-PG is converted into phosphoenolpyruvate (PEP) in the presence of the enzyme enolase. Enol phosphates such as PEP have the desired high phosphoryl group transfer potential. In the presence of the enzyme pyruvate kinase, PEP donates its phosphoryl group to ADP, resulting in the formation of two moles of ATP and two moles of pyruvate per mole of glucose metabolised. Thus, although two moles of ATP have been consumed by the early reactions of the Embden Meyerhof pathway, four moles of ATP are generated by subsequent reactions resulting in a net gain of two moles of ATP per mole of glucose metabolised. Pyruvate is subsequently converted into lactate under the influence of the enzyme lactate dehydrogenase.

The Rappaport Luebering Shunt

1,3-DPG, in addition to its direct conversion to 3-PG, can be converted in the presence of the enzyme diphosphoglycerate mutase into 2,3-diphosphoglycerate (2,3-DPG). This diversion from the main Embden Meyerhof pathway is called the Rappaport Luebering shunt and is of prime physiological importance because of the role that 2,3-DPG plays in controlling the oxygen affinity of haemoglobin. The unique role of 2,3-DPG in red cells is underlined by its high concentration within these cells. Most other cells of the body contain only traces of the substance.

2,3-DPG can be converted to 3-PG under the influence of the enzyme 2,3-diphosphoglycerate phosphatase, thus completing the shunt. However, the co-product of this reaction is free phosphate rather than ATP.

Gustav Embden was Director of the Physiological Institute at the Municipal Hospital of Frankfurt Sachsenhausen and was greatly interested in muscle metabolism. He and his co-workers performed much of the pioneering work on the glycolytic pathway that was later to bear his name. Unfortunately, he died prematurely of a pulmonary embolism in 1933 at the age of 49. He left behind many unsolved mysteries about the metabolism of glucose by muscle cells.

Although a fellow countryman, Otto Meyerhof was not an associate of Embden. Working at the University of Heidelberg, he was awarded the Nobel prize for his work on anaerobic muscle metabolism in 1922. It was he who recognised that the same glycolytic pathway which operated in muscle cells also operated in red cells. It was not until 1949, however, that the complete EM Pathway was elucidated and published.

The mode of 2,3-DPG formation within red cells was elucidated by Rappaport and Luebering one year later.

The Hexose Monophosphate Pathway

The hexose monophosphate pathway generates reducing potential for the red cell in the form of nicotinamide adenine dinucleotide phosphate (NADPH) which is an essential component of the glutathione cycle as shown in Figure 11.2. Reduced glutathione (GSH) is the most important antioxidant within red cells. Under normal circumstances, hexose monophosphate pathway activity consumes about 5% of the glucose-6-phosphate formed as the first step of glycolysis. However, the rate of activity can be increased by a factor of up to 30 times when required to deal with an increased level of oxidants.

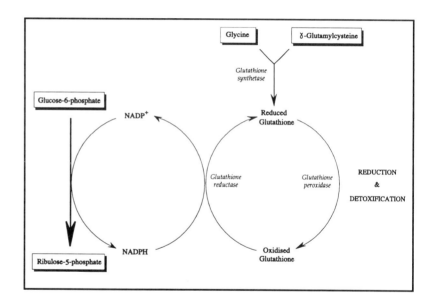

Figure 11.2 *The glutathione cycle*

Reducing power is required by the red cell for three main reasons:

- **combating membrane lipid oxidation.** Oxidation and peroxidation of membrane lipids would cause an increase in membrane rigidity and permeability and so render the red cell liable to destruction in the spleen.

- **reduction of methaemoglobin.** Oxidation of the ferrous (Fe II) iron in haem to the ferric (Fe III) form results in the formation of methaemoglobin which is incapable of oxygen transport. Small quantities of methaemoglobin are constantly formed within the red cell. It is obviously essential that an accumulation of methaemoglobin is prevented by its rapid reduction to functional haemoglobin.

- **detoxification of oxidants**. In the process of methaemoglobin formation, highly reactive oxygen radicals such as superoxide and hydroxyl radical are formed which lead to the generation of the powerful oxidant, hydrogen peroxide. Ingestion of oxidant drugs such as primaquine also results in the formation of hydrogen peroxide. Detoxification of these substances via the glutathione cycle is essential if severe oxidant damage to the cell is to be avoided.

The Reaction Steps of the Hexose Monophosphate Pathway

The first reaction of the hexose monophosphate pathway involves the **dehydrogenation** of G-6-P to form 6-phosphogluconate (6-PG) via an intermediate called 6-phosphoglucono-δ-lactone. The conversion of G-6-P into 6-phosphoglucono-δ-lactone is the rate determining step of the hexose monophosphate pathway and is catalysed by the enzyme glucose-6-phosphate dehydrogenase (G-6-PD). This reaction is accompanied by the generation of NADPH.

6-PG is then **decarboxylated** in the presence of the enzyme 6-phosphogluconate dehydrogenase to form ribulose-5-phosphate (Ru-5-P) and, in the process, another mole of NADPH is formed. Thus, for each mole of glucose which enters the hexose monophosphate pathway, two moles of NADPH are generated. NADPH formation is the physiologically relevant role of this pathway in red cells.

Ru-5-P is subsequently converted into ribose-5-phosphate (R-5-P) under the influence of the enzyme phosphopentose isomerase. R-5-P is used by other cells in the synthesis of nucleotides and nucleic acids. In red cells, however, R-5-P is converted into F-6-P and G-3-P in the presence of the enzymes transaldolase and transketolase respectively. These substances are then metabolised via the Embden Meyerhof pathway.

The conversion of G-6-P to Ri-5-P constantly consumes NADP$^+$ and generates NADPH. The NADPH thus formed acts as a reducing agent in the reduction of oxidised glutathione (GSSG) in the presence of the enzyme glutathione reductase. In this process, $NADP^+$ is formed which is then utilised in the generation of more Ri-5-P. Reduced glutathione (GSH) is required for the detoxification of oxidants as described above. In this process, GSH is cycled back to GSSG.

The Purine Salvage Pathway

Red cells are incapable of *de novo* synthesis of purines because the enzyme 5' phosphoribosyl-1-pyrophosphate (PRPP) amidotransferase is absent. However, an active purine salvage pathway exists which can generate ATP from preformed bases. Adenine can penetrate red cells where, in the presence of PRPP and the enzyme adenine phosphoribosyl transferase, it is converted to adenosine monophosphate (AMP). AMP can then be phosphorylated to form first ADP and then ATP in the presence of the enzyme adenylate kinase.

The existence of the purine salvage pathway in red cells is exploited in the storage of blood for transfusion. The addition of adenine to the storage medium provides a supplementary source of fuel for ATP synthesis and so prolongs the useful life of the stored red cells. However, purine salvage is of doubtful physiological significance.

Suggested Further Reading

Surgenor, D.M. (ed.) (1974). *The Red Blood Cell* (2nd ed.). New York: Academic Press.

Devlin, T.M. (ed.) (1992). *Textbook of Biochemistry with Clinical Correlations* (3rd ed.). New York: Wiley-Liss.

Dacie, J. (1985). *The Haemolytic Anaemias* (3rd ed.). Edinburgh: Churchill Livingstone.

Disorders of Red Cell Metabolism

As described in the previous chapter, the mature red cell has lost its nucleus and mitochondria and so depends almost completely upon glycolysis via the Embden Meyerhof pathway for the fulfilment of its energy requirement and on the hexose monophosphate pathway for its reducing power. Thus, a defect or a deficiency of any of the enzymes which catalyse these pathways can have serious deleterious effects on the overall economy of the cell and may lead to a shortening of red cell lifespan. By common agreement, the definition of an enzyme deficiency relates to suboptimal activity of the enzyme: both quantitative and qualitative enzyme disorders are encompassed by this term.

Disorders of the Embden Meyerhof Pathway

Failure of the Embden Meyerhof pathway is associated with deficiency of ATP within the red cell with a consequent collapse of energy-dependent processes such as cation pump activity. The result, in most cases, is a shortening of red cell lifespan (deficiencies of glyceraldehyde-3-phosphate dehydrogenase, phosphoglycerate mutase and enolase typically are not associated with haemolysis). Defects of the Embden Meyerhof pathway are manifest as a **congenital non-spherocytic haemolytic anaemia (CNSHA)** of highly variable severity. This clinical heterogeneity arises partly because of the great variety of mutations which are encountered but, as explained later in this chapter, is also related to the position of the affected enzyme relative to the Rappaport-Luebering shunt.

Abnormalities of all of the enzymes of the Embden Meyerhof pathway have been described, although most are extremely rare. The most common defect, pyruvate kinase deficiency, accounts for more than 90% of cases of glycolytic enzyme deficiency which are associated with haemolysis.

SAQ 1

What is the product of the Rappaport-Luebering shunt?

Pyruvate Kinase Deficiency

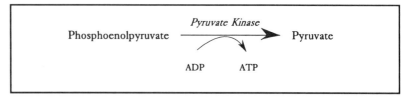

Figure 12.1 *The catalytic action of pyruvate kinase*

Pyruvate kinase (PK) catalyses the conversion of phosphoenol pyruvate (PEP) to pyruvate. Pyruvate kinase exists in several isoenzyme forms in different tissues of the body. In most tissues, PK exists as a homotetramer. For example, in the liver, PK is composed of four identical L subunits; in muscle and brain tissue it is composed of four identical M_1 subunits and in kidney, white cells and platelets four identical M_2 subunits. In red cell precursors, PK is an M_2 homotetramer but, as the cell matures, M_2 subunit synthesis is replaced by L and L′ subunit synthesis. In reticulocytes, the predominant form of PK is an L homotetramer. This form of PK is known as the R_1 isoenzyme. In mature red cells the predominant form of PK is an L_2L_2' heterotetramer. This form of PK is known as the R_2 isoenzyme. L and M subunits are encoded by different genes. Thus, a deficiency of red cell PK is not reflected in white cells and platelets. Each form of PK can exist in two different molecular conformations which are analogous to the T and R forms of tetrameric haemoglobin. Similarly, small amounts of PEP promote binding of more substrate in a manner analogous to haem:haem interaction.

Pyruvate kinase deficiency was first recognised in 1960 by Dr William Valentine and colleagues at the University of California in Los Angeles. Detailed investigation of several families with congenital non-spherocytic haemolytic anaemia pointed to a deficiency of this enzyme as the most likely cause of their condition. Interestingly, the original paper describing this important discovery was submitted for publication (in *Science*); it was rejected as being of limited interest!

Pyruvate kinase deficiency is inherited as an autosomal recessive trait, being expressed only in homozygotes and compound heterozygotes. Many different mutant forms of PK exist: most individuals who express disease are compound heterozygotes for two different variant enzymes. It is this genetic heterogeneity which is the major determinant of the clinical variability of this disorder. Dysfunctional variants of PK may have low overall enzyme activity, low affinity for the substrate phosphoenol pyruvate, may be unduly sensitive to inhibition by ATP or may fail to interact with the allosteric effector molecule fructose-1,6-diphosphate which is normally a strong activator of PK.

Pathophysiology

The clinical severity of pyruvate kinase deficiency is highly variable, ranging from a severe CNSHA to a clinically silent, compensated form. In most cases, there is a moderate reduction in haemoglobin concentration to 6-10 g/dl. The haemoglobin concentration usually is stable but intercurrent infection occasionally may precipitate an aplastic crisis in which bone marrow erythropoietic activity is arrested temporarily. Some degree of jaundice and splenomegaly is almost always present. Neonatal jaundice is relatively common and, occasionally, may be severe enough to require an exchange transfusion. As explained in Chapter 10, prolonged hyperbilirubinaemia can result in the formation of pigment gallstones and the development of cholecystitis at a relatively young age. In common with other chronic haemolytic conditions, there is an increased incidence of folate deficiency in affected individuals.

Although most individuals with PK deficiency are moderately anaemic, clinical symptoms of anaemia may be minimal or absent. This apparent anomaly is explained by the position of PK in the EM pathway. Deficiency of PK causes an accumulation of PEP and other intermediates from higher up the EM pathway. Most importantly, the concentration of red cell 2,3-DPG may treble. As explained in Chapter 6, 2,3-DPG binds to β globin chains thereby stabilising the haemoglobin molecule in the low oxygen affinity configuration. Thus, although the haemoglobin concentration is reduced in PK deficiency, the capacity for oxygen delivery to the tissues is greatly increased and the effects of the anaemia are minimised. There have been a number of reports of PK-deficient individuals with haemoglobin concentrations of 8 g/dl or less who regularly indulge in middle-distance running!

There are no characteristic features of red cell morphology associated with pyruvate kinase deficiency. Moderate reticulocytosis usually is present and irregularly contracted red cells (pyknocytes) may be seen, but these are not diagnostic.

The severity of the anaemia is diminished by splenectomy but, paradoxically, the reticulocyte count rises following this operation. This apparent anomaly can be explained by consideration of normal splenic function and of the conditions which red cells experience as they pass through the spleen. Enzyme-deficient red cells are sequestered by the spleen because their rigid membranes impair their ability to traverse the narrow gaps in the splenic cords of the red pulp. PK-deficient reticulocytes have a residual capacity to generate ATP by oxidative phosphorylation and so have a selective advantage over circulating mature red cells which have lost this

---

SAQ 2

Which 2 reactions provide the major means of control over the rate of glycolysis?

ability. However, the hypoxic conditions experienced during passage through the spleen extinguishes this advantage and reticulocytes are sequestered in the same way as mature cells. Splenectomy restores the selective survival advantage of the reticulocyte and leads to their accumulation in the peripheral blood.

Hexokinase Deficiency

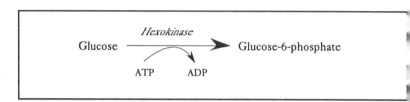

Figure 12.2 *The catalytic action of hexokinase*

Hexokinase catalyses the phosphorylation of glucose to form glucose-6-phosphate (G-6-P) in the presence of divalent metal ions such as Mg^{2+}. The inhibition of hexokinase activity by the product of this reaction provides an important mechanism for the control of the rate of glycolysis. Hexokinase exists as a monomer of molecular weight 100,000. Three isoenzymes have been identified (Hk-1, Hk-2 and Hk-3). It is unknown whether these are encoded by separate genes or represent post-translational modifications of a single gene product. Red cells have been shown to contain Hk-1 and Hk-2 isoenzymes while white cells and platelets contain Hk-1 and Hk-3. Hexokinase deficiency has no clinically significant effect on platelet or white cell function. Hexokinase activity diminishes rapidly with increasing red cell age. This phenomenon leads to a reduction in glycolytic activity and a relative lack of ATP within senescent red cells and is thought to contribute to their demise.

Hexokinase deficiency is extremely rare but most reported cases have shown an autosomal recessive mode of inheritance. Occasional examples of autosomal dominant inheritance have also been reported.

The sequelae of hexokinase deficiency are similar to those for PK deficiency in most respects. However, because hexokinase acts above the Rappaport-Luebering shunt, deficiency leads to an increased haemoglobin oxygen affinity due to lack of 2,3-DPG. This is manifest as severe symptoms of anaemia in the presence of a moderately reduced haemoglobin concentration.

Phosphoglucose Isomerase Deficiency

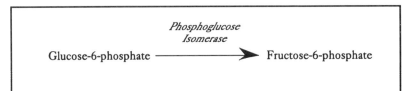

Figure 12.3 *The catalytic action of phosphoglucose isomerase*

Phosphoglucose isomerase (PGI) catalyses the isomerisation reaction which converts glucose-6-phosphate to fructose-6-phosphate. The enzyme exists as a homodimer of molecular weight 120,000. Only one form of PGI exists so deficiency of this enzyme affects a wide range of tissues. However, most tissues other than red cells retain the capacity for continued synthesis of the enzyme and so are only minimally affected. As a result, the clinical sequelae of PGI deficiency mirror those of PK deficiency.

Haemolysis in PGI deficiency does not appear to be the result of a lack of ATP. Instead, recycling of fructose-6-phosphate through the hexose monophosphate pathway is profoundly abnormal, leading to a susceptibility to oxidative damage within the red cell.

SAQ 3

Which 2 reactions in the early stages of the EM pathway consume ATP?

Phosphofructokinase Deficiency

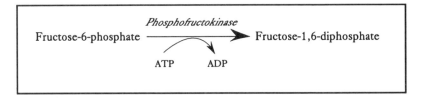

Figure 12.4 *The catalytic action of phosphofructokinase*

Phosphofructokinase (PFK) catalyses the phosphorylation of fructose-6-phosphate to form fructose-1,6-diphosphate. Red cell PFK is a heterotetramer, composed of varying combinations of two non-identical subunits (designated L and M). Muscle PFK is an M4 homotetramer. Most reported cases of PFK deficiency have been the result of deficiency or dysfunction of M subunits, resulting in a severe myopathy. Red cell PFK concentration, as measured *in vitro* frequently is only minimally reduced because, when M subunits are in short supply, L4 homotetramers are formed. However, L4 homotetramers are highly susceptible to the inhibitory action of ATP on PFK, resulting in a relatively severe functional deficiency *in vivo*.

Aldolase Deficiency

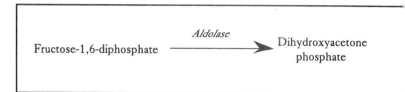

Figure 12.5 *The catalytic action of aldolase*

Aldolase catalyses the cleavage of fructose-1,6-diphosphate to form dihydroxyacetone phosphate and glyceraldehyde-3-phosphate. Only two reports of aldolase deficiency currently exist. The first case to be described was the product of a consanguineous marriage and presented with CNSHA, facial malformations and mental and growth retardation. No defect of aldolase was demonstrated in either parent. The second case involved two members of a Japanese family who exhibited severe aldolase deficiency resulting in a severe CNSHA but were otherwise normal. In this case both parents exhibited intermediate levels of red cell aldolase, suggesting an autosomal recessive mode of inheritance.

SAQ 4

Which 2 reactions in the later stages of the EM pathway produce ATP?

Triose Phosphate Isomerase Deficiency

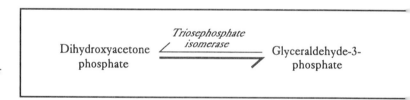

Figure 12.6 *The catalytic action of triose phosphate isomerase*

Triose phosphate isomerase (TPI) catalyses the interconversion of dihydroxyacetone phosphate to glyceraldehyde-3-phosphate. Red cell TPI exists as a homodimer, with each subunit having a molecular weight of 53,000. TPI deficiency is associated with haemolysis, splenomegaly, severe spasticity and premature death. The enzyme is deficient in a range of tissues including white cells, muscle, serum and cerebrospinal fluid. Most reported cases have shown clear evidence of an autosomal recessive mode of inheritance. In contrast to the extreme rarity of TPI deficient homozygotes, the incidence of the asymptomatic heterozygous state has been estimated to be up to 5 cases per 1000 in Caucasians and possibly 10 times higher in American blacks. The most likely explanation for this apparent disparity is that most homozygotes die *in utero*. The biochemical defect induced by TPI deficiency can be partially offset by increased activity of the hexose monophosphate pathway which can generate glyceraldehyde-3-phosphate by alternative means.

Phosphoglycerate Kinase Deficiency

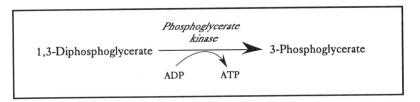

Figure 12.7 *The catalytic action of phosphoglycerate kinase*

Phosphoglycerate kinase (PGK) catalyses the dephosphorylation of 1,3-diphosphoglycerate in the presence of ADP to form 3-phosphoglycerate and ATP. PGK deficiency is associated with congenital haemolytic anaemia and, in some cases, neurological disorders such as motor dysfunction, seizures and even tetraplegia. The disorder is inherited in an X-linked recessive fashion.

Disorders of the Hexose Monophosphate Pathway

Defects of the hexose monophosphate pathway result in an increased susceptibility of the red cell to oxidant stress. All are rare except deficiency of glucose-6-phosphate dehydrogenase (G-6-PD) which is by far the most common red cell enzymopathy, affecting almost 1% of the world's population.

Glucose-6-Phosphate Dehydrogenase Deficiency

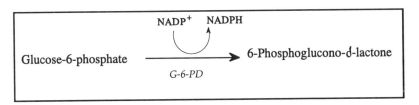

Figure 12.8 *The catalytic action of glucose-6-phosphate dehydrogenase*

G-6-PD catalyses the dehydrogenation of glucose-6-phosphate (G-6-P) to form 6-phosphoglucono-δ-lactone with the simultaneous reduction of nicotinamide adenine dinucleotide phosphate (NADP) to

The widespread use of anti-malarial prophylactic drugs in US soldiers in World War II led to the observation that pamaquine triggered an acute and severe, but self-limited haemolytic anaemia in about one in ten blacks. US military-funded studies of a group of "volunteers" from the Stateville Penitentiary, Illinois showed that this phenomenon was caused by an intracorpuscular red cell defect. However, it was not until 1956 that this form of drug-induced haemolysis was traced to a deficiency of G-6-PD by Dr Paul Carson and colleagues.

The self-limited nature of the haemolysis is explained by the higher concentration of G-6-PD present in juvenile erythrocytes. The marked reticulocyte response which follows the primary haemolytic episode effectively raises the circulating G-6-PD level, and thereby reduces the sensitivity of the circulating red cells to oxidant stress.

form reduced nicotinamide adenine dinucleotide phosphate (NADPH). Red cell G-6-PD exists as a cylindrical homodimer of molecular weight 108, 000. Deficiency of G-6-PD has been reported in most populations of the world but is most commonly seen in Western and Central Africa, the Mediterranean region, the Middle East and SE Asia. For example, in some parts of Saudi Arabia, almost one third of the population carry an abnormal G-6-PD gene. In common with thalassaemia and sickle cell disease, G-6-PD deficiency is associated with malarial areas because female carriers have increased resistance to malarial infection.

The gene which encodes G-6-PD is located on the tip of the q arm of the X chromosome, close to the factor VIII gene. The normal form of G-6-PD is, for historical reasons, designated G-6-PDB or Gd^B and the normal gene is denoted Gd^B. This form of G-6-PD is present in 99% of Caucasians and in about 70% of blacks. A functionally normal variant G-6-PD isoenzyme, Gd^A is found in about 20% of blacks.

G-6-PD deficiency results from the synthesis of structurally abnormal enzyme variants which have impaired stability or catalytic activity. More than 350 different G-6-PD variants have been described but only a relative few are associated with clinically severe disease. The most common variant of G-6-PD is found in about 10% of blacks and is designated Gd^{A-}. All other abnormal G-6-PD variants are designated by their area of greatest incidence eg Gd^{Med} is most prevalent in the Mediterranean region, India and SE Asia while Gd^{Canton} is most prevalent in Chinese populations.

G-6-PD deficiency is inherited in a sex-linked recessive manner ie it is transmitted by symptomless female heterozygotes to affected male **hemizygotes**. Because of the relatively high incidence of aberrant genes in some populations, female homozygotes are not uncommon.

Pathophysiology

As described in the previous chapter, the red cell is protected from oxidative damage by the constant regeneration of reduced glutathione (GSH) via the glutathione cycle. The continuous supply of NADPH required to drive the glutathione cycle is provided by the hexose monophosphate pathway. Thus, red cells which are deficient in G-6-PD develop a secondary deficiency of GSH and are highly susceptible to oxidative damage. This can lead to a reduction in red cell lifespan in three ways:

- cross-linking and aggregation of membrane cytoskeletal proteins causes a decrease in red cell deformability thereby promoting sequestration in the liver and spleen.

- peroxidation of membrane lipids also causes a loss of deformability and, in extreme cases, may result in intravascular haemolysis.

- oxidation of thiol and other groups in globin chains leads to the aggregation and precipitation of denatured globin within the cell, forming **Heinz bodies**. These inclusion bodies bind to the inner aspect of the red cell membrane and are "pitted" from the cell during its passage through the spleen, resulting in the formation of "bite" cells and premature haemolysis.

Despite the large number of G-6-PD variants, individuals with G-6-PD deficiency typically exhibit one of two patterns of haemolysis: chronic non-spherocytic haemolytic anaemia (CNSHA) or episodic haemolysis.

Chronic Non-spherocytic Haemolytic Anaemia

CNSHA is associated with extremely unstable or severely dysfunctional G-6-PD variants. A large number of such variants exist but all are rare; many have only been described in a single family. This form of G-6-PD deficiency presents as a life-long decompensated haemolytic anaemia of variable severity which does not respond to splenectomy. The condition may be complicated by sporadic hyper-haemolytic episodes or aplastic crises which may be triggered by infection or by ingestion of oxidant drugs.

Episodic Haemolysis

The most common G-6-PD variants are not associated with chronic haemolysis. Instead, they are characterised by episodes of acute haemolysis induced by increased oxidant stress. In the vast majority of cases of G-6-PD deficiency, red cell enzyme activity is sufficient to combat the oxidative stresses imposed by every day life and red cell survival is almost normal. However, exposure to increased oxidant stress exposes the inability of the red cell to respond by increasing hexose monophosphate pathway activity and leads to acute intravascular haemolysis. Broadly, three sets of triggers of acute haemolysis in G-6-PD deficient individuals have been identified:

- **ingestion of oxidant drugs** can trigger acute intravascular haemolysis in G-6-PD deficient individuals. A wide range of drugs have been implicated as shown in Table 12.1. Most of the offending drugs are taken up by the red cell where they mediate the transfer of electrons from intracellular reducing agents such as NADPH and GSH to molecular oxygen, thereby forming superoxide, hydrogen peroxide and hydroxyl radicals within the red cell. The inability of G-6-PD deficient red cells to detoxify these powerful oxidants leads to acute intravascular haemolysis.

- **ingestion of the common broad bean**, *Vicia fava*, may trigger acute intravascular haemolysis in individuals with some types of G-6-PD deficiency. This form of haemolysis is known as **favism** and is associated particularly with the Gd^{Med} variant of G-6-PD. The Gd^{A-} variant is not associated with favism. The substance present in broad beans which elicits the haemolysis is thought to be **divicine**. Haemolysis is most common following ingestion of fresh, raw broad beans but has been reported following ingestion of cooked, dried and frozen beans. At least one report exists of haemolysis in a breast-fed infant following maternal ingestion of broad beans.

- **infection** is a relatively common trigger of acute intravascular haemolysis in G-6-PD deficient individuals. Haemolysis is seen most commonly following pneumococcal infection or viral hepatitis. The exact mechanisms which trigger haemolysis remain obscure but release of oxidants from activated neutrophils, ingestion of antimicrobial drugs, hyperthermia and acidosis probably all contribute.

In the absence of acute haemolysis, the blood of a G-6-PD deficient individual appears essentially normal. During a haemolytic crisis, however, moderate anisocytosis, bite cells and occasional spherocytes typically are present. Heinz bodies may be present in acute

---

SAQ 5

Which three amino acids are required for the *de novo* synthesis of glutathione?

Drug Family	Drug Name
Antimalarials	Primaquine
	Pamaquine
Sulphonamides and sulphones	Sulphanilamide
	Sulphapyridine
	Sulphamethoxazole
	Salazopyrin
	Septrin
	Dapsone
	Thiazolesulphone
Nitrofurans	Nitrofurantoin
Miscellaneous	Nalidixic acid
	Phenylhydrazine
	Aspirin

Table 10.1 *Drugs commonly implicated as triggers of acute haemolysis in G-6-PD deficiency*

drug-induced haemolysis or favism but are seldom seen otherwise. Methaemoglobinaemia may be present but seldom is severe.

G-6-PD deficiency is the most common cause of neonatal jaundice worldwide. Normal neonatal red cells typically have suboptimal activity of the glutathione cycle and so, when a deficiency of G-6-PD is superimposed upon this, are highly susceptible to oxidant-induced haemolysis. However, the degree of jaundice observed frequently is more severe than expected, due to the relative inability of the neonatal liver to conjugate bilirubin and, possibly, to a deficiency of hepatic G-6-PD. In some cases, the cause of acute haemolysis in a G-6-PD deficient neonate can be traced to an oxidant drug used by the mother during labour or to the use of sulphonamides to combat neonatal infection. In most cases, however, no trigger can be identified.

6-Phosphogluconate Dehydrogenase Deficiency

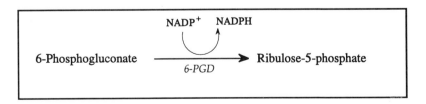

Figure 12.9 *The catalytic action of 6-phosphogluconate dehydrogenase*

6-phosphogluconate dehydrogenase (6-PGD) catalyses the conversion of 6-phosphogluconate to ribulose-5-phosphate with the production of NADPH. Several variants of this enzyme have been reported but none have been associated with haemolysis. True deficiency of 6-PGD is extremely rare. The degree of haemolysis associated with deficiency of 6-PGD is highly variable, but can be severe.

Reduced Glutathione Synthesis

Deficiency of either of the two enzymes which catalyse the *de novo* synthesis of glutathione in red cells is associated with haemolysis due to oxidative damage. Glutamyl-cysteine synthetase deficiency is a rare autosomal recessive trait which, in homozygotes, is associated with moderately severe decompensated haemolysis, progressive neurological damage and amino aciduria. Heterozygotes are clinically normal. Glutathione synthetase deficiency also is inherited as an autosomal recessive trait. When deficiency of this enzyme is restricted to red cells, a relatively mild, fully compensated haemolysis results. Deficiency of glutathione synthetase in all tissues of the body is associated with severe glutathione deficiency, metabolic acidosis, decompensated haemolysis, hyperbilirubinaemia, 5-oxoprolinuria and, in some cases, neurological deficit.

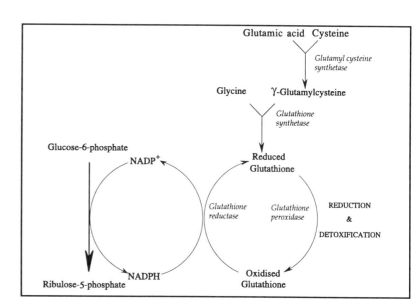

Figure 12.10 *The glutathione cycle*

Glutathione Peroxidase Deficiency

Glutathione peroxidase catalyses the oxidation of glutathione and the simultaneous destruction of peroxides. The concentration of this enzyme within red cells shows remarkable ethnic variation: the diagnosis of a deficiency must be made with extreme caution. True deficiency of glutathione peroxidase is inherited as an autosomal recessive trait and is extremely rare. All authenticated cases have been associated with chronic haemolysis which is exacerbated by ingestion of oxidant drugs.

Glutathione Reductase Deficiency

Glutathione reductase catalyses the reduction of oxidised glutathione with the coincident oxidation of NADPH to NADP. Acquired deficiency of this enzyme is relatively common and is caused by suboptimal synthesis of the cofactor flavin adenine nucleotide (FAD). True deficiency of glutathione reductase is inherited as an autosomal recessive trait and is associated with an increased incidence of cataracts and with episodes of acute haemolysis which are triggered by oxidative stress. The true incidence of hereditary glutathione reductase deficiency is difficult to determine because of confusion with the much more common acquired form.

Pyrimidine 5' Nucleotidase Deficiency

As a reticulocyte matures, residual ribosomal RNA is broken down by the action of ribonuclease enzymes and purine and pyrimidine nucleotides are released into the cytoplasm. The enzyme pyrimidine 5' nucleotidase catalyses the hydrolysis of the pyrimidine nucleotides CMP and UMP to form cytidine and uridine which can diffuse out of the cell. Thus, pyrimidine 5' nucleotidase deficiency is characterised by the accumulation of pyrimidine nucleotides within the cell. Why this accumulation should trigger haemolysis is unclear. Some workers believe that the pyrimidine nucleotides act as competitive inhibitors of glycolysis by competing with adenine nucleotides for enzyme binding sites. Pyrimidine 5' nucleotidase deficiency appears to be inherited as an autosomal recessive trait and is rather less common than pyruvate kinase deficiency, but is more common than the other glycolytic enzymopathies.

Pyrimidine 5' nucleotidase deficiency is accompanied by incompletely compensated haemolysis, jaundice and splenomegaly. The cardinal feature of this condition, however, is basophilic stippling of the red cells which is only otherwise seen in thalassaemia and lead poisoning. Interestingly, lead is a powerful inhibitor of pyrimidine 5' nucleotidase activity.

Suggested Further Reading

Surgenor, D.M. (ed.) (1974). *The Red Blood Cell* (2nd ed.). New York: Academic Press.

Dacie, J. (1985). *The Haemolytic Anaemias* (3rd ed.). Edinburgh: Churchill Livingstone.

Answers to Self Assessment Questions

1. 2,3 DPG

2. The conversion of glucose to glucose-6-phosphate which is catalysed by hexokinase and, more importantly, the phosphorylation of fructose-6-phosphate to form fructose-1,6-diphosphate which is catalysed by phosphofructokinase are both rate-limiting steps.

3. The two phosphorylation reactions described in answer 2 both consume ATP.

4. The formation of 3-phosphoglycerate from 1,3-diphosphoglycerate and the conversion of phosphoenolpyruvate to pyruvate both result in the generation of ATP.

5. Glutathione is synthesised from glutamic acid, cysteine and glycine.

The Immune System: an Overview

The immune system encompasses all of the myriad mechanisms used by the body to afford protection against potentially harmful foreign substances. Knowledge and understanding of the mechanisms of immunity is expanding rapidly. A comprehensive review of the science of immunology is well beyond the scope of this book (and of this author!). Instead, this chapter presents a summary of the most important features of the immune system and its operation. The interested reader is referred to the suggested further reading at the end of this chapter.

Immune mechanisms can be considered under two broad headings:

- those mechanisms which are present from birth. These usually are non-specific mechanisms which operate early in the immune response and are grouped under the heading **innate immunity**.

- those mechanisms which are specific to the foreign agent, and which require prior exposure to that agent for their full expression. These are grouped under the heading **acquired immunity**. The mechanisms of acquired immunity generally operate later in the immune response and act as a supplement to the protection afforded by innate mechanisms.

Innate Immunity

The mechanisms of innate immunity are primarily concerned with the prevention of entry of microorganisms and other potentially noxious substances into the body and with the first line of defence following entry to the tissues.

Protection against the entry of microorganisms into the tissues is afforded by a number of mechanisms:

Ancient Greek concepts of disease centred upon imbalances between the four humours that were thought to constitute the body viz blood, phlegm, black bile and yellow bile. This concept led to the widespread use of phlebotomy and purgation in an attempt to restore the proper balance and effect a cure.

Although now considered naive, these concepts have left their mark on our everyday language. An excess of black bile (produced by the spleen) was associated with depression of mood. The word melancholy (literally black bile) to describe such a state is still in common use. We also talk of enraged people "venting their spleen", obviously to release the excess of black bile stored there. Excessively calm people are today described as phlegmatic. The popular treatment for excessive passion, or "hot-bloodedness" was administration of cucumber seeds which gives rise to the modern cliche "as cool as a cucumber".

- **Physical barriers to infection.** Intact skin and mucous membranes together form an effective physical barrier to the entry of microorganisms into the body.

- **Chemical actions.** Various body secretions exert a wide range of antimicrobial effects ranging from acidic pH to the action of hydrolytic and proteolytic enzymes.

- **Physical actions.** The respiratory and gastro-intestinal tracts are coated with a layer of sticky mucus which traps invading microorganisms. The accumulation of infected mucus is prevented by its constant propulsion towards external openings by ciliated cells. Colonisation of the urethra is minimised by the lavaging action of urination. The gut is similarly protected by defaecation.

Despite all of these antimicrobial activities, the body inevitably is colonised in infancy by a variety of non-pathogenic microorganisms, each occupying their own ecological niche. For example, the gut is colonised by anaerobic genera and the vagina is colonised by lactobacilli. These microorganisms form the **commensal flora** of the body. Their numbers are maintained below pathogenic levels by the various mechanisms outlined above. The commensal flora help to inhibit the establishment of other, potentially pathogenic, microorganisms and so a successful symbiotic relationship with the host exists. The microorganisms of the commensal flora are only non-pathogenic when occupying their specific ecological niche, invasion of other tissues can cause disease.

If all of the above mechanisms fail to prevent the establishment of pathogenic microorganisms in the tissues, the action of the two most important non-specific defence mechanisms is triggered viz the alternative pathway of Complement activation and phagocytosis. The alternative pathway of Complement activation is described later in this chapter, along with the classical pathway.

Phagocytosis

The phagocytic cells of the body form the first line of defence against the establishment of invading microorganisms once the epithelial or mucosal barrier has been breached. There are three important types of phagocytic cell within the body: neutrophils, circulating monocytes and fixed tissue macrophages. The most important of these in the context of first line defence against microbial invasion are the neutrophils. Circulating monocytes are relatively long-lived cells which play an important role in the removal of certain types of microorganism from the tissues and also in the processing and presentation of antigen to T lymphocytes. The fixed tissue macrophages are derived from blood monocytes and are an important component of the reticuloendothelial system which is responsible for the clearance of foreign particulate matter from the body and for the selective destruction of senescent or abnormal blood cells.

Neutrophil Function

Under normal conditions, peripheral blood neutrophils belong to one of two pools which are approximately equal in size. Those neutrophils which circulate freely in the bloodstream constitute the **circulating pool**. The remaining neutrophils slowly trundle along in loose association with the vascular endothelium, and constitute the **marginated pool**. There is no functional or morphological difference between the neutrophils in the circulating and marginated pools, and individual cells are free to cross from one pool to the other.

The presence of microorganisms in tissue causes the release of a variety of substances which are stimulatory to neutrophils. Some of these substances are released directly by the microorganisms eg bacterial lipopolysaccharide while others result from the activation of immune mechanisms at the site of infection. Examples of the latter group include Complement components such as C5a and soluble mediators released by lymphocytes and tissue macrophages such as interleukin 1 (IL-1) and tumour necrosis factor (TNF). These substances diffuse outwards, creating a concentration gradient which is centred on the site of infection. The diffusing substances quickly reach and enter neighbouring capillaries where they cause the immobilisation of the marginated neutrophils in that area. This effect is caused by the simultaneous expression of adhesion molecules such as Mo1 (CD11b) and LFA-1 (CD11a) by the stimulated neutrophils and of receptors for these molecules by adjacent vascular endothelial cells (eg ICAM-1). Further, stimulation of the vascular endothelial cells causes relaxation of their intercellular

Ilya Metchnikov, a professor of zoology at Messina, had been interested in the activities of itinerant amoeboid cells of marine sponges for some years. He had defined their role in the digestive processes of the creature and had christened the cells "phagocytes" (from the Greek *phagein*, to eat). However, the thought had begun to form in his mind that these cells might also play a role in defence against injury or microbial invasion. He tested this idea by inserting a number of rose thorns beneath the skins of larval starfish, surmising that this insult would spur the phagocytes to attempt to remove the thorn. The next day showed that the predicted accumulation of phagocytes around the thorns had indeed taken place. Metchnikov felt that this was compelling evidence for the defensive role of phagocytes. This new concept was not universally accepted. The popular theory of the day was that bacteria actively sought to invade leucocytes because they provided a safe haven from the defence mechanisms of the body!

junctions which facilitates the egress of the adherent neutrophils, a process known as **diapedesis**.

The various substances which are elaborated at sites of infection and inflammation which stimulate neutrophil motility are known collectively as **chemotactic factors**. The most important of these is the Complement fragment C5a, but a wide range of metabolic products of bacteria and leucocytes are also stimulatory. Occupation of neutrophil surface receptors by chemotactic factors serves to orient movement towards the source of the stimulant. In this way, neutrophils are guided by the concentration gradient of the chemotactic factor towards the site of infection, a process called **chemotaxis**. In the absence of a concentration gradient neutrophil locomotion is accelerated but random, a condition called **chemokinesis**.

Movement of neutrophils is mediated by the assembly and disassembly of submembranous actin filaments, which is directed by the actions of a trio of actin-modulating proteins, acumentin, gelsolin and profilin. Briefly, occupation of neutrophil surface receptors by chemotactic factors induces a localised efflux of calcium ions which favours the assembly of actin into long double helices, with the consequent projection of a lamellipod in the direction of movement. The lamellipod adheres to the surface along which the neutrophil is crawling. Adhesion of the lamellipod is followed by contraction of the remainder of the cell towards the leading edge, a phenomenon mediated by the interaction of myosin with the actin duplex. Thus, the neutrophil edges forwards by a process akin to the movement of a caterpillar.

Neutrophils are incapable of recognising individual microorganisms as targets for ingestion. Instead, they rely on prior treatment of the surfaces of the invading microorganism by IgG antibody or fragments of the Complement component C3, a process called **opsonisation**. Neutrophils possess specific surface receptors for C3 fragments (Mo1) and for the F_c portion of IgG. Opsonisation provides a mechanism for the non-specific recognition by neutrophils of the huge variety of microorganisms. Encapsulated microorganisms are only poorly opsonised and so are less susceptible to phagocytosis. This is an important factor in the pathogenicity of such microorganisms.

Binding of an opsonised microorganism to neutrophil surface receptors simultaneously triggers a number of important biochemical pathways which culminate in the ingestion and destruction of the microorganism. As described above, receptor occupation stimulates localised polymerisation of actin, thereby providing the propulsive force required for ingestion of the microorganism. As shown in Figure 13.1, internalisation of the receptor-bound microorganism is achieved by the extension of pseudopods on either side of the microorganism, which fuse at the distal pole of the microorganism, thereby enclosing it in a **phagocytic vesicle**. This process is known as **phagocytosis** or "cell-eating". An analogous process is used to internalise soluble molecules or particles of less than 1 µm in diameter, but is then known as **pinocytosis** or "cell-drinking".

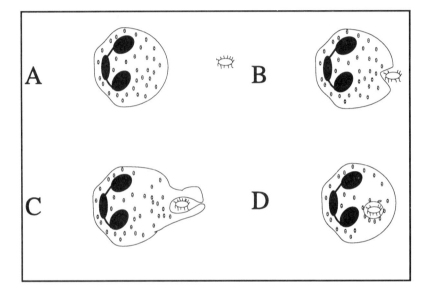

Figure 13.1 *The mechanism of neutrophil phagocytosis*
A neutrophil crawls toward opsonised bacterium
B attachment of bacterium to neutrophil surface receptor and invagination of neutrophil membrane
C extension of pseudopods which fuse at distal pole of bacterium
D emptying of granular contents into phagocytic vesicle

Immediately following ingestion, the secondary granules of the neutrophil fuse with the membrane of the phagocytic vesicle and discharge their contents into it, a process known as **degranulation**. This is followed by the fusion and discharge of primary granules. Neutrophil granules contain a bewildering array of antimicrobial substances which, together, constitute the oxygen-independent microbicidal mechanisms. Some of the contents of neutrophil granules are listed in Table 13.1.

One of the most striking changes in neutrophil behaviour following binding of an opsonised microorganism to its surface receptors is a marked increase in oxygen uptake, a phenomenon known as the **respiratory burst**. The biochemical basis for the respiratory burst is

Primary Granules	Secondary Granules
elastase	lysozyme
cathepsins B, D & G	collagenase
myeloperoxidase	lactoferrin
lysozyme	transcobalamin I
N-acetylglucuronidase	histaminase
β glucuronidase	Complement activator
β glycerophosphatase	fMLP receptors
α mannosidase	plasminogen activator
defensins	cytochrome b$_{-245}$
antibacterial cationic proteins	C3b receptors
kinin-generating enzyme	protein kinase C inhibitor
C5a inactivating factor	monocyte chemotactic
phospholipase A$_2$	factor

Table 13.1 *The constituents of neutrophil primary (azurophilic) and secondary (specific) granules*

the single electron reduction of oxygen to form the highly reactive species superoxide (O_2^-).

$$2O_2 + NADPH \longrightarrow 2O_2^- + NADP^+ + H^+ \quad (1)$$

Superoxide is extremely unstable and so rapidly undergoes dismutation to form hydrogen peroxide (H_2O_2).

$$2O_2^- + 2H^+ \longrightarrow H_2O_2 + O_2 \quad (2)$$

Hydrogen peroxide is detoxified via the glutathione cycle as described in Chapter 11. The greatly increased availability of $NADP^+$ derived from reaction 1 and stimulation of the glutathione cycle results in greatly increased hexose monophosphate shunt activity. In turn, increased HMP shunt activity increases the production of NADPH which is required in reaction 1.

The reactive species which are actually responsible for killing ingested organisms are generated from superoxide and hydrogen peroxide by a complex series of secondary reactions.

$$O_2 + H_2O_2 \longrightarrow OH^\bullet + OH^- + O_2 \quad (3)$$

Hydroxyl radical ($OH^\bullet$) is known to attack DNA, inducing similar damage to ionising radiation such as strand breaks and oxidation of bases.

$$Cl^- + H_2O_2 \longrightarrow HOCl + H_2O \qquad (4)$$

Hypochlorous acid (HOCl) exerts a number of toxic effects on actively metabolising cells such as destruction of the biologic activity of nucleotides such as ATP.

$$RNH_2 + HOCl \longrightarrow RNHCl + H_2O \qquad (5)$$

Chloramines (RNHCl) formed from polar amines such as taurine are long-lived and biologically harmless. In contrast, those formed from non-polar amines such as spermidine are soluble in cell membranes and extremely toxic.

The antimicrobial products of the respiratory burst together constitute the oxygen-dependent microbicidal mechanisms of the neutrophil.

Signal Transduction Pathways in Neutrophils

As described above, occupation of surface receptors provides the stimulus for a range of neutrophil activities. The process whereby receptor occupation is translated within the neutrophil into cell movement is an example of **signal transduction** or **stimulus response coupling**. Binding of an agonist such as a chemotactic factor to its surface receptor induces an allosteric change in the receptor which results in the association of a cytoplasmic GTP-binding protein and the enzyme phospholipase C with the receptor (Figure 13.2).

SAQ 1

Which of the following neutrophil products are effective under anaerobic conditions?

A. Myeloperoxidase
B. Hydroxyl radical
C. Lactoferrin
D. Lysozyme
E. Hydrogen peroxide

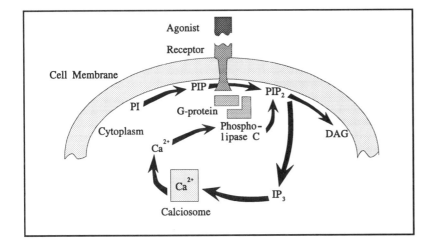

Figure 13.2 *Phosphoinositide turnover in neutrophils.*
PI - phosphatidylinositol
PIP - phosphatidylinositol phospate
PIP$_2$ - phosphatidylinositol diphosphate
IP$_3$-inositol triphosphate
DAG - diacylglycerol

Normally, phospholipase C requires the presence of a higher concentration of calcium ions than is present in the cytoplasm of unstimulated neutrophils. However, association with the G-protein and the surface receptor promotes the activity of phospholipase C at cytoplasmic calcium ion concentrations. The action of phospholipase C on membrane phosphatidylinositol diphosphate (PIP_2) liberates inositol triphosphate (IP_3) which diffuses into the cytoplasm, leaving diacylglycerol (DAG) at the plasma membrane. IP_3 stimulates the release of calcium ions from calciosomes, thereby stimulating actin assembly and cell movement as described above and further promoting the activity of phospholipase C. The diacylglycerol is attacked by an enzyme called phospholipase A_2, producing arachidonic acid which is converted to a series of compounds called **leucotrienes** which are important mediators of inflammation (Figure 13.3).

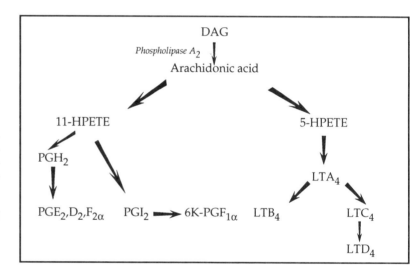

Figure 13.3 *Arachidonic acid metabolism in neutrophils results in the formation of both prostaglandins and leucotrienes. Normally, leucotriene formation dominates.*
DAG - diacylglycerol
11-HPETE - 11 hydroxypentaeonic acid
5-HPETE - 5 hydroxypentaeonic acid
PGH$_2$- prostaglandin H$_2$ etc
LTA$_4$- leucotriene A$_4$ etc

Acquired Immunity

In vertebrates, the protection afforded by the relatively crude mechanisms of innate immunity is augmented by a battery of activities which are specifically targeted against the invading microorganism. These mechanisms are mediated by the activities of lymphocytes and include the synthesis of specific antibody, the promotion of cytolysis by Complement and cell-mediated cytotoxicity. These diverse activities are grouped under the heading of acquired or

adaptive immunity. There are four cardinal features which distinguish acquired from innate immune mechanisms:

- **Prior exposure**. The mechanisms of acquired
immunity require prior exposure to the inducing
substance or **immunogen** for their full expression.
The primary contact with the immunogen is known
as **immunisation**.

- **Specificity**. In contrast to innate mechanisms, the
mechanisms of acquired immunity are always
highly specific to the immunogen.

- **Memory**. The primary response to immunisation
typically is short-lived but part of the process
involves the generation of specific memory
lymphocytes which are primed to react with the
immunogen. Secondary exposure to the immunogen elicits a rapid and more substantial response.
The ability to mount an anamnestic response forms
the rationale for the practice of vaccination.

- **Discrimination between "self" and "non-self"**.
Perhaps the most important feature of acquired
immunity is the ability to distinguish accurately
between host and foreign molecules and to mount
an assault upon the latter.

For the purposes of clarity, it is convenient to consider the mechanisms of immunity as either humoral or cell-mediated mechanisms.
This should not be taken to imply that the mechanisms operate in
isolation from one another. On the contrary, each activity forms a
tiny part of a highly integrated response to tissue damage which
includes the coagulation, fibrinolytic and kinin systems in addition
to those described in this chapter.

Humoral Mechanisms of Immunity

Humoral immunity is mediated by soluble **antibodies** which are
synthesised and secreted by plasma cells in response to foreign
antigen. The antibodies produced bind specifically to the inducing
antigen and mediate a range of biological effects which culminate
in the removal of the antigen.

In 1957, Glick and his colleagues were trying to define the function of the Bursa of Fabricius in chickens. The Bursa was known to be at its largest relative to body weight soon after hatching and to atrophy rapidly thereafter. This implied that its function was only vital early in development so it was decided to investigate the effect of Bursectomy in the first week of life.

Frustratingly, the Bursectomised birds demonstrated no readily discernible defect: the experiment was considered to have been fruitless. The matter might well have ended there but for a chronic shortage of resources for teaching purposes (some things never change!). The adult birds were recruited for a student practical exercise designed to demonstrate the synthesis of antibody in response to Salmonella infection. When the Bursectomised birds were the only ones to fail to synthesis antibody, Glick surmised that an intact Bursa is a prerequisite for the capacity to synthesise antibody later in life. This apparently arcane observation can be seen in retrospect to have been one of the most important made in the definition of the B lymphocyte as the mediator of humoral immunity.

This simplistic summary begs an extremely important question: how is specificity of response effected? The answer to this question forms the bedrock upon which much of modern immunology rests - **clonal selection**. The theory of clonal selection states that contact with foreign antigen does not elicit *de novo* synthesis of antibody; rather, it stimulates expansion of a pre-existing clone of cells which synthesise antibody which has the requisite specificity. This theory fits with all existing data about the ontogeny and behaviour of B lymphocytes and is now universally accepted. Although the theory was originally proposed to explain the specificity of B lymphocyte action, it is now realised that specificity of T lymphocyte action is achieved by similar means.

As described, the theory of clonal selection requires that:

- B lymphocytes are produced which exhibit an astonishing diversity of surface membrane receptors which are capable of binding to the vast range of foreign antigens which may be encountered.

- individual B lymphocytes carry surface receptors of a single specificity.

- occupation of the surface receptor by antigen stimulates proliferation and differentiation of the B lymphocyte to form a clone of plasma cells which synthesise and secrete specific antibody and a clone of immunologically primed memory cells.

- there must be some means of preventing the development of lymphocytes which carry surface receptors which recognise host antigens.

Generation of Diversity

The surface receptors on B lymphocytes which recognise and bind to foreign antigen are actually membrane-bound antibodies. Before the complex mechanisms involved in the generation of antibody diversity can be appreciated, it is essential to understand the basic structure of antibodies.

Antibody Structure

Antibodies belong to a family of plasma proteins called the **immunoglobulins**. The different members of the immunoglobulin family share a similar monomeric structure. As shown in Figure 13.4, the main structure of the immunoglobulin molecule is formed by two identical polypeptide chains which are about 430 amino acids in length and are designated the "heavy" or H chains. The pair of H chains are linked by a disulphide bridge. The remainder of the structure is formed by a pair of identical "light" or L chains which are about 220 amino acids long: one L chain is bound to each H chain by a disulphide bridge.

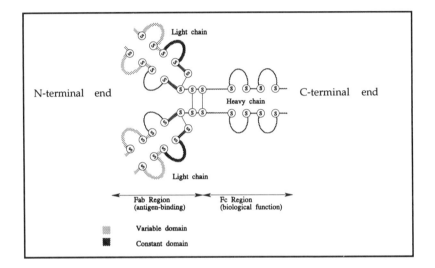

Figure 13.4 *The monomeric structure of immunoglobulin*

There are two different types of L chain, which are designated κ and λ. Each immunoglobulin molecule will include either κ chains or λ chains, never both. There are five different types of H chain, which are designated α, δ, ε, γ and μ. The "class" to which an immunoglobulin molecule belongs is determined by the H chains which it contains. The five different classes of immunoglobulin are designated IgA, IgD, IgE, IgG and IgM respectively. Each class of immunoglobulin is characterised by different biological, biochemical and physical properties which determine its function (Table 13.2).

The antigen-binding sites are located at the N-terminal ends of the H and L chains and it is here that the diversity between immunoglobulin molecules is concentrated. The hypervariable regions of the H and L chains are designated V_H and V_L respectively. Similarly, the constant regions of the H and L chains are designated C_H and C_L respectively.

	IgG	IgM	IgA	IgD	IgE
Molecular weight (x10³)	150	900	160	180	200
Subclasses	4	2	2	1	1
Serum concentration (mg/ml)	12	1	2	0.04	0.00002
Half-life (days)	23	5	6	3	2
Placental passage	Yes	No	No	No	No
Complement activation	+	+++	No	No	No
Fc receptor binding	++	No	No	No	No
Rate of synthesis (mg/kg body weight/day)	28	6	9	0.4	2.5

Table 13.2 *Properties of the immuno-globulins*

Molecular Basis of Antibody Diversity

The total genome in humans is thought to include about 10^5 genes. It has been estimated that a normal healthy individual synthesises somewhere between 10^6 and 10^8 different antibody molecules! It is immediately apparent that each antibody molecule cannot be coded for by an individual gene: some alternative mechanism for the generation of this huge diversity must exist. The breakthrough in our understanding of antibody diversity was made by Tonegawa in the early 1980s when he demonstrated that immunoglobulin genes can rearrange themselves during lymphocyte differentiation.

Arrangement and Rearrangement of L Chain Genes

As described above, L chains consist of two major domains, the constant region (C) and the variable region (V). The constant regions of κ and λ chains are coded for by single genes on chromosomes 2 and 22 in man. However, synthesis of the variable regions is considerably more complex. The variable regions are coded for by two distinct gene segments: a V_L segment which codes for the N-terminal 95 amino acid residue segment of the variable region and a J_L joining segment which codes for the remaining 13 amino acid residues of the variable region. DNA sequencing has shown that between 100 and 200 V_κ and 5 J_κ genes exist. The genetic diversity of λ chains is somewhat less with about 40 V_λ and 6 J_λ genes being present. The synthesis of a κ light chain is shown schematically in Figure 13.5. The initial step involves the random selection of

SAQ 2

Which class of immunoglobulin is likely to be implicated in a case of haemolytic disease of the newborn due to ABO incompatibility?

a single V_κ gene and a single J_κ. These are then brought into apposition with the C_κ gene by the rearrangement of the germline DNA within the developing B lymphocyte. The rearranged genes are then transcribed into mRNA in the normal manner. This process of rearrangement means that up to 1,000 different κ chains can be transcribed from only 206 genes, and that up to 240 λ chains can be transcribed from only 47 genes.

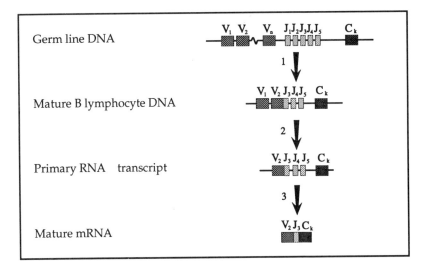

Figure 13.5 *Gene rearrangement in the synthesis of an immunoglobulin light (kappa) chain. V=variable segment gene, J=joining segment gene, C=constant segment gene.*
1. DNA rearrangement
2. Transcription
3. Splicing

Arrangement and Rearrangement of H Chain Genes

Heavy chain genes are located on chromosome 14 in man. Although the basic principles for assembly and rearrangement of heavy chains are similar to those for light chains, there are two important differences:

- the variable region of heavy chains is constructed from three, not two, gene segments. These are designated V, D and J gene segments. There are about 200 V genes, 12 D genes and 6 J genes in man as shown in Figure 13.6.

- the constant region of heavy chains is coded by 9 different genes as shown in Figure 13.6. Which of these C genes is used determines the immunoglobulin class. For example, if the μ gene is used the resulting immunoglobulin will be an IgM.

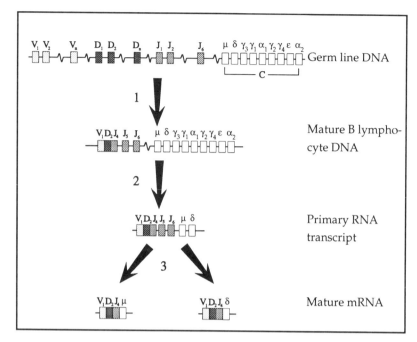

Figure 13.6 *Gene rearrangement in the synthesis of an immunoglobulin heavy chain. V=variable segment gene, D=diversity segment gene, J=joining segment gene, C=constant segment gene.*
1. DNA rearrangement
2. Transcription
3. Splicing

There are two germ line DNA rearrangements required in the synthesis of a heavy chain. The first rearrangement results in the selection of one D and one J gene and places them together. The second rearrangement results in the addition of a V gene to the DJ segment, thereby determining the antigenic specificity of the heavy chain. The resultant VDJ segment is transcribed along with the two C genes which are in close proximity viz the μ and δ genes. The resultant primary transcript can be spliced to form two different products as shown in Figure 13.6. Thus, an unstimulated B lymphocyte may express both IgM and IgD immunoglobulins with identical antigenic specificity.

Although the antigenic specificity of the immunoglobulin that a given B lymphocyte can synthesise is irrevocably determined by the particular V, D and J segments which are brought into apposition, the *class* of immunoglobulin can be changed, a phenomenon known as **isotype switching**. At the 5′ end of each C gene except the δ gene there is a region of repeating base sequences called a switch or S region as shown in Figure 13.7. B lymphocytes are capable of rearranging their DNA by aligning the VDJ segment with the S region of any of the downstream C genes as shown in Figure 13.7. In this process, the intervening C region DNA is deleted and so the cell

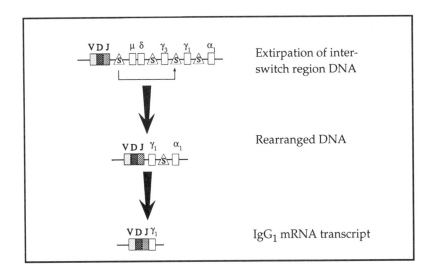

Extirpation of inter-switch region DNA

Rearranged DNA

IgG$_1$ mRNA transcript

Figure 13.7 *The mechanism of immunoglobulin isotype switching in B lymphocytes*

loses the ability to synthesise immunoglobulin of those classes. For example, after the rearrangement shown in Figure 13.7, the cell can never synthesise IgM or IgD immunoglobulin but could undergo further isotype switching to synthesise any of the downstream classes of immunoglobulin.

Complement

The synthesis and attachment of specific antibody to invading microorganisms does not directly lead to their destruction. Rather, it acts as a "label" which identifies them as targets for destruction. For example, microorganisms which are coated with specific IgG antibody are more susceptible to phagocytosis by neutrophils and macrophages. Another important effector mechanism which is activated by antigen:antibody complexes is the Complement system. Complement consists of a series of plasma proteins which, when activated, lead to lysis of target cells.

The Classical Pathway of Complement Activation

The classical pathway of Complement activation (Figure 13.8) involves the sequential activation of nine plasma proteins, designated C1-C9 and requires the presence of antigen:antibody complexes for its initiation. The cascade of Complement activation is analogous to the coagulation cascade described in Chapter 21. The nine proteins involved in the classical pathway of Complement activation can be grouped into three functional units:

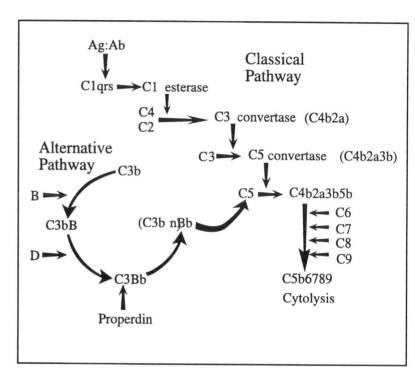

Figure 13.8 *The classical and alternative pathways of Complement activation*

- **the recognition unit**, which consists of C1q, C1r and C1s

- **the activation unit**, which consists of C4, C2 and C3

- **the membrane attack unit**, which consists of C5-C9

The recognition unit is the C1 macromolecule which consists of three subunits C1q, C1r and C1s held together by calcium ions. The C1q part of the molecule binds to the Fc region of IgG and IgM antibodies that are bound to cellular antigens. Binding of C1q to antibody induces a conformational change in the molecule causing activation of the C1r sub-unit which then activates the C1s subunit by cleaving a peptide from it. The resultant complex, which remains bound to the target cell surface, is called **C1 esterase**.

C1 esterase cleaves a small peptide from C4, thereby causing its activation. The small fragment is designated C4a, while the larger remaining fragment is designated C4b. By convention, minor cleavage products of Complement proteins are designated as "a" fragments (eg C5a) while the major fragments are designated as "b" fragments (eg C5b). The exception to this rule is C2, where the major fragment is designated C2a. C4b binds to the target cell membrane in close proximity to the C1 esterase, and cleaves C2. C2a fuses with C4b, which is then dislodged from the C1 esterase complex and binds directly to the target cell membrane. The C4bC2a complex is called **C3 convertase**. In this way, the C1 esterase complex is free to activate many molecules of C4. C3 convertase acts on C3, splitting it into fragments C3a and C3b. The C3b combines with the C3 convertase complex, forming **C5 convertase**, which is responsible for the initiation of the membrane attack complex.

In a similar manner to the above, C5 convertase cleaves C5 into fragments C5a and C5b, and C5b attaches to the target cell membrane alongside the C5 convertase complex. C6 and C7 are not cleaved but bind to the C5b, forming a new complex C5bC6C7 which then directs the insertion of C8 and C9 into the target cell membrane, thereby forming hydrophilic transmembrane channels through which water, potassium ions and sodium ions can pass. This disturbs the osmotic balance of the cell and leads to cytolysis.

The minor fragments of Complement are not directly involved in cytolysis, but do have an important role to play in immune function. For example, C3a and C5a act as anaphylotoxins, causing the release of histamine from tissue mast cells and localised oedema at the site of infection. C5a is the most potent chemotactic factor for neutrophils known, while C3b is an important opsonin for neutrophils. This demonstrates that the separation of immune function into innate and acquired mechanisms is artificial. In practice, both innate and acquired mechanisms cooperate extensively in the destruction of invading microorganisms.

The Alternative Pathway of Complement Activation

The alternative pathway of Complement activation (Figure 13.8) developed earlier in evolution than the classical pathway and is independent of specific antibody for its initiation. The alternative pathway can also be considered in terms of recognition, activation and membrane attack units.

The Complement fragment C3b exists in trace amounts in normal plasma, and functions as the recognition unit for the alternative pathway. C3b can be activated via the alternative pathway by a variety of substances present at the site of microbial infection such as lipopolysaccharide, cell wall components of some bacteria and yeasts and bacterial endotoxin.

In the presence of an activating substance C3b complexes with factor B to form C3bB. This complex is then attacked by factor D to form C3bBb which functions as a C3 convertase and cleaves C3 to form C3a and C3b as in the classical pathway. The C3bBb complex is stabilised by the presence of a plasma protein called properdin. This increased stability facilitates the formation of $(C3b)_nBb$ complexes which function as a C5 convertase. Thus, the C3bBb complex represents the activation unit of the alternative pathway. The membrane attack unit of the alternative pathway is similar to that for the classical pathway.

Cell-mediated Mechanisms of Immunity

Cellular immunity is mediated by T lymphocytes. The mechanism of activation of T lymphocytes bears many similarities to the activation of B lymphocytes. In particular, activation is antigen-specific, requiring contact between foreign antigen and a pre-existing surface receptor on the T lymphocyte which is specific for the inducing antigen. In contrast to B lymphocyte function, however, T lymphocytes are not activated by contact with free antigen; they require the antigen to be "processed" and presented in a suitable way by accessory cells called antigen-presenting cells (APC). In outline, the APC incorporates free antigen and breaks it down into a series of smaller peptides. Some of these peptides bind to molecules which are coded for by the genes of the major histocompatibility complex (MHC), and are then displayed on the surface of the APC in a form suitable for the activation of T lymphocytes. The role of the major histocompatibility complex in immunity is considered in detail later in this chapter.

T Lymphocyte Subsets

There are four main subsets of mature T lymphocytes which are defined in terms of their function and the presence of the adhesion molecules CD4 and CD8. As explained in Chapter 2, developing T lymphocytes transiently express both CD4 and CD8 but, by the time of their release as circulating cells, express only one or the other molecule on their surface membranes.

About 65% of peripheral blood T lymphocytes are CD4$^+$. CD4 is thought to promote contact between T lymphocytes and antigen-presenting cells by binding to MHC class II proteins (explained later in this chapter) expressed on the surface of the antigen-presenting cell. This has the dual effect of promoting recognition of antigen by the T lymphocyte and ensuring that IL-1 which is released by the antigen-presenting cell finds its target. There are two subsets of CD4$^+$ T lymphocytes: T helper lymphocytes (T$_H$) which help and induce activation of B lymphocytes, and those which take part in delayed-type hypersensitivity (T$_{DTH}$). T$_H$ lymphocytes secrete IL-2 which acts as a T lymphocyte growth factor, IL-3 which promotes the growth and maturation of various blood cell precursors, γ-interferon which activates macrophages and GM-CSF which is a growth factor for neutrophils and monocytes. T$_{DTH}$ lymphocytes are known to secrete a number of factors which are chemotactic for macrophages, stimulate activation of macrophages and inhibit migration away from the reaction site. The multiplicity of interactions between T and B lymphocytes described here serves as a reminder of the highly integrated nature of the immune response.

CD8 is thought to bind to MHC class I proteins on the target cell, thereby promoting recognition of foreign antigen. There are two subsets of CD8$^+$ T lymphocytes: T suppressor lymphocytes (T$_s$) which act as a brake on T$_H$ lymphocytes and cytotoxic T lymphocytes (T$_C$) which release cytolytic substances such as perforin directly onto the target cell to which they are bound.

SAQ 3

Which of the following interleukins is not a T lymphocyte product?

A. IL-1
B. IL-2
C. IL-4
D. IL-5

The T Lymphocyte Receptor

The antigen-specific T lymphocyte receptor (TcR) comprises an antigen-recognising molecule (Ti) in non-covalent association with an invariant polypeptide complex (CD3) as shown in Figure 13.9. The structure and function of the antigen-recognising molecules of T lymphocytes are analogous to those of the surface immunoglobulin receptors of B lymphocytes. The diversity of Ti molecules is accounted for by the same processes of germ line DNA rearrangement as those described earlier which account for antibody diversity. It is likely that the immunoglobulin genes and the Ti genes have evolved from a common ancestral gene. Both sets of genes are said to belong to the **immunoglobulin gene superfamily**.

The Ti molecule comprises two polypeptide chains linked by disulphide bridges. Four different polypeptide chains, designated α, β, δ

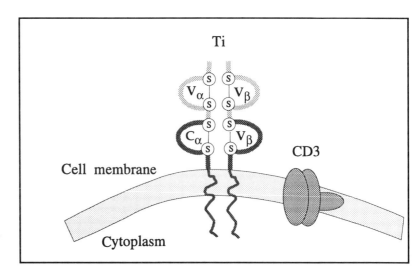

Figure 13.9 *The structure of the T lymphocyte receptor*

and γ, have been identified as components of Ti molecules. There are only two different Ti structures, however, because α chains are always found in association with β chains and γ chains are always found in association with δ chains. The $Ti_{\alpha\beta}$ configuration predominates; only about 10% of T lymphocytes carry $Ti_{\gamma\delta}$ molecules. The function of T lymphocytes which carry $Ti_{\gamma\delta}$ molecules remains obscure.

The genes which code for Ti_{β} and Ti_{γ} chains are located on chromosome 7, while those for Ti_{α} and Ti_{δ} are located on chromosome 14. The Ti_{δ} gene cluster is nested completely within the Ti_{α} gene cluster. The Ti_{α} cluster comprises about 50 variable (V) segments, about 50 joining (J) segments and a single constant (C) segment. It does not possess a diversity (D) segment. This organisation is analogous to that for immunoglobulin light chains. Conversely, the Ti_{β} locus comprises about 70 V segments, about 13 J segments, 2 D segments and two C segments, an arrangement analogous to that of immunoglobulin heavy chains.

The pattern and timing of Ti gene rearrangement is closely regulated. The most undifferentiated lymphocytes found in the thymus have their Ti genes in the germ line configuration. The next stage of differentiation involves the simultaneous rearrangement of the Ti_{γ} and Ti_{β} gene clusters. If the result of Ti_{γ} gene rearrangement is capable of expression, Ti_{δ} gene rearrangement ensues. If the result of the Ti_{δ} gene rearrangement is capable of expression, the cell will carry a $Ti_{\gamma\delta}$ receptor: no further gene rearrangement occurs. Con-

SAQ 4

Which of the following are T lymphocyte markers?

A. CD2
B. Surface immunoglobulin
C. CD3
D. CD8
E. Fcγ receptors

versely, if the result of either Ti_γ or Ti_δ gene rearrangement is non-functional, Ti_α gene rearrangement commences and the cell carries a $Ti_{\alpha\beta}$ receptor.

The Role of the Major Histocompatibility Complex

The major histocompatibility complex (MHC) is a group of closely linked genes located on the short arm of chromosome 6 as shown in Figure 13.10. The MHC directs the synthesis of three different classes of proteins, designated MHC classes I, II and III. MHC proteins of classes I and II belong to the immunoglobulin superfamily, and function as a third set of antigen-recognising proteins. MHC class III proteins are Complement components (C2, C4 and factor B) as described earlier in this chapter. The products of the MHC class I and II genes are designated as HLA antigens: the class I proteins are designated HLA-A, HLA-B and HLA-C while the class II proteins are designated HLA-DP, HLA-DQ and HLA-DR. The MHC class I and II genes are highly polymorphic ie each gene exists in a number of different forms or **alleles**. The product of each allele is identified with a numbered suffix eg HLA-B27. The MHC is inherited as a complete unit and is expressed codominantly ie each individual expresses MHC genes from both parents. The consequence of this is that there is considerable variety in the MHC proteins which individuals express. This is why transplant donors must be "tissue-typed" and matched to the recipient if rejection is to be avoided.

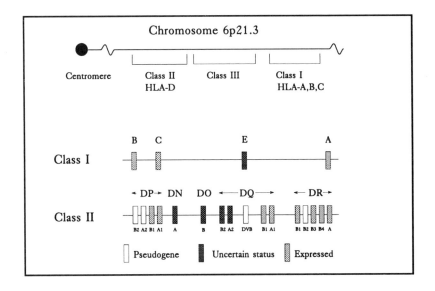

Figure 13.10 *The structure of the major histocompatibility complex (MHC)*

MHC class I molecules are present on almost all nucleated cells in the body. As shown in Figure 13.11, MHC class I molecules consist of three domains (designated α_1, α_2 and α_3) complexed with an invariant protein of similar domain structure called β_2 microglobulin. In effect, the molecule behaves as if it is composed of four domains. The differences between different class I alleles are localised to the cleft between the α_1 and α_2 domains which forms the peptide binding site.

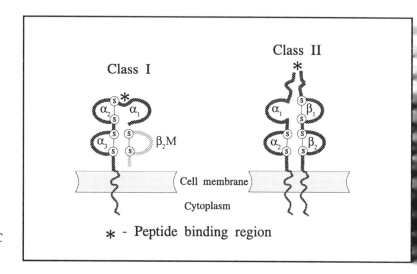

Figure 13.11 *The structure of MHC class I and II molecules*

MHC class II molecules are expressed by antigen-presenting cells such as B lymphocytes, dendritic cells and, following exposure to γ-interferon, macrophages. The structure of a typical MHC class II protein is shown in Figure 13.11. As shown, each molecule consists of two peptide chains which are designated α and β, each of which contains two domains (designated α_1, α_2 and β_1, β_2 respectively). The peptide binding site is situated between the α_1 and β_1 domains. Variation in the amino acid sequences between MHC class II alleles is largely confined to the region of the peptide binding site.

MHC molecules play an important role in the development of the T lymphocyte repertoire and, subsequently, control the cellular cooperation necessary for an effective specific immune response. The role of MHC molecules in cellular cooperation is described in more detail later in this chapter.

As described in Chapter 2, the thymus gland is extremely active as a site of production of T lymphocytes in the early months of life.

SAQ 5

Which of the following belong to the immunoglobulin superfamily?

A. MHC class I molecules
B. Ti
C. MHC class III molecules
D. CD10

However, the vast majority of T lymphocytes produced there die in the process of maturation and are never released into the circulation. It is thought that all immature T lymphocytes are predestined to undergo apoptosis in the thymus unless they are specifically selected for "rescue". The first stage of selection occurs in the thymic cortex where $Ti^+ CD3^+ CD4^+ CD8^+$ thymocytes are exposed to MHC class I and II molecules on the surfaces of cortical epithelial cells. Those cortical T lymphocytes which carry receptors capable of recognising self MHC molecules are granted a reprieve and thus continue to mature. The majority of cortical T lymphocytes do not bind to self MHC molecules and so undergo apoptosis. This process is known as **positive selection** and ensures that mature circulating T lymphocytes can only recognise peptide antigens expressed in association with self MHC class I or II molecules on the surface of antigen-presenting cells. Further, each T lymphocyte can interact only with the specific MHC allele to which it was exposed in the thymic cortex during its maturation. This phenomenon is known as **MHC restriction**. Mature $Ti^+ CD3^+ CD4^+$ lymphocytes are capable of interacting only with MHC class II molecules and are said to be MHC class II restricted. Similarly, mature $Ti^+ CD3^+ CD8^+$ lymphocytes are capable of interacting only with MHC class I molecules and are said to be MHC class I restricted.

As the cortical T lymphocytes mature, they become either $Ti^+ CD3^+ CD4^+$ or $Ti^+ CD3^+ CD8^+$ cells and migrate into the thymic medulla. Here, they come into contact with antigen-presenting cells which carry processed host antigens in association with self MHC molecules. Those T lymphocytes which recognise and bind to self antigen are destroyed. This process is known as **negative selection**. The mechanism of destruction of self-reacting medullary T lymphocytes is poorly understood. Thus, T lymphocytes which pass both positive and negative selection criteria are capable of recognising peptide antigen only when it is bound to self MHC molecules but are not autoreactive.

Cellular Cooperation in the Activation of the Specific Immune Response

An optimal specific immune response requires the interaction and cooperation of antigen-presenting cells, B lymphocytes and T lymphocytes.

Activation of T_H and B Lymphocytes

As described earlier, T lymphocytes do not respond to free antigen. Instead, they require antigen to be presented to them in association with MHC class I or II molecules on the surfaces of antigen-presenting cells (APC) such as macrophages and B lymphocytes. These cells are capable of internalising and partially degrading protein antigens. The resulting peptide fragments bind to MHC molecules which are recycled from the cell surface, forming an antigen:MHC complex which subsequently is expressed on the cell surface. Exogenous antigens are bound specifically to MHC class II molecules while endogenous antigens such as viral proteins produced by infected cells bind specifically to MHC class I molecules.

The combination of processed peptide antigen:MHC class II complex is capable of binding specifically to the Ti-CD3 complex on the surface of T_H (CD4+) lymphocytes, as shown in Figure 13.12. This interaction occurs with a relatively low affinity and is insufficient to trigger activation of the T_H lymphocyte. Contact between the T_H lymphocyte and the APC subsequently is stabilised by the strong association between the accessory molecule CD4 and the MHC class II molecule and also by the simultaneous expression of adhesion molecules and their receptors by both cells.

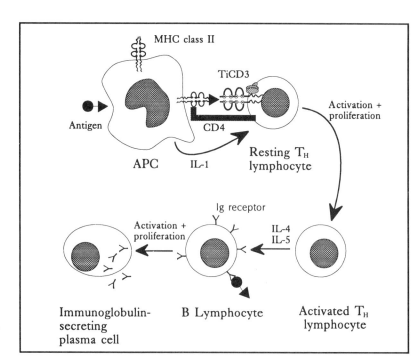

Figure 13.12 *The mechanism of activation of B and T helper lymphocytes*

Once the T_H lymphocyte and APC are fully engaged, activation of the T_H lymphocyte is elicited by the synthesis and localised secretion of IL-1 by the APC. T_H lymphocyte activation is accompanied by the synthesis and secretion of a range of lymphokines, the expression of lymphokine receptors on the cell surface and, ultimately, by clonal proliferation. Two T_H subsets exist which are designated T_{H1} and T_{H2}. Activated T_{H1} lymphocytes secrete γ-interferon and IL-2 which are required for the activation of cytotoxic T_c lymphocytes, NK cells and macrophages. In contrast, activated T_{H2} lymphocytes secrete IL-4 and IL-5 which are required for the activation of B lymphocytes.

At the same time as the events outlined above are taking place, the inducing protein antigen will bind specifically to the surface immunoglobulin receptors of B lymphocytes. As above, the process of receptor occupation is insufficient to elicit activation of the cell, but the secretion of IL-4 and IL-5 by activated T_{H2} lymphocytes prompts both clonal proliferation and differentiation into antibody-secreting plasma cells as shown in Figure 13.12. On subsequent exposure to the offending antigen, the expanded antigen-specific B lymphocyte clone is capable of usurping the role of the macrophage as the APC, thereby prompting an accelerated and more substantial secondary immune response.

Some antigens, such as bacterial lipopolysaccharide, are capable of provoking B lymphocyte activation independently of T_H lymphocyte activation. Such T-independent antigens typically are large polymeric molecules which contain multiple repeating copies of antigenic determinants and so are capable of binding to several immunoglobulin receptors simultaneously. This cross-linking and "capping" of the surface immunoglobulin receptors provokes B lymphocyte activation directly. The response to T-independent antigens differs from the T-dependent response in that only IgM antibody is synthesised and subsequent exposure to the offending antigen does not elicit an accelerated secondary immune response or class switching.

Activation of Cytotoxic T_c Lymphocytes and Macrophages

The expression of endogenous protein antigen in association with MHC class I molecules, for example on the surface of virus-infected cells, promotes the binding of resting CD8+ T_c lymphocytes as shown in Figure 13.13. The initial weak interaction between the T

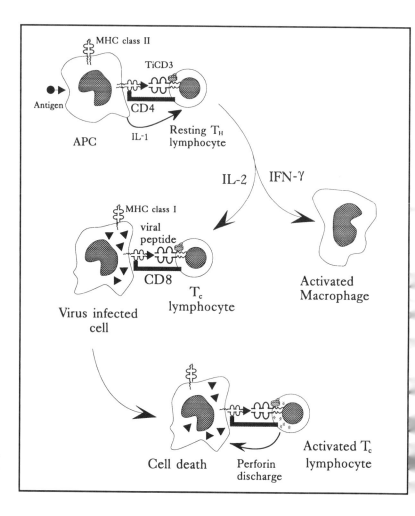

Figure 13.13 *The mechanism of activation and action of cytotoxic T lymphocytes and macrophages*

lymphocyte receptor and the APC is strengthened by the binding of CD8 on the T_c lymphocyte to the MHC class I molecules on the APC and the expression of adhesion molecules in a manner analogous to the engagement of T_H lymphocytes to MHC class II molecules. Once engagement is complete, the T_c lymphocyte is stimulated to undergo proliferation and differentiation by the binding of IL-2 to specific receptors expressed on the cell surface. IL-2 is secreted by activated T_H lymphocytes.

Activated mature T_c lymphocytes bind specifically via their Ti-CD3 receptors to the MHC class I:viral peptide antigen complexes expressed on the surface of virus-infected cells as shown in Figure 13.13. Once the T_c lymphocyte and its target are fully engaged, the cytoplasmic granules in the T_c lymphocyte migrate towards the target cell and discharge their contents onto it. These granules contain a range of monomeric molecules known as **perforins** which, in the presence of Ca^{2+} ions, polymerise within target cell membranes, resulting in the destruction of the target cell in a manner analogous to the action of Complement. Having dealt the target cell a lethal blow, the T_c lymphocyte disengages itself and seeks out a new victim. It is thought that NK cells use a similar mechanism to destroy their target cells.

Activated T_H lymphocytes also secrete macrophage chemotactic factor which recruits monocytes and macrophages to the immune focus and γ-interferon (IFN-γ) which elicits the activation of macrophages. Activated macrophages largely are responsible for the ingestion and destruction of certain types of bacteria, tumour cells and intracellular parasites such as *Leishmania* and *Listeria*.

In most cases, the mechanisms outlined above result in the clearance of the inducing foreign antigen with minimal collateral damage to normal host tissue. However, when a foreign antigen is resistant to the mechanisms of cell-mediated immunity, persistent activation of macrophages and T_c lymphocytes can lead to severe damage to normal host tissue. This phenomenon is known as **delayed-type hypersensitivity** and is the mechanism which mediates contact dermatitis, transplant rejection and graft versus host disease.

Activated T_c lymphocytes are not the only lymphocytes which possess the ability to kill cells directly. Natural Killer (NK) cells belong to the morphologically defined class of large granular lymphocytes (LGL). The lineage of NK cells remains the subject of debate. Certainly, they lack the surface markers which define T and B lymphocytes and macrophages, although they possess IgG Fc receptors. The exact mechanisms by which NK cells exert their cytotoxic effect remains obscure but does not require prior immunisation and is not MHC restricted. NK cells are thought to be important in host defence against the establishment of tumours.

Suggested Further Reading

Roitt, I.M. (1988). *Essential Immunology (6th edn). Oxford: Blackwell Scientific Publications.*

Brenner, M.K. and Hoffbrand, A.V. (1989). Normal lymphocytes and their benign disorders. In *Postgraduate Haematology*. (3rd edn) (eds A.V. Hoffbrand and S.M. Lewis). Oxford: Butterworth-Heinemann.

Roitt, I., Brostoff, J. and Male, D. (1988). *Immunology,*. London: Gower Medical Publishing.

Answers to Self-Assessment Questions

1. A, C, D.

2. IgG as it is the only class of immunoglobulin which crosses the placental barrier.

3. A. IL-1 is a macrophage product.

4. A, C, D.

5. A, B.

Disorders of the Immune System

Disorders of the immune system, or immunodeficiencies, are characterised by an increased susceptibility to infection, often with organisms normally considered to be of relatively low pathogenicity, and a predisposition to the development of certain tumours. As described in the previous chapter, the immune system consists of a multitude of highly integrated and mutually dependent defence mechanisms. Optimal defence of the body requires the proper functioning of each component of the system, since a defect in one component can contribute to a more generalised loss of immunity. The various immunodeficiency states are classified as primary immunodeficiency where the fundamental defect lies within one or more components of the immune system and secondary immunodeficiency where the immune deficit is a side effect of some other primary disorder such as diabetes or leukaemia. For the purposes of this chapter, the primary immunodeficiencies are classified according to the component of the immune system which is primarily affected, even though this belies the complexity of the pathogenesis of these disorders. Familiarity with the content of Chapter 13 is assumed in this chapter.

Disorders of Innate Immunity

The most significant component of innate immunity against microbial infection is provided by the phagocytic cells of the body. As described in the previous chapter, there are three important types of phagocytic cell within the body viz neutrophils, circulating monocytes and fixed tissue macrophages. The most important of these in the context of first line defence against microbial invasion are the neutrophils.

Optimal defence against the establishment of microbial infection once the epithelial or mucosal barrier has been breached requires sufficient numbers of functionally intact neutrophils. Thus, a deficiency of neutrophil numbers or a defect of neutrophil function leads to a susceptibility to bacterial and fungal infection.

The reference range for neutrophil count is affected by a wide range of variables such as sex (women typically have slightly higher WBC than men although the WBC falls sharply during menstruation), time of sampling (neutrophil counts are highest in the afternoon), exercise (WBC rises with vigorous exercise), cigarette smoking (WBC is higher in smokers) and ethnic origin (Caucasian and Asian WBC are higher than those in blacks).

SAQ 1

What is the most important component of innate immunity against bacterial infection?

In the early years of this century, a number of case reports appeared which described a syndrome of acute and severe neutropaenia with pharyngitis and rapid progression to collapse, septicaemia and death. Most cases occurred in middle aged women.

It was not until 1933 that a link between drug ingestion and neutropaenia was established when Watkins suggested that aminopyrine ingestion could be to blame in many cases. Further evidence that aminopyrine was linked directly to acute neutropaenia was provided a year later by Madison and Squiers who showed that withdrawal of aminopyrine from neutropaenic individuals reduced the mortality rate significantly. Because of these findings, aminopyrine rapidly fell into disfavour and the incidence of drug-induced neutropaenia subsided. As memories of the catastrophic side effects of aminopyrine faded, a chemically related analgesic, dipyrone, found favour with the medical profession. This led to a new wave of drug-induced neutropaenia, including a number of patients who had previously recovered from aminopyrine-induced neutropaenia, and resulted in many deaths.

Quantitative Disorders of Neutrophils

Neutropaenia is defined as a fall in the circulating neutrophil count below that expected in a normal individual of the same age, sex and racial origin and is commonly seen in a wide range of conditions as shown in Table 14.1.

Neutropaenia in Infections

Transient neutropaenia is observed in a wide range of acute non-pyogenic infections, particularly where some degree of myelosuppression is present such as in malnutrition or following cytotoxic chemotherapy. Typically, the neutrophils in such cases show prominent primary granulation ("toxic" granulation) and nuclear hyposegmentation (left shift). The pathogenesis of the neutropaenia in these infections remains the subject of debate but increased neutrophil margination, increased neutrophil losses due to utilisation, Complement activation via the alternative pathway and suppression of granulopoiesis by the infecting organism probably all play a role.

Drug-induced Neutropaenia

As described in Chapter 15, the cytotoxic drugs used to treat malignant disease are non-specific; they attack normal cells as well as malignant cells. Because of this, some degree of neutropaenia is unavoidable during cytotoxic chemotherapy. Therapy-induced neutropaenia contributes to the high incidence of infectious complications seen in malignant disease, and limits the doses of cytotoxic agents that can be used. In most cases, temporary withdrawal of cytotoxic treatment in neutropaenic individuals permits the gradual recovery of normal granulopoiesis and the restoration of a normal neutrophil count. This process can be accelerated by the administration of recombinant human haemopoietic growth factors.

In contrast to the cytotoxic drugs which invariably induce marrow hypoplasia, a large number of drugs have been reported to cause neutropaenia in a minority of people taking them. In most cases, the cause of this idiosyncratic response to the drug is unknown, although immune mechanisms appear to be implicated in the induction of the acute form of drug-induced neutropaenia. Among the drugs most frequently implicated in the occasional induction of

Bacterial & Viral Infections

> *Salmonella typhi*
> *Salmonella paratyphi*
> Septicaemia
> Hepatitis A (infectious hepatitis)
> Varicella zoster (chicken pox)
> Measles
> Rubella (German measles)
> Yellow fever
> Dengue
> HIV (AIDS)

Rickettsial Infections

> *Rickettsia tsutsugamushi* (scrub typhus)
> *Rickettsia rickettsii* (Rocky Mountain spotted fever)
> Rickettsial pox

Protozoal Infections

> *Plasmodia spp* (malaria)
> *Leishmania donovanii* (kala-azar)
> *Borrelia recurrentis* (relapsing fever)

Chemical & Physical Agents

> Cytotoxic drugs (Chapter 15)
> Sulphonamides
> Idiosyncratic reactions to various drugs
> Ionising radiation
> Benzene (Chapter 20)

Haematological Disorders

> Aplastic and hypoplastic anaemias (Chapter 20)
> Megaloblastic anaemia (Chapter 4)
> Hypersplenism

Cachexia & Debilitated States

Anaphylactoid Shock

Rare Congenital Types

> Cyclic neutropaenia
> Familial benign neutropaenia
> Chronic hypoplastic neutropaenia
> Infantile genetic agranulocytosis
> Primary splenic neutropaenia
> Chronic idiopathic neutropaenia
> Reticular dysgenesis
> Immune neutropaenia

Broadly, susceptibility to microbial infection is inversely proportional to the neutrophil count. There is no predisposition to infection with neutrophil counts above $2.0 \times 10^9/l$, but as the count falls below $1.0 \times 10^9/l$, bacterial infections become progressively more common. As the neutrophil count approaches $0.5 \times 10^9/l$, fungal superinfections become likely and even commensal bacteria are potentially pathogenic. Absolute neutropaenia is incompatible with life in the absence of strenuous prophylactic measures.

Table 14.1 *The major causes of neutropaenia*

neutropaenia are the chemically related analgesics aminopyrine and phenylbutazone, the tranquiliser chlorpromazine and a wide range of antimicrobial drugs such as the sulphonamides, chloramphenicol and the penicillins. Acute drug-induced neutropaenia is associated with a severe susceptibility to infection and, if untreated, may result in death. In most cases, withdrawal of the offending drug causes remission of the symptoms and the gradual restoration of a normal neutrophil count.

Rare Congenital Neutropaenias

Numerous isolated case reports exist of extremely rare congenital neutropaenias. The investigations carried out on the affected infants have varied enormously and it is difficult to assess the relationship, if any, between these reported conditions. This section describes a selection of the better characterised congenital neutropaenias.

Cyclic Neutropaenia

Cyclic neutropaenia is a rare congenital disorder which is characterised by recurrent neutropaenia with oral ulceration, pharyngitis with lymphadenopathy and, in severe cases, pneumonia. The neutrophil count in affected individuals follows a regular cyclic pattern with a fixed period. In most cases, bouts of neutropaenia occur at about three weekly intervals and last for about four days. Examination of the bone marrow reveals that a sharp fall in the numbers of CFU-GM present and an arrest of granulopoietic activity occurs about 1 week before the neutropaenic phase. These changes remit spontaneously after a few days and the neutrophil count climbs back into the lower reaches of normality for about 2-3 weeks before the cycle repeats itself.

Careful temporal studies of affected individuals have revealed that a lesser degree of cycling of B lymphocytes, eosinophils, monocytes, red cells and platelets also is present. The widespread nature of these cyclic changes suggests that cyclic neutropaenia results from a defect in the regulation of haemopoiesis at the pluripotential stem cell level. A single reported case of the transmission of cyclic neutropaenia between siblings following allogeneic bone marrow transplant for acute lymphoblastic leukaemia adds weight to this theory. Further weight is added by the results of a series of experiments in dogs with a similar condition (see sidebox).

The discovery of an autosomal recessive form of cyclic neutropaenia in grey collie dogs has facilitated studies to try to determine the cause of the condition. Canine cyclic neutropaenia is associated with loss of hair pigmentation and a shorter periodicity of about 12 days but is otherwise similar to the human condition. These studies have shown that the survival of neutrophils is normal in affected dogs and that this does not change during the neutropaenic phase; that the plasma and urine concentrations of various haemopoietic growth factors cycles with a similar periodicity to the changes in cell count and that transplantation of bone marrow from normal dogs to affected recipients effectively cured the condition while transplantation from affected dogs to normal recipients transmitted the condition. All of this evidence points to the existence of some regulatory defect of haemopoiesis which operates at the pluripotential stem cell level.

Cyclic neutropaenia usually is a congenital abnormality although occasional reports exist of the development of this condition in later life. In most cases, the mode of inheritance is uncertain but a minority show clear evidence of autosomal dominant inheritance. Typically, cyclic neutropaenia is relatively benign, requiring only antimicrobial therapy to treat the minor infections which occur during the neutropaenic phase of the cycle.

Kostmann's Infantile Genetic Agranulocytosis

Infantile agranulocytosis is a rare, autosomal recessive trait which is characterised by profound neutropaenia despite the presence of normal numbers of CFU-GM in the bone marrow which are capable of terminal differentiation in culture, vacuolation of neutrophil precursors and a severe susceptibility to infection. Early attempts at treatment with steroids and haematinics were ineffective: most affected infants died from overwhelming infection within the first year of life. Recent work has suggested that infantile agranulocytosis is caused by a failure of synthesis of a haemopoietic growth factor. Attempts to treat this condition with recombinant human G-CSF have shown early promise.

Familial Benign Neutropaenia

Familial benign neutropaenia is a rare condition which is inherited in an autosomal dominant fashion and is characterised by chronic mild neutropaenia with a compensatory increase in the cell count of the other leucocytes and a relatively mild clinical course. Bone marrow examination typically reveals mild granulocytic hypoplasia but normal erythropoietic and thrombopoietic activity.

Reticular Dysgenesis

Reticular dysgenesis is a rare condition of unknown aetiology which is characterised by a selective and complete absence of leucopoiesis. Affected infants lack any identifiable granulocyte, monocyte or lymphocyte precursors in the bone marrow and lymphoid organs, and so are extremely immunosuppressed. Interestingly, erythropoiesis and thrombopoiesis appear to be normal in this condition.

Immune Neutropaenia

Several cases have been described of isoimmune neutropaenia caused by the transplacental passage of maternal antibodies directed against foetal neutrophil antigens such as NA1 and NA2. Affected infants are born with profound neutropaenia, a late granulocytic maturation arrest and skin infections are common. Isoimmune neutropaenia is analogous in many respects to haemolytic disease of the newborn caused by foetomaternal incompatibility of red cell antigens as described in Chapter 10. This condition remits within the first few weeks of life as maternal antibodies disappear from the neonatal circulation. A small number of case reports exist of isoimmune neutropaenia caused by the transplacental passage of a maternal autoantibody directed against shared foetomaternal neutrophil antigens.

Autoimmune neutropaenia is caused by the presence of circulating antibodies directed against host neutrophil antigens. The condition is seen most commonly in early infancy where it is manifest as a variable degree of chronic neutropaenia with an apparent late granulocytic maturation arrest. However, studies have shown that the neutrophil precursors are capable of terminal differentiation and that the apparent maturation arrest is caused by the selective immune destruction of mature neutrophils. Several cases of spontaneous remission of autoimmune neutropaenia in early childhood have been reported. In most cases, the antigenic target of the autoantibody is unknown.

Recent work has suggested that chronic benign neutropaenia of infancy, which originally was thought to be a separate disorder of unknown aetiology, is caused by an autoimmune mechanism.

Qualitative Disorders of Neutrophils

Inherited disorders of every stage of neutrophil function have been described, many of which cause a severe predisposition to microbial infection. However, most of these disorders are rare. The total incidence of clinically significant primary defects of neutrophil function is about 1 per 100,000. In contrast, secondary disorders of neutrophil function are relatively common.

Defects of Margination

The earliest observable response of neutrophils to stimulation is an increase in margination. Adherence to vascular endothelium in this way is a prerequisite for diapedesis so that the excited neutrophils can begin their journey towards the site of infection.

Leucocyte Adhesion Deficiency Syndrome

Leucocyte adhesion deficiency syndrome is a rare autosomal recessive or X-linked recessive disorder of neutrophil margination and adherence caused by a deficiency of any of a family of three leucocyte membrane adhesion molecules. As shown in Table 14.2, each of these adhesion molecules is a heterodimer composed of a common β subunit (CD18) and a specific α subunit (CD11a, CD11b or CD11c) and each has a specific function. CD11a/CD18 strengthens the binding of activated Tc lymphocytes and NK cells to their target cells and promotes the binding of neutrophils to surfaces to enable chemotaxis to occur. This adhesion molecule is located on the neutrophil surface and is not upregulated following stimulation of the cell. CD11b/CD18 forms the neutrophil C3b receptor and therefore mediates the ingestion of opsonised particles, degranulation and activation of the respiratory burst as well as promoting neutrophil binding to surfaces. This molecule is stored in the specific granules of the neutrophil and is released to the membrane surface following stimulation by chemotactic factors. This mechanism enables the neutrophil to respond rapidly to contact with chemotactic factors by augmenting its adhesive capacity, thereby promoting chemotaxis and phagocytosis. The alternative mechanism for receptor upregulation, *de novo* synthesis, would take too long to be effective. The function of CD11c/CD18 is unknown.

SAQ 2

Which of the following cells are CD4+

A. NK cells
B. T_s lymphocytes
C. T_H lymphocytes
D. T_{DTH} lymphocytes
E. Small cortical thymocytes

Adhesion Molecule	Synonym	Molecular Weight	Present on	Function
CD11a/CD18	LFA-1	177,000/ 94,000	All leucocytes	Promotion of neutrophil function, binding of T_C lymphocytes and NK cells to targets
CD11b/CD18	Mo1 Mac1	155,000/ 94,000	Neutrophils monocytes NK cells	C3b receptor, promotes adhesion, chemotaxis and phagocytosis
CD11c/CD18	p150,95	150,000/ 94,000	Neutrophils monocytes	Function unknown Possible C3d receptor

Table 14.2 *Structure and function of neutrophil adhesion molecules*

Hyperimmunoglobulin E syndrome is also known as Job's syndrome after a character in the Old Testament of the Bible whose strength of faith was tested by a series of disasters wrought by Satan. Job was a wealthy landowner who had 10 healthy children, owned 7,000 sheep, 3,000 camels, 1,000 oxen, 500 donkeys and had many servants.

In the first test of his faith, Job's oxen and donkeys were stolen by a neighbouring tribe, the Sabeans; his sheep were incinerated by a firestorm and his camels were stolen by a second neighbouring tribe, the Chaldeans. All of his servants were killed during these attacks. Finally, all of his children were killed when their house collapsed under the force of a mighty wind from the desert. In short, Job lost almost everything that was dear to him in the space of one day. Despite this, his faith did not waver.

In the second test of his faith..

"Satan went out from the presence of the Lord and afflicted Job with painful sores from the soles of his feet to the top of his head."

Again, Job's faith remained unbroken and Satan finally admitted defeat. As a reward, Job's wealth was returned to him twice over and he had 10 more children. Job died a happy and contented man at the age of 140 years.

Leucocyte adhesion deficiency syndrome affects neutrophils, monocytes and lymphocytes and is manifest as a susceptibility to severe, often life-threatening bacterial and viral infections, especially of the skin, middle ear and oropharynx. Delayed separation of the umbilical cord has been noted in many affected infants. The peripheral blood neutrophil count is normal or raised but these cells do not accumulate at sites of infection. *In vitro* testing reveals that the neutrophils of affected individuals have defective adherence, chemotaxis, phagocytosis, degranulation and impaired respiratory burst activity. The susceptibility to viral infections is explained by the presence of these adhesion molecules on T and B lymphocytes and monocytes.

Defects of Chemotaxis

Optimal chemotaxis requires that the neutrophil possesses sufficient surface receptors for the inducing chemotactic factor and also sufficient surface adhesion molecules to enable it to crawl over cell surfaces towards the site of infection. It is the lack of adhesion molecules that causes the chemotactic defect in leucocyte adhesion deficiency syndrome.

Specific Granule Deficiency

Specific granule deficiency is a rare, autosomal recessive disorder which is characterised by impaired neutrophil chemotactic and microbicidal function, nuclear hyposegmentation, absence of specific cytoplasmic granules and a susceptibility to skin infections, especially with *Staphylococcus aureas* and *Candida albicans*. The microbicidal defect is caused by the absence of specific granule contents such as lactoferrin. The chemotactic defect is the main contributor to the susceptibility to infection and is caused by the inability of affected neutrophils to upregulate their chemotactic receptors following stimulation. The normal storage site of chemotactic receptors is the secondary granules. The phagocytic capacity and respiratory burst activity of affected neutrophils appears to be normal.

Hyperimmunoglobulin E Syndrome

The earliest descriptions of hyperimmunoglobulin E syndrome all involved red-haired, fair-skinned girls and the condition originally was thought to be restricted to such individuals. This is now known to be untrue: hyperimmunoglobulin E syndrome affects both sexes and has been described in many different races. This extremely rare condition is characterised by impaired neutrophil chemotaxis with normal phagocytic and microbicidal function, a raised serum concentration of IgE which commonly is directed against *Staphylococcus aureas*, recurrent "cold" abscesses, infected eczema and pulmonary infections. The primary defect in this condition is unknown, but most workers believe that the defect of neutrophil function is a secondary phenomenon.

Defects of Opsonisation

A deficiency of IgG or Complement components reduces the opsonisation of invading microbes, thereby reducing the ability of neutrophils to recognise them as targets for phagocytosis. These forms of immunodeficiency are described later in this chapter.

Defects of Microbial Killing

Chronic Granulomatous Disease of Childhood

Chronic granulomatous disease (CGD) is characterised by a failure of the post-phagocytic respiratory burst in neutrophils and other phagocytic cells. It is associated with recurrent pulmonary and skin infections with the progressive formation of necrotic granulomas and hepatosplenomegaly. The most common infecting organisms are *Staphylococci spp, Serratia marescens, Klebsiella spp, Aerobacter spp* and *Salmonella spp*. In the absence of aggressive antimicrobial therapy and prompt drainage of abscesses, CGD typically is fatal in early childhood.

As described in the previous chapter, perturbation of the neutrophil membrane such as occurs during phagocytosis triggers the cell to undergo a sudden burst of respiration which culminates in the formation of a series of toxic oxygen radicals, the most important of which is superoxide. Activation of the respiratory burst is mediated by an enzyme system known as the **NADPH oxidase**. The NADPH oxidase, which was thought to be restricted to phagocytic cells but is now known to be present in a range of other cells, functions as an electron transport system and consists of both plasma membrane and cytosolic components. The electron donor for the oxidase system is NADPH. The plasma membrane-associated component is known as cytochrome b_{-245} or b_{558} and exists as a heterodimer

SAQ 3

Which Complement fragment is most closely associated with:

A. opsonisation
B. chemotaxis

consisting of an α subunit of molecular weight 22,000 (p22-*phox*) and a β subunit of molecular weight 91,000 (gp91-*phox*). The genes which encode the α and β subunits are located at 16p24 and Xp21.1 respectively. A reserve supply of cytochrome b$_{-245}$ is stored in neutrophil secondary granules. A number of cytosolic components of the NADPH oxidase system have been identified, the best characterised of which are known as p47-*phox* and p67-*phox*. These proteins are encoded by genes located at 7q11.23 and 1q25 respectively.

Perturbation of the neutrophil membrane stimulates the migration of the cytosolic components towards the cell membrane, thereby permitting the assembly of the NADPH oxidase system and activation of the respiratory burst. The precise nature and behaviour of the various cytosolic components of the NADPH oxidase system and the manner of their association with cytochrome b$_{-245}$ is incompletely understood at present.

CGD is caused by a failure of some component of the NADPH oxidase system with a consequent failure of superoxide generation and an inability to kill ingested bacteria and fungi effectively. All of the other components of neutrophil function are normal in CGD. Broadly, four types of CGD are recognised:

- **X91 CGD** is the most common form of the disease, accounting for about 55% of cases. This form is inherited as an X-linked recessive trait and is associated with a complete (X91°), or partial (X91⁻) deficiency of cytochrome b$_{-245}$. X91 CGD is caused by a mutation of the gene which encodes the β subunit (gp91-*phox*) of cytochrome b$_{-245}$. The absence of the α subunit is presumed to be a secondary phenomenon. Female carriers of this form of CGD have two populations of circulating neutrophils: one population is entirely normal, the other is deficient in cytochrome b$_{-245}$. A number of rare variants of this form of CGD have been described which are characterised by the presence of a normal membrane concentration of a dysfunctional cytochrome b$_{-245}$. These variants are designated X91^{+} CGD.

- **A47 CGD** also is a relatively common form, accounting for about one third of cases. This form is caused by a mutation of the p47-*phox* gene and is

SAQ 4

What is the main source of NADPH within the red cell?

characterised by an autosomal recessive mode of inheritance and a complete absence of p47-*phox* (A47° CGD). The concentration of cytochrome b$_{-245}$ in the neutrophil membrane typically is normal but the cell is still incapable of generating superoxide in response to phagocytic or soluble stimuli.

- **A22 CGD** accounts for about 5% of cases of CGD and is characterised by an autosomal recessive mode of inheritance and a relatively mild clinical course. This form of CGD is caused by mutations of the gene which encodes the α subunit (p22-*phox*) of cytochrome b$_{-245}$ leading to a complete deficiency of cytochrome b$_{-245}$ (A22° CGD) or a normal membrane concentration of a dysfunctional cytochrome (A22$^+$ CGD). The absence of cytochrome b$_{-245}$ in both X91° and A22° CGD suggests that stability of the cytochrome requires the coincident expression of both components.

- **A67 CGD** has a similar incidence to A22 CGD and is caused by mutations of the p67-*phox* gene on chromosome 1. The molecular defects which lead to this form of CGD are unknown.

Chediak-Higashi-Steinbrinck Anomaly

Chediak-Higashi-Steinbrink (CHS) anomaly is a generalised disorder of lysosomal granules which is inherited as an autosomal recessive trait. CHS is characterised by partial albinism of the eyes and skin with silvery hair and an aversion to bright light; the presence of abnormally large lysosomal granules in granulocytes, melanocytes, and most other granule-containing cells of the body; a bleeding tendency and a susceptibility to recurrent respiratory and skin infections, most commonly with *Staphylococci* and other gram-positive bacteria.

The cause of CHS is unknown. The abnormal lysosomes in neutrophils are formed by the coalescence of primary granules. Neutrophil phagocytosis and respiratory burst activity appear to be normal in affected individuals but delivery of lysosomal enzymes from the abnormal granules is delayed, leading to a microbicidal defect. A range of other neutrophil functional defects have been described, including a deficiency of cathepsin G and elastase,

SAQ 5

Where are cathepsin G and elastase stored by neutrophils?

The mucopolysaccharidoses are caused by a deficiency of an enzyme required for the breakdown of mucopolysaccharides such as dermatan sulphate, heparan sulphate, keratan sulphate and chondroitin-6-sulphate. They are all inherited disorders and are characterised by the presence of coarse facial features, skeletal dysplasia, corneal clouding, mental retardation and a greatly reduced life expectancy.

Hunter's Syndrome is caused by deficiency of the enzyme iduronate sulphatase.

Hurler's Syndrome is caused by deficiency of the enzyme α-L-iduronidase.

Sanfillipo's Syndrome is clinically homogeneous but can be caused by deficiency of any of 4 different enzymes viz heparan N-sulphamidase, N-acetyl-α-D-glucosaminidase, heparin N-acetyl transferase and N-acetyl-α-D-glucosamine sulphatase.

Maroteaux-Lamy Syndrome is caused by the coincident deficiency of both aryl sulphatase B and galactosamine sulphatase.

impaired chemotactic response and failure of microtubule assembly. The bleeding tendency results from defective platelet function.

Most affected individuals die in the first few years of life from infection or haemorrhage. In the months leading up to their death, most experience a progressive worsening of their condition with lymphadenopathy, hepatosplenomegaly, peripheral neuropathy pancytopaenia and a deterioration of immune function.

Myeloperoxidase Deficiency

Myeloperoxidase deficiency probably is inherited in an autosomal dominant fashion and is the most common inherited defect of neutrophils, with an incidence of about 1 in 2000. Myeloperoxidase plays an important role in the intracellular killing of fungi such as *Candida spp* and *Aspergillus spp* and deficient neutrophils can be shown to have a grossly impaired fungicidal capacity *in vitro*. A small number of cases of candidiasis and aspergillosis in myeloperoxidase deficient individuals have been reported. However, because of the variety of myeloperoxidase-independent microbicidal mechanisms available to the neutrophil, there is no clinically significant susceptibility to infection in most cases.

Glucose-6-Phosphate Dehydrogenase Deficiency

Severe deficiency of G-6-PD is associated with an impairment of neutrophil bactericidal function. This defect is only seen when the level of neutrophil G-6-PD activity falls below 5% of normal.

Miscellaneous Defects

The following neutrophil defects typically are not associated with a significant degree of dysfunction.

Alder-Reilly Anomaly

The Alder-Reilly anomaly is characterised by the presence of enlarged cytoplasmic granulation in all types of leucocytes. These abnormal granules have been shown to be rich in mucopolysaccharide and are most frequently seen in the mucopolysaccharidoses such as Hunter's, Hurler's, Sanfillipo and Maroteaux-Lamy syndromes. There is no apparent defect of neutrophil function associated with this condition.

May-Hegglin Anomaly

May-Hegglin anomaly is a rare autosomal dominant condition which is characterised by the presence of basophilic inclusions in the cytoplasm of the neutrophils called **Döhle bodies**, giant platelets with a diameter of up to 20 µm and, in about a third of cases, thrombocytopaenia. Most affected individuals have no bleeding tendency despite the presence of the large, dysfunctional platelets and no increased susceptibility to infection. The Döhle bodies appear to consist mainly of RNA and are derived from the rough endoplasmic reticulum of the cell.

Döhle bodies are also seen in a variety of bacterial and viral infections and following severe burns. The two forms can be distinguished by the fact that, in infection, the Döhle bodies are few in number, are restricted to the neutrophil series and frequently are accompanied by toxic granulation, whereas in May-Hegglin anomaly they are more numerous and are present in all types of granulocyte.

Jordan's Anomaly

Jordan's anomaly has only ever been described in two families, both of whom showed prominent vacuolation of blood and bone marrow leucocytes. There were no apparent abnormalities of erythropoiesis or thrombopoiesis nor was there an obvious predisposition to infection in any of the affected family members. In one family, both affected individuals developed a progressive muscular dystrophy while in the other a non-infectious skin disease called icthyosis accompanied the disorder. The cause of this familial disorder is unknown.

Pelger-Huët Anomaly

Pelger-Huët anomaly is a relatively common autosomal dominant condition which is characterised by a failure of nuclear segmentation in granulocytes and megakaryocytes. Heterozygotes have a marked predominance of bilobed nuclei in peripheral blood neutrophils, the so-called "pince-nez" configuration. Homozygotes have a complete absence of neutrophil nuclear segmentation. Neither form of this condition appears to be associated with a susceptibility to infection or any measurable defect of neutrophil function. It is important that this benign condition should be differentiated from the left shift of neutrophils seen in severe infections.

Pince-nez are spectacles which have no legs, but are fixed to the nose by means of a spring clip. They appear to be worn only by stereotypical scientists in Hollywood and old British films. These characters always perch their pince-nez on the very tips of their noses and peer over the top of them in an extremely condescending manner at lesser mortals (ie non-scientists!). This unappealing trait is supposed, by film-makers, to represent the apparently universal dual idiosyncrasies of all scientists namely, intellectual superiority and eccentricity.

Disorders of Acquired Immunity

The primary disorders of acquired immunity may, for the purposes of discussion, be divided into those which predominantly affect humoral immunity, those which predominantly affect cell-mediated immunity and combined immunodeficiencies. As described previously, the immune system functions in a highly integrated manner and it must be remembered that such divisions are simplistic. Disorders of acquired immunity typically are manifest as a susceptibility to infection or an increased incidence of certain malignant or autoimmune conditions.

Disorders of Humoral Immunity

The primary disorders of humoral immunity are characterised by a deficiency of immunoglobulin or Complement components. Typically these conditions are manifest as a susceptibility to infection with encapsulated organisms due to failure of opsonisation.

Bruton's Agammaglobulinaemia

Bruton's agammaglobulinaemia is an X-linked recessive condition which is characterised by B lymphopaenia, a failure of immunoglobulin gene rearrangement and a consequent arrest of B lymphoid maturation at the pre-B lymphocyte stage, leading to an inability to mount an antibody response to antigenic challenge. The T lymphocyte compartment is normal in size and function in this condition.

Female carriers of Bruton's agammaglobulinaemia have normal numbers of circulating B lymphocytes and have no observable immunological deficit. This can be explained by the fact that those lymphoid stem cells which, early in embryonic life, have their abnormal X chromosome inactivated have a selective growth advantage over those which express the aberrant gene. A few case reports exist of females with a condition similar to Bruton's agammaglobulinaemia. This is thought to reflect the existence of an extremely rare autosomal recessive variant of this condition.

The inability to synthesise endogenous immunoglobulin is present at birth in affected infants but passively acquired maternal immunoglobulin affords some protection from infection in the early months of life. However, by the age of 6 months, this protection is lost and the typical pattern of recurrent pyogenic infections of the respiratory tract, sinuses, middle ear and skin becomes established. The most common infecting organisms are encapsulated bacteria which are resistant to phagocytosis such as *Haemophilus influenzae, Staphylococcus aureas, Streptococcus pneumoniae* and *Pseudomonas aeruginosa.* Treatment for this condition consists of immunoglobulin replacement therapy, prophylactic antimicrobial chemotherapy and the prompt and aggressive treatment of established infections. Vaccination using attenuated live organisms is contra-indicated. Failure to treat chronic and deep-seated infections effectively can lead to progressive pulmonary damage.

In addition to the susceptibility to infection, Bruton's agammaglobulinaemia is associated with a variety of collagen vascular disorders and conditions which mimic autoimmune diseases such as rheumatoid arthritis, dermatomyositis and haemolytic anaemia but in the absence of detectable autoantibodies. The pathogenesis of these complications is obscure.

Hypogammaglobulinaemia with Raised IgM Concentration

This condition is characterised by a selective deficiency of the immunoglobulins IgG, IgA and IgE in the presence of an increased concentration of IgM and IgD. It is inherited as an X-linked recessive disorder and is associated with a similar clinical pattern to Bruton's agammaglobulinaemia. Recent studies have shown that the B lymphocytes of affected individuals are not incapable of synthesising IgG, IgA and IgE, suggesting that this disorder arises as a result of a lack of T lymphocyte control of the immunoglobulin isotype switching mechanism. Other aspects of T lymphocyte function are normal. Rare autosomal variants of this condition have been described.

Selective Immunoglobulin Deficiencies

Selective IgA deficiency is, by far, the most common immunoglobulin deficiency, affecting almost 0.2% of the world's population. In the vast majority of cases, IgA deficiency is not associated with any obvious immune deficit. In some cases, however, mild recurrent respiratory tract infections, and a tendency to develop autoimmune conditions such as rheumatoid arthritis and systemic lupus erythematosus are observed.

Selective deficiency of one or more IgG subclass is associated with susceptibility to recurrent infection. As described in the previous chapter, the different types of immunoglobulin have distinct biological functions: IgG_1 is associated with antibodies directed against protein antigens and antiviral antibodies; IgG_2 is associated with antibody directed against polyvalent polysaccharide antigens; IgG_3 is associated with antibody directed against protein antigens and IgG_4 is associated with antiparasitic antibodies. Armed with this knowledge, the outcome of selective IgG subclass deficiency is predictable. For example, selective deficiency of IgG_2 is associated with recurrent middle ear and sinus infections involving encapsulated bacteria such as *Haemophilus influenzae*, *Neisseria meningitidis* and *Streptococcus pneumoniae*. Antibody responses to other protein antigenic challenges is normal.

Selective IgM deficiency is characterised by recurrent bacterial infections and a susceptibility to blood-borne dissemination of infection. This disorder is thought to be caused by T lymphocyte-mediated suppression of IgM synthesis rather than an inability to synthesise IgM.

Selective IgE deficiency is associated with lymphopaenia and recurrent pulmonary infections leading to chronic lung disease.

Transient Hypogammaglobulinaemia of Infancy

This relatively benign condition is caused by the delayed onset of endogenous immunoglobulin synthesis due to a functional deficiency of T_H lymphocytes. It is a self-limiting condition: most cases have resolved by the age of 2 years. Interestingly, the incidence of transient hypogammaglobulinaemia is higher in families with immunodeficiency states such as severe combined immunodeficiency (SCID).

Deficiency of Complement Components

Hereditary deficiencies of virtually all of the components of the Complement system have been described. All are rare disorders which, with the sole exception of C1 esterase inhibitor deficiency, are inherited in an autosomal recessive fashion. C1 esterase inhibitor deficiency results in a disorder called **angioneurotic oedema** and is inherited in an autosomal dominant fashion. In contrast to the rarity of inherited deficiencies of the Complement system, acquired deficiency of one or more Complement components is a relatively common finding in a range of autoimmune disorders. The clinical outcome of an inherited Complement deficiency can be predicted by studying the interactions between the two Complement activation pathways. A deficiency involving C1, C2 or C4 is clinically mild because the resulting defect of the classical pathway of Complement activation can be offset by the activity of the alternative pathway. These deficiencies are associated with a collection of disorders which mimic the autoimmune disorder systemic lupus erythematosus. Deficiency of any component of the non-specific alternative pathway is associated with a relatively severe susceptibility to infection, particularly with *Neisseria spp.*

Angioneurotic oedema is characterised by recurrent swelling in the submucosal tissue of the gastrointestinal and respiratory tracts and of the skin. These swellings may be triggered by a variety of stimuli such as minor trauma, exercise and exposure to cold or heat, and cause a variety of symptoms such as abdominal cramps, bowel disturbances and respiratory embarrassment which may be life-threatening.

Disorders of Cell-mediated Immunity

The primary disorders of cell-mediated immunity typically are manifest as a susceptibility to fungal and viral infection due to the failure of T_H lymphocyte function and of T_c lymphocytes to kill virus infected cells.

DiGeorge Syndrome

DiGeorge syndrome is an acquired disorder which arises as a result of faulty development of the third and fourth pharyngeal pouches in embryonic life leading to an absence, or incomplete development, of thymus and parathyroid glands. This disorder is thought to be caused by a variety of insults such as intra-uterine infections or excessive maternal alcohol intake during the first trimester of pregnancy.

DiGeorge syndrome is highly variable in severity but, in its most severe form, is characterised by facial malformations, anatomical abnormalities of the heart and great vessels, hypocalcaemia and defective T lymphocyte function which is manifest as an extreme susceptibility to viral, fungal and bacterial infections. At the other extreme, affected infants may have only minimal immunodeficiency and hypoparathyroidism. In all cases, B lymphocyte number and function is normal. However, the ability to mount an antibody response is impaired because of the absence of T_H lymphocytes.

The treatment for DiGeorge syndrome requires reconstitution of the T lymphocyte compartment. This can be achieved either by transplantation of foetal thymus gland or, more commonly nowadays, by bone marrow transplantation. These dangerous and expensive procedures cannot be justified in those infants with inoperable cardiac or other abnormalities.

Acquired Immunodeficiency Syndrome

SAQ 6

What unique property distinguishes retroviruses?

Acquired immunodeficiency syndrome (AIDS) was first recognised as a new and distinct condition in 1981. In the ensuing 13 years, this syndrome has generated more hysteria, had more written about it and had more money spent on it than any other disease in history. A full description of AIDS and its sequelae is beyond the scope of this book. This section is confined to a brief summary of some of the most important aspects of this syndrome.

Most workers believe that the causative agent of AIDS is one or other of the human immunodeficiency viruses (HIV-1 and HIV-2), but a small number of scientists dissent from this view. These retroviruses bind specifically via the envelope glycoprotein gp120 to CD4 molecules on the surfaces of lymphocytes, monocytes and macrophages. Primary infection of a cell with HIV results in the incorporation of viral DNA into the host genome. Infected cells may remain dormant for some time, but sooner or later they are stimulated and then synthesise new infective virions which burst forth from the cell and propagate the infection. HIV infection of T_H lymphocytes results in derangement of their function and, eventually, prompts their destruction. The early stages of HIV infection are characterised by a gradual loss of T_H lymphocytes and an exaggeration of the humoral response, which is manifest as an increased incidence of autoimmune conditions such as ITP and isoimmune neutropaenia. Disease progression is marked by worsening T_H lymphopaenia and a progressive loss of both cell-mediated and humoral immune responses. Infected monocytes and macrophages are not killed by HIV infection. These cells appear to act as a viral reservoir, transporting virus throughout the body and are thought to contribute to the propagation of the infection by releasing large amounts of IL-1 and tumour necrosis factor. HIV has also been shown to infect brain glial cells, fibroblasts and epithelial cells.

The time taken to develop symptoms of immunodeficiency following HIV infection varies tremendously and may be as long as 10 years. The reason for this variability is unclear but recent evidence has suggested that MHC status may play a part in resistance to disease progression. HIV-associated disease progresses through a number of clinically defined stages before full-blown AIDS is manifest as shown in Table 14.3

Group	Subgroup	Defining features
I		Acute infection produces an illness similar to infectious mononucleosis with anti-HIV seroconversion
II		Asymptomatic infection associated with progressive loss of immune function
III		Persistent generalised lymphadenopathy ie 2 or more lymph nodes >1 cm in diameter which persist for more than 3 months. Other causes must be excluded
IV	A	Constitutional disease eg unexplained loss of >10% of body weight or persistent unexplained fever or diarrhoea
	B	Neurological disease such as unexplained dementia, myelopathy or peripheral neuropathy
	C	Opportunistic infections secondary to defective cell-mediated immunity eg *Pneumocystis carinii* pneumonia, *Cryptosporidium, Toxoplasma gondii, Strongyloides stercoralis, Candida spp, Mycobacteria spp, Herpes zoster & simplex,* CMV, oral hairy leucoplakia
	D	Kaposi's sarcoma, NHL or primary lymphoma of the brain
	E	Other groups not defined above

Table 14.3 *Clinical staging of AIDS*

HIV infection is associated with a variety of haematological complications which increase in frequency and severity as the disease progresses. The most frequently observed complications include anaemia, granulocytopaenia, lymphopaenia, thrombocytopaenia, antiphospholipid syndrome and a tendency to develop lymphoid malignancies such as NHL and HD.

The degree of anaemia typically is mild in the early stages of HIV infection but may become severe enough to require blood transfusion in full-blown AIDS. In untreated cases, anaemia usually is normocytic and normochromic and is secondary to T lymphocyte-mediated suppression of CFU-GEMM and BFU-E. The anaemia of chronic disease may also play a role, particularly during infections and in secondary malignant conditions. A failure to synthesise erythropoietin in response to tissue hypoxia has also been reported in a number of cases. The treatment of HIV disease frequently exacerbates the degree of anaemia. Azidothymidine (AZT) is used to inhibit viral replication but is severely myelotoxic. The development of severe anaemia, granulocytopaenia and thrombocytopaenia frequently limit the use of this agent. Several of the antimicrobial agents used to treat the recurrent infections which punctuate the course of this disease also are myelotoxic. Finally, although red cell autoantibodies are common in AIDS, significant AIHA is not.

Granulocytopaenia is present in up to three quarters of AIDS cases and is secondary to T lymphocyte-mediated suppression of CFU-GEMM and CFU-GM which is exacerbated by the secretion of IL-1 and tumour necrosis factor by HIV-infected monocytes and macrophages. As described above, treatment with AZT also is associated with severe neutropaenia. In addition to the neutropaenia, defects of all phases of neutrophil function have been reported. Neutrophil autoantibodies commonly are present during the course of HIV infection, but do not appear to contribute to the development of neutropaenia.

Autoimmune thrombocytopaenia is a feature of about 50% of AIDS cases, although bleeding is seldom a problem except in haemophiliacs. AITP may develop fairly early in the course of HIV infection, and may even be the presenting feature.

Up to two thirds of HIV-positive individuals develop an antiphospholipid antibody at some stage of their disease. Unlike the classical lupus inhibitor, these antibodies are not associated with a thrombotic tendency. There is some evidence that the development of antiphospholipid antibodies and *Pneumocystis carinii* pneumonia may be related.

About 5% of cases of full-blown AIDS develop non-Hodgkin's lymphoma. The incidence of this complication is expected to rise as the success of antiretroviral and antimicrobial chemotherapy improve. Involvement of the CNS and other extranodal sites is much more common in AIDS-related lymphomas which also are more aggressive and more refractory to treatment than in HIV-negative individuals. Treatment of AIDS-related NHL is further complicated by the tendency to panhypoplasia described above.

Wiskott-Aldrich Syndrome

Wiskott-Aldrich syndrome is an X-linked recessive disorder which is characterised by recurrent viral and bacterial infections, thrombocytopaenia and eczema. The pattern of recurrent cytomegalovirus, herpes simplex and *Pneumocystis carinii* infections and periodic bleeding secondary to thrombocytopaenia is clearly established by the age of 6 months. Wiskott-Aldrich syndrome typically follows a downward spiral with a progressive worsening of immune status secondary to T lymphopaenia and T lymphocyte dysfunction and a concomitant increase in the frequency and severity of infections. Most affected boys die in the first few years of life, most commonly from disseminated infection. In addition to the bleeding and infectious problems, there is an increased incidence of aggressive lymphoid malignancies associated with this condition.

Despite the identification of numerous characteristic immunological abnormalities and the localisation of the aberrant gene responsible for Wiskott-Aldrich syndrome to Xp11.1, the pathogenesis of this condition remains obscure.

Short-limbed Dwarfism with Immunodeficiency

Short-limbed dwarfism with immunodeficiency describes a collection of disorders which are characterised by stunted growth of arms and legs secondary to metaphyseal and epiphyseal dysplasia, fine, sparse hair and a variety of T and B lymphocyte abnormalities. The T lymphocyte abnormalities described in association with short-limbed dwarfism include T lymphopaenia, impaired delayed hypersensitivity response and delayed rejection of foreign tissue grafts. In most cases, immune status deteriorates over time, leading to an increase in infectious complications. However, the recurrent viral and bacterial infections which punctuate this condition typically are relatively mild and seldom are life-threatening. Most affected individuals have normal B lymphocyte function.

Combined Humoral and Cell-mediated Immunodeficiency

Severe Combined Immunodeficiency

Severe combined immunodeficiency (SCID) is a highly disparate group of inherited conditions whose defining feature is a severe defect of both T and B lymphocyte function, leading to devastating viral and opportunistic infections. The most common infectious complications include *Pneumocystis carinii* pneumonia, disseminated candidiasis, herpes simplex, adenovirus and cytomegalovirus infections. The only currently viable treatment for SCID is bone marrow transplantation, although gene replacement therapy holds long-term promise.

The X-linked recessive form of SCID is caused by an aberrant gene on Xq13 which precludes T lymphocyte development, resulting in thymic aplasia, absolute T lymphopaenia and hypoplasia of the lymph nodes. Any circulating B lymphocytes present are incapable of mounting any form of immune response in the absence of T lymphocytes. The mode of action of the normal equivalent of the SCID gene is poorly understood, at present.

Several different forms of SCID exist which are inherited in an autosomal recessive manner. The most common of these is deficiency of the purine degradation enzyme **adenosine deaminase (ADA)**. Deficiency of this enzyme is estimated to account for almost 50% of autosomal recessive cases of SCID. The gene for ADA resides on chromosome 20.

Within the cell, ADA catalyses the deamination of adenosine and deoxyadenosine to form inosine and deoxyinosine respectively. ADA deficiency, therefore, is accompanied by the intracellular accumulation of deoxyadenosine and, more importantly, its metabolite deoxyadenosine triphosphate (dATP). This latter substance acts as a powerful inhibitor of the enzyme ribonucleotide reductase which is uniquely responsible for the production of deoxynucleotides for DNA synthesis. The resulting dearth of deoxynucleotides leads to a severe impairment of DNA synthesis. T lymphocyte precursors are particularly susceptible to the toxic effects of dATP accumulation for two reasons:

- T lymphocyte precursors have a relatively high concentration of the enzyme deoxycytidine kinase in comparison to other cells. Normally, this enzyme catalyses the phosphorylation of deoxycytidine but, in the presence of a large excess of deoxyadenosine, it will act preferentially on this substrate. Thus, the accumulation of the toxic metabolite, dATP, is enhanced in T lymphocyte precursors.

- the activity of the nucleotidase enzymes which dephosphorylate dATP is relatively low in T lymphocyte precursors. Thus, dATP removal is slower in T lymphocyte precursors.

Another enzyme of the purine degradation pathway is implicated as a cause of autosomal recessive SCID viz **purine nucleoside phosphorylase (PNP)**. The PNP gene resides on chromosome 14. PNP catalyses the conversion of inosine and deoxyinosine to form hypoxanthine and also guanosine and deoxyguanosine to form guanine. Thus, in a similar way to ADA deficiency, PNP deficiency results in the intracellular accumulation of the toxic metabolite dGTP with gross impairment of DNA synthesis.

Common Variable Immunodeficiency

The term common variable immunodeficiency (CVID) encompasses a number of acquired disorders which are characterised by panhypogammaglobulinaemia, an impaired ability to mount an antibody response to antigenic challenge and recurrent bacterial infections. Most affected individuals are young adults, although CVID has been described in all age groups. A variety of immune defects have been described in association with this disorder, including T and B lymphocyte dysfunction, an increase in the number of T_s lymphocytes, circulating autoantibodies directed against both T and B lymphocytes and an increased incidence of autoimmune diseases such as systemic lupus erythematosus (SLE), idiopathic thrombocytopaenic purpura (ITP), autoimmune haemolytic anaemia (AIHA) and pernicious anaemia (PA). Immunoglobulin replacement therapy remedies the susceptibility to bacterial infection.

Bare Lymphocyte Syndrome

There are two forms of bare lymphocyte syndrome, both of which are inherited in an autosomal recessive fashion. In MHC class I deficiency, there is a complete absence of MHC class I (HLA-A, B and C) molecules on leucocyte surfaces but MHC class II (HLA-DR) molecules are expressed normally. In the less common MHC class II deficiency, HLA-DR expression is absent, while MHC class I expression is normal. Because MHC molecules have a controlling influence in T lymphocyte development and also function as recognition molecules for antigen presentation, the result of bare lymphocyte syndrome is a profound deficiency of both humoral and cell-mediated immunity and the familiar pattern of severe, recurrent viral, fungal and bacterial infections. However, in contrast to all forms of SCID, the circulating lymphocyte count typically is normal and lymph nodes are normal in size.

Ataxia Telangiectasia

Ataxia telangiectasia is inherited in an autosomal recessive fashion and is characterised by a progressive loss of control over motor function leading to jerky, uncoordinated movements (ataxia), the development of visible malformations of the capillaries in the skin and mucous membranes (telangiectases), chromosomal fragility and combined immunodeficiency with recurrent viral and bacterial infections. The chromosomal breakpoints are non-random. More than half occur close to the immunoglobulin heavy chain gene complex on chromosome 14 or the T lymphocyte receptor gene complexes on chromosomes 7 and 14. The aberrant gene responsible for ataxia telangiectasia is located at 11q22-33. The product of the normal counterpart of the ataxia telangiectasia gene remains to be identified but it seems likely that it is involved in the process of repair at sites of genetic recombination. Absence of this gene product causes a failure of immunoglobulin superfamily gene rearrangement and leads to a maturation arrest in both T and B lymphocyte precursors. The consequence of this is a gross impairment of both T and B lymphocyte function, lymphopenia, disturbances of immunoglobulin concentration and impairment of delayed hypersensitivity.

In addition to the progressive motor dysfunction and the infectious complications, ataxia telangiectasia is associated with an excess incidence of lymphoid and other malignant conditions.

Suggested Further Reading

Roitt, I.M. (1988). *Essential Immunology, (6th edn)*. Oxford: Blackwell Scientific Publications.

Brenner, M.K. and Hoffbrand, A.V. (1989). Normal lymphocytes and their benign disorders. In *Postgraduate Haematology* (3rd edn) (eds A.V. Hoffbrand and S.M. Lewis). Oxford: Butterworth-Heinemann.

Roitt, I., Brostoff, J. and Male, D. (1988). *Immunology*. London: Gower Medical Publishing.

Seligman, M. and Hitzig, W.H. (eds) (1980). *Primary Immunodeficiencies*. New York: Elsevier-North Holland Biomedical Press.

DeVita, V.T., Hellman, S. and Rosenberg, S.A. (eds) (1988). *AIDS: Etiology, Diagnosis, Treatment and Prevention*. Philadelphia: J.B. Lippincott.

Answers to Self-Assessment Questions

1. Intact skin and mucous membranes form a physical barrier to the entry of microorganisms into the tissues. Conditions which are associated with disruption of this barrier such as burns and eczema predispose strongly to bacterial infection.

2. T_H, T_{DTH} carry CD4 molecules on their membranes, but not CD8 molecules. Small cortical thymocytes carry both CD4 and CD8 molecules.

3. Neutrophils carry specific receptors for the Complement fragment C3b, making it a powerful opsonin. The most important chemotactic factor is C5a.

4. NADPH is derived from the hexose monophosphate shunt.

5. Cathepsin G and elastase are stored in neutrophil primary granules.

6. Retroviruses are capable of reverse transcription ie converting viral RNA into DNA for incorporation into the host genome.

Malignant Disorders of the Blood: an Overview

Malignant disorders of the blood are characterised by an untram-melled clonal proliferation of haemopoietic cells. Numerous classi-fication schemes exist for this group of disorders. In this book, the different haemopoietic malignancies are grouped under one of the following headings:

- the acute leukaemias

- the chronic leukaemias

- the myelodysplastic syndromes

- the non-leukaemic lymphoproliferative disorders

- the non-leukaemic myeloproliferative disorders

The specific characteristics of each group is considered in detail in the following chapters. This chapter concentrates on topics which are important across the spectrum of haemopoietic malignancy.

The Acute Leukaemias

Acute leukaemias are characterised by an uncontrolled prolifera-tion of poorly differentiated cells (blasts). The acute leukaemias are divided on the basis of the predominant haemopoietic lineage involved into **acute lymphoblastic leukaemia (ALL)** and **acute non-lymphoblastic leukaemia (ANLL)**. The most widely used system of classification of the acute leukaemias is the French-American-British or **FAB system**. The FAB system classifies indi-vidual cases of acute leukaemia according to their morphological appearance on Romanowsky-stained bone marrow smears. This system is described in detail in the next chapter. Briefly, ALL is divided into three subtypes designated L1, L2 and L3 and ANLL is divided into seven subtypes designated M1-M7. A further sub-type of ANLL, M0, is characterised by an absence of cytochemical reac-tivity.

The division of the leukaemias into acute and chronic types describes the natural history of the diseases in the absence of treatment. In these circumstances, acute leukaemia typically is fatal within weeks or months of diagnosis. In contrast, sur-vival in chronic leukaemia is measured in years. Modern treatment methods have made the distinction in sur-vival time between acute and chronic leukaemias much less clear, however. In general, the acute leukaemias have proved to be more amenable to treatment than the chronic types. For example, acute lymphoblastic leukaemia of childhood is now considered to be a curable disease whereas conventional cyto-toxic chemotherapy for chronic myeloid leukaemia is palliative and does not signif-icantly influence survival.

The Chronic Leukaemias

Chronic leukaemias differ from acute types in that the predominant cell type shows some characteristics of maturity. The need for a standardised system of classification for the chronic leukaemias is not so great since they usually are easily recognisable on the basis of cell morphology and cytochemistry. There are four subtypes of chronic leukaemia: **chronic lymphocytic leukaemia (CLL); pro-lymphocytic leukaemia (PLL); hairy cell leukaemia (HCL)** and **chronic myeloid leukaemia (CML)**. A fifth type, chronic myelomonocytic leukaemia (CMML) is considered with the myelodysplastic syndromes.

The Myelodysplastic Syndromes

The myelodysplastic syndromes can be thought of as preleukaemic conditions. They are classified according to FAB criteria into **refractory anaemia (RA), refractory anaemia with sideroblasts (RAS), refractory anaemia with excess of blasts (RAEB), refractory anaemia with excess of blasts in transformation (RAEB-t)** and **chronic myelomonocytic leukaemia (CMML)**. The classification criteria are described in Chapter 18.

The Non-leukaemic Lymphoproliferative Disorders

This diverse group of conditions includes **multiple myeloma (MM)** and related plasma cell disorders, **Hodgkin's disease (HD)** and the **Non-Hodgkin's lymphomas (NHL)**. These conditions and their classification are considered in Chapter 19.

The Non-leukaemic Myeloproliferative Disorders

There are three different non-leukaemic myeloproliferative disorders viz **primary proliferative polycythaemia (PPP), primary thrombocythaemia** and **myelofibrosis**. These conditions are considered in Chapter 19.

Epidemiology of Haemopoietic Malignancy

Epidemiology is a statistical approach to the study of disease incidence, distribution and aetiology. It involves statistical surveys of defined populations to determine the incidence of the disease under study and factors such as age, sex, race, occupation and socioeconomic status which may influence the disease incidence. **Descriptive studies** such as this are designed to discern statistically significant *associations* between the disease and one or more of the factors under study. For example, suppose that a descriptive study revealed a clear association between disease X and exposure to an imaginary pesticide, DPD. Although tempting, it cannot be concluded that exposure to DPD *causes* disease X, that requires the performance of **analytical studies**.

Analytical studies in this case would attempt to quantify the risk of developing disease X in those exposed to DPD and to determine whether the association can be considered to be cause and effect. This is accomplished using both **retrospective case control studies** which compare the incidence of exposure to DPD in confirmed cases of disease X with that in a carefully matched, disease-free control group, and **prospective cohort studies** which follow a disease-free group to determine the incidence of disease X. The incidence of the disease in those exposed to DPD can then be compared to the incidence in those not so exposed. Similarly, failure to develop disease X following exposure to DPD can be determined.

Definitive evidence that DPD is a cause of disease X would ideally include a statistically significant excess of the disease in those exposed in both retrospective and prospective studies, evidence of a dose effect, evidence that removal of exposure diminishes the incidence of the disease and evidence that the disease can be induced experimentally in animals by exposing them to DPD. Such complete evidence is difficult to obtain in many cases.

Epidemiological studies of the haemopoietic malignancies have always been difficult to perform because of the relative rarity of the conditions and the problems of misdiagnosis and misclassification. However, the use of objective classification systems such as the FAB system for the acute leukaemias and myelodysplastic syndromes have increased concordance between investigators sufficiently to permit the gathering of reliable international data.

Acute Leukaemia

The most reliable data for the incidence of acute leukaemia in the UK come from the *Leukaemia/Lymphoma Atlas of the United Kingdom* which was prepared under the auspices of the Leukaemia Research Fund.

As shown in Figure 15.1, ALL is most common in childhood with a peak incidence at age 4 or 5 years.

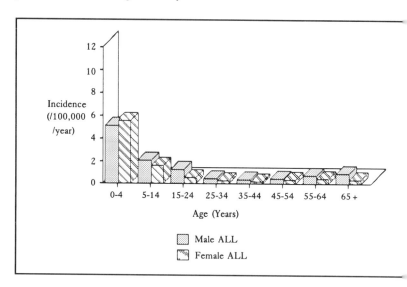

Figure 15.1 *Age- and sex-related incidence of ALL in the UK*

Childhood ALL is more common in the developed countries of the world (Figure 15.2) whereas in relatively underdeveloped countries lymphoma predominates in this age group. For example, in Uganda, lymphoma is about 15-20 times more common in the under 14's than leukaemia.

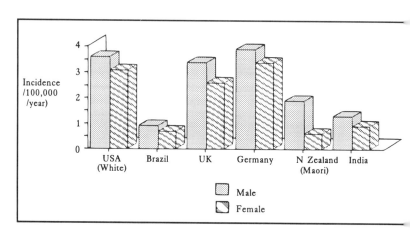

Figure 15.2 *The incidence of childhood ALL in developed and developing countries (age-matched 0-14 years)*

In contrast to ALL, the incidence of ANLL is greatest in middle to old age, being most common in males over the age of 65 (Figure 15.3). Although ALL predominates in young children, ANLL also shows a minor peak incidence in children under the age of 5 years.

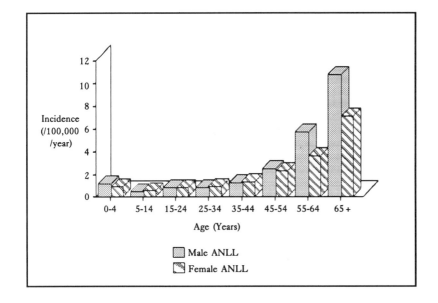

Figure 15.3 *Age- and sex-related incidence of ANLL in the UK*

Chronic Leukaemia

As shown in Figure 15.4, CLL is very rare below the age of 30 years but then increases sharply with increasing age. There is little difference in the overall incidence of CLL in white and black populations but the disease has a much lower frequency in Asians over the age of 55 years. For example, in Canada and Scandinavia CLL forms about one third of all leukaemias whereas in Japan this figure is reduced to less than 5% of the total.

CLL is more common in men than in women with most countries having a male:female ratio of between 1.5 and 2.5. The excess of CLL is most remarkable in Australia where the male:female ratio is as high as 4.7.

Figure 15.4 shows that CML is primarily a disease of middle to old age but a small peak in incidence is discernible in most studies in white boys under the age of 5 years. In this younger age group, most cases are the Philadelphia chromosome negative juvenile vari-

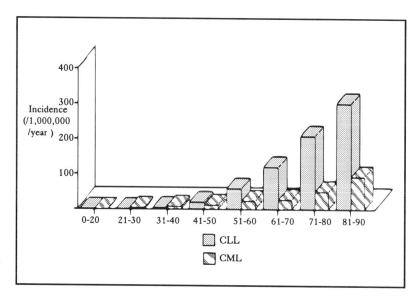

Figure 15.4 *Age-related incidence of CML and CLL in the UK*

ant of CML. The incidence of classical CML begins to rise in adolescence and then increases steadily with age. Variation of CML incidence with ethnic background is much less impressive than for CLL although the disease appears to be more common in young blacks than whites. CML is slightly more common in men than in women. Most studies have shown a male:female ratio for CML of between 1.0 and 2.0. The age standardised international incidence of both CLL and CML is shown in Figure 15.5.

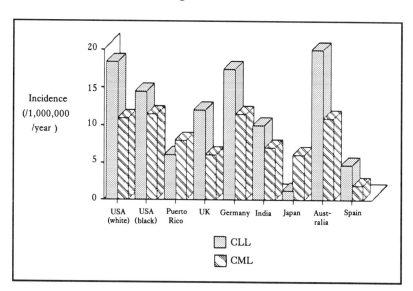

Figure 15.5 *The age standardised incidence of CLL and CML in developed and developing countries*

The incidence of both CML and CLL and the median survival times have stayed remarkably stable over the last 20 years or so. Studies which show an increased incidence of either disease are thought to reflect improved diagnosis and increased access to health care.

Non-leukaemic Lymphoproliferative Disorders

Hodgkin's disease (HD) has an overall incidence of about 2.5 per 100,000/year in the UK and has a bimodal age distribution as shown in Figure 15.6. HD is relatively uncommon in children in developed countries such as the UK, the most commonly affected age group being young adults in the third decade of life. A second peak incidence occurs in those over the age of 55 years in most studies, but some workers doubt the validity of this observation. A different age distribution is common in developing countries, where the highest incidence of HD occurs in children and a second, smaller peak occurs in the elderly. HD is a rare condition in young adults in developing countries.

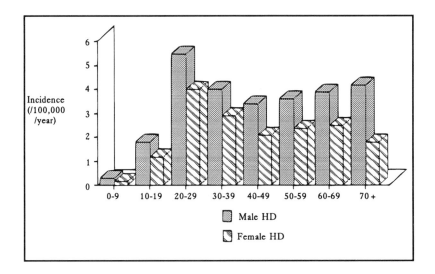

Figure 15.6 *The age- and sex-related incidence of Hodgkin's disease in the UK*

Overall, HD is slightly more common in males with most studies showing a male:female ratio of about 1.5. This sex difference is most pronounced in childhood and the elderly.

Socioeconomic status is an important risk factor in all forms of lymphoma (HD and NHL), with higher socioeconomic status being associated with an increased incidence. The fact that lymphomas are more common in whites than blacks in developed countries probably reflects the role of socioeconomic conditions rather than a true racial difference. The incidence of the lymphomas is rising in the developed countries of the world.

Epidemiological studies of non-Hodgkin's lymphoma (NHL) have been greatly hampered by confusion over the classification of this heterogeneous group of disorders. Reliable data are available for most developed countries but the picture in developing countries is much less clear. Overall, NHL is about four times more common than HD. The incidence of NHL rises with age, most obviously after the age of 40 years: these disorders are rare in children.

Multiple myeloma (MM) is predominantly a disease of old age, with a median age at diagnosis of 70 years. The disorder is more common in men with a male:female ratio of about 1.5. In contrast to HD and NHL, MM is much more common in blacks than whites and socioeconomic status does not appear to be an important factor. The incidence of MM appears to be rising in the developed world; reliable statistics generally are unavailable for most developing countries.

Aetiology of Haemopoietic Malignancy

As explained above, much of our current understanding of the aetiology of haemopoietic malignancy has been derived from epidemiological studies. Such studies are notoriously difficult to perform, bedevilled as they are by the rarity of the conditions under study, by lack of reliable historical data and by the confounding influences of socioeconomic factors such as access to health care. The results of such studies must always be interpreted with caution.

Although exposure to certain environmental conditions, drugs and chemicals has been shown to be associated with the development of haematological malignancy, proof that this is cause and effect often is lacking. In addition, only a relatively small proportion of individuals exposed to these carcinogenic factors actually develops a malignant condition, suggesting that other factors such as genetic constitution may be operating.

The following factors are widely regarded as being involved in the aetiology of haemopoietic malignancy:

- ionising radiation

- therapeutic drugs

- chemicals

- viruses

- familial and genetic factors

Ionising Radiation

The atomic bombs which were dropped on Hiroshima and Nagasaki have provided incontrovertible evidence that exposure to doses of ionising radiation in excess of 1 Gray (Gy) is leukaemogenic. An increased incidence of CML, ALL, ANLL and MM in survivors of these horrific events was identified in 1948, and a long-term follow-up study commenced two years later. The frequency of these forms of leukaemia continued to increase for a further 10 years. After this period, the incidence of CML returned to normal. ANLL and ALL are still more common in this unfortunate group of people than in those not exposed. The excess risk is greater in males and increases with increasing age at the time of exposure.

Confirmatory evidence that the observed excess of leukaemia was attributable to the effects of the atomic bombs was provided by the dual observations that the risk of developing leukaemia was inversely related to the distance from the hypocentre of the explosion and that survivors of the Hiroshima bomb, which emitted a greater level of neutron radiation than that dropped on Nagasaki, were more likely to develop leukaemia. There was no observable increase in the incidence of CLL or lymphoma observed in either group of survivors. Both of these conditions are relatively rare in Japan.

Chronic exposure to therapeutic X irradiation also has been associated with an increased incidence of leukaemia, aplastic anaemia and solid tumours in heavily exposed tissue. The risk of leukaemogenesis is especially high if alkylating agents are used concurrently. Retrospective studies of cause of death in medical staff showed an excess of fatal leukaemia in radiologists prior to 1940. This excess disappeared following the introduction of adequate shielding and dosage monitoring in such staff. Foetal exposure to X-rays in the

The biological damage inflicted by ionising radiation largely is determined by the dosage which is defined in terms of the amount of energy transferred to the irradiated tissue. Dosage is expressed in Gray where 1 Gray is equivalent to the absorption of 1 joule of energy per kilogram of irradiated tissue. The older unit of dosage was the rad. 1 Gy = 100 rad.

Several factors influence the sensitivity of tissues to radiation damage as discussed in the text.

A new, UK Government-sponsored study of the Sellafield controversy was launched in 1993. The study is being carried out by the independent Committee on the Medical Aspects of Radiation in the Environment (COMARE) and is investigating 3 aspects of the controversy viz the epidemiology of malignant disease in the region of Sellafield and other nuclear installations; a review of the exposure to radiation of the local people (there is considerable doubt over the accuracy of past figures) and a review of the possibility that fathers exposed to radiation during their work in nuclear installations may pass on a susceptibility to leukaemia in their children.

The third arm of the study is a follow up to the Gardner report which found evidence for such a link. The study has been called into question by other workers in the field and by the apparent lack of such an excess of leukaemia in the children of the survivors of the Hiroshima and Nagasaki atomic bombs.

first trimester of pregnancy has been shown to be associated with an increased incidence of ALL and other malignancies in infancy.

The effect of long-term, low-level exposure to natural background ionising radiation or, more controversially, living near or working in nuclear reprocessing plants or other nuclear installations remains undetermined. Much attention has centred on the village of Seascale in Cumbria which lies close to the nuclear reprocessing plant at Sellafield. A 1984 Government Committee of Inquiry concluded that a cluster of ALL existed in the children of the area and that further study was needed. It has subsequently been shown that the excess risk appears to be restricted to children born in the area; no excess risk was found in children who moved into the area after birth. A recent study linking childhood ALL to fathers who work in the nuclear industry has added to the controversy. There is no conclusive proof that this cluster is radiation-induced.

It is unlikely that epidemiological methods will ever be able to provide definitive proof of the existence or otherwise of a leukaemogenic effect at such low levels of exposure. Any effect which might exist would almost certainly be very small and therefore would be difficult to extract from other possible aetiological factors.

Sporadic reports of an association between low frequency non-ionising radiation such as that encountered near high-tension power lines and leukaemia exist. Biological and epidemiological evidence for any such effect is highly controversial.

Therapeutic Drugs

As described later in this chapter, treatment of established malignancy often involves the administration of cytotoxic drugs. The use of one particular group of cytotoxic drugs, the **alkylating agents**, is associated strongly with an increased incidence of secondary ANLL. The median length of time from initiation of therapy and the development of ANLL is about 4 years. Some other cytotoxic agents, eg epipodophyllotoxin, have been implicated in the development of secondary ANLL, but the association is not so clear as for the alkylating agents. Therapy-induced ANLL is most commonly observed following melphalan therapy for multiple myeloma and busulphan therapy for lung or ovarian carcinoma. A recent study has suggested that there is an increased risk of developing NHL following intensive multi-drug cytotoxic chemotherapy.

Therapy-induced ANLL differs from *de novo* ANLL in a number of important respects:

- at least 90% of therapy-induced ANLL cases have cytogenetic abnormalities. The most common findings are monosomy 5, 5q-, monosomy 7 and 7q-. Less than 60% of *de novo* cases bear cytogenetic abnormalities and chromosomes 5 and 7 are involved less commonly.

- more than two thirds of cases of therapy-induced ANLL are preceded by a preleukaemic phase which is marked by severe dysplastic changes and ineffective haemopoiesis. A preleukaemic phase occurs in less than one quarter of *de novo* cases. Interestingly, ANLL secondary to epipodophyllo-toxin therapy does not appear to be associated with a preleukaemic phase.

- therapy-induced ANLL typically is refractory to treatment: the mean survival time from diagnosis is 4 months compared to 20 months in *de novo* cases.

> **SAQ 1**
>
> Which haemopoietic growth factors are encoded by genes on chromosomes 5 and 7?

The mechanism of induction of leukaemia following therapy with alkylating agents remains unknown. Early suggestions that the development of secondary ANLL is a part of the natural history of primary malignancy which has been revealed by the success of cytotoxic chemotherapy in prolonging life now seem unlikely. The hypothesis that immunosuppression secondary to treatment promotes the establishment of malignant clones which would normally be destroyed also seems unlikely because congenital and acquired immunodeficiency states are associated with an excess of lymphoid rather than myeloid malignancy.

The most likely explanation for the induction of ANLL by alkylating agents lies with their known mutagenic properties. Alkylating agents are strongly electrophilic molecules which bind avidly to nucleophilic sites on DNA. They are capable of alkylating the nitrogen and oxygen molecules of all four bases, phosphodiester bonds and the 2' oxygen atom of ribose. The action of alkylating agents on

The evidence for the harmful effects of smoking tobacco is widely known and must now be regarded as incontrovertible. In 1991, smoking-related deaths topped 68,000 in the UK alone. However, much less well known are the apparent benefits of smoking tobacco. Epidemiologists have known since the late 1960's that smokers have a lower incidence of the brain disorders Parkinson's disease and Alzheimer's disease, the inflammatory gut disorder ulcerative colitis and rheumatoid arthritis. The mechanisms of protection against these disorders, if indeed such protection genuinely exists, remain obscure.

DNA can result in inappropriate base pairing, the introduction of strand breaks, complex rearrangements and the deletion of part or all of a chromosome. As described later in this chapter, evidence is accumulating that mutations which alter the expression of normal cellular oncogenes can result in malignant change.

Chloramphenicol therapy is widely reported to be associated with aplastic anaemia and leukaemia. A number of other drugs have been suggested as possible leukaemogens, including phenylbutazone, phenytoin and dapsone, but conclusive proof of such an effect is lacking.

Chemicals

A large number of different chemicals have been suggested as possible inducers or promoters of haemopoietic malignancy but, in most cases, the evidence is unconvincing. The exception is benzene which has been confirmed as a leukaemogen. Chronic exposure to benzene and its derivatives is associated with an increased incidence of aplastic anaemia and ANLL. Most cases have resulted from prolonged occupational exposure to relatively high concentrations of benzene, in some cases spanning over 20 years. However, recent reports of an excess of ANLL in male cigarette smokers have raised the possibility that chronic exposure to the low levels of aromatic compounds found in tobacco smoke may be leukaemogenic. Some studies have also shown a small excess of CLL and CML in exposed workers but these findings are controversial.

Epidemiological studies of rates of haemopoietic malignancy in different occupations have revealed a slight excess incidence of myeloma, NHL, ANLL and CML in agricultural workers, possibly related to increased exposure to animal insecticides and phenoxyacetic acid herbicides. Similar studies have shown an excess of CLL and NHL in rubber industry workers, ALL in the children of nuclear industry workers, CML in welders and NHL in anaesthetists and those exposed to halomethane compounds. None of these associations are universally accepted as proven cases of cause and effect.

Viruses

Viruses are the smallest and simplest macromolecular structures which possess sufficient genetic information to permit self-duplication. They are incapable, however, of independent reproduction. Instead, viruses must infect a host cell and insert their genes into the DNA of the infected cell, thereby "hijacking" the host cell to reproduce viral particles. Ultimately, the infected host cell ruptures, releasing scores of newly produced virus particles which propagate the infection.

There is a wealth of evidence for viral induction of leukaemia and solid tumours in animals, including higher primates (see sidebox). These oncogenic viruses can be divided into two types, the DNA viruses (papovaviruses, adenoviruses and herpesviruses) and the RNA viruses, including **retroviruses**. Examples of the involvement of DNA viruses in the induction of human tumours include **human papillomavirus (HPV)** in cervical neoplasia, **Epstein-Barr virus (EBV)** in Burkitt's lymphoma, Hodgkin's disease and nasopharyngeal carcinoma and **hepatitis B virus (HBV)** in primary hepatoma. The only convincing evidence for retroviral induction of neoplasia in humans comes from studies of the retrovirus **human T lymphotropic virus I (HTLV-I)**. The accumulated evidence for the role of this virus in the aetiology of an unusual form of acute T cell leukaemia/lymphoma (ATL) in Southern Japan and the Caribbean is compelling.

The retroviral genome is composed of two identical strands of RNA which are linked near to the 5′ end. Three genes contribute to viral replication: *gag* which codes for structural proteins which are located in the interior of the virus; *pol* which codes for the polymerase, **reverse transcriptase**, which is responsible for transcription of viral RNA into viral DNA for random insertion into host DNA and *env* which codes for the viral envelope glycoproteins. Some retroviruses also possess an oncogene (*v-onc*) which is responsible for the malignant transformation of the infected host cell. The life-cycle of a typical retrovirus is shown schematically in Figure 15.7.

Retroviruses can induce malignant transformation of host cells in three ways:

- retroviruses which contain an oncogene can induce malignant transformation in host cells by insertion of the viral oncogene into the host cell genome.

SAQ 2

What benign condition is associated with EBV infection in developed countries?

The earliest demonstration that leukaemia could be transmitted between animals was made in 1908 at the Royal Veterinary School in Copenhagen by V Ellermann and O Bang. They showed that injecting leukaemic cells from chickens with avian myeloblastosis into healthy birds caused the development of the condition in the healthy birds. Further experiments showed that the same effect could be obtained by injecting carefully filtered, cell-free extracts. Three years later, P Rous showed that solid tumours could be induced in chickens by the injection of cell-free extracts from similarly afflicted birds.

These observations were not extended to mammals until 1936 when JJ Bittner demonstrated the transmission of murine mammary carcinoma through maternal milk. The earliest clear demonstration of leukaemia induction by the injection of cell-free extracts was made in 1951 by L Gross in New York who used new-born mice. Attempts to induce leukaemia in adult mice were unsuccessful.

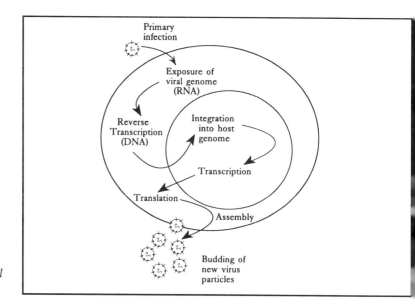

Figure 15.7 *The life-cycle of a typical retrovirus*

This mechanism, known as **direct mutagenesis** typically leads to an acute and rapidly progressive tumour.

- the most commonly encountered mechanism of retroviral transformation involves the insertion of the viral DNA at a specific point in the host DNA, enabling the viral regulatory sequences to influence the expression of host cellular proliferation genes. This mechanism, known as **insertional mutagenesis,** is associated with a relatively long latency period and only a minority of infected animals develop neoplasia.

- HTLV-I differs in that the point of insertion of viral DNA into host DNA varies widely. HTLV-I is thought to be capable of transforming host T lymphocytes by a process known as **trans-activation.** A viral protein designated **tax** has been shown to trans-activate the genes which encode the IL-2 receptor, IL-3, IL-4, GM-CSF and the oncogene *fos.*

A second retrovirus, HTLV-II, has been isolated from the malignant cells of two individuals with the extremely rare T cell variant of HCL. The role of this virus, if any, in the induction of THCL remains unclear.

Numerous epidemiological studies have suggested a possible role for infectious agents in human haemopoietic malignancy. The observation of an increased incidence of myeloma, NHL, ANLL and CML in agricultural workers raises the possibility that contact with oncogenic animal viruses may be involved. However, exhaustive studies of pet owners, slaughterhouse workers and children bitten by animals have failed to provide consistent confirmation of this observation.

The apparent phenomenon of "clustering" of cases of leukaemia has attracted considerable interest over the years. Numerous epidemiological studies have shown an excess of leukaemia in a restricted geographical location. Most reported clusters have involved ALL of childhood, but occasional reports of CML clusters exist.

One possible explanation for this phenomenon is the horizontal transmission of an infectious agent such as a virus. It seems likely that no single virus which directly causes ALL in children exists. Instead, the *pattern* of common childhood infections may be implicated. Children in developed countries typically are protected from infections in the early months of life, leading to an abnormally restricted immunological repertoire which may be susceptible to malignant change when faced with the barrage of common viral and bacterial infections which characterise infancy.

This hypothesis fits well with the observed excess of ALL in the children of the developed world. The characteristic peak incidence of ALL in children aged 0-5 only developed in the UK since the 1920's. There is also some evidence that childhood ALL temporarily is more common following a "population-mixing" event such as the rapid expansion of a small village into a new town. It is suggested that the disruption of the spectrum of infections which inevitably accompanies a major influx of population is implicated in this excess of childhood ALL.

Burkitt's lymphoma (BL) is an NHL which is manifest as tumours of the jaw and abdomen with extensive extranodal involvement, especially of the kidneys, thyroid, ovaries and testes. It is endemic to areas of high humidity in tropical Africa and Papua New Guinea. Virtually all cases of African BL have definitive evidence of Epstein-Barr virus (EBV) infection and one of three chromosomal translocations involving the c-*myc* oncogene and the immunoglobulin genes: (t(8;14)(q24;q32); t(8;22)(q24;q11); or t(2;8)(p12;q24)). Sporadic cases of BL have been reported in many other locations around the world, but only a minority of these have shown evidence of EBV infection.

Although the leukaemia cluster at Sellafield has the greatest notoriety, the existence of a similar cluster near Dounreay in the north of Scotland has been known for some time. The proximity of the cluster to a nuclear power station at this site has raised the suspicion that radiation discharges may be to blame. However, proponents of the viral aetiology theory point to the sudden influx of population experienced by this tiny, isolated community following the expansion of the North Sea oil industry as an alternative explanation.

EBV is a very common virus worldwide but infection in developed countries causes the self-limiting lymphoproliferative condition **infectious mononucleosis**. This relatively mild condition is associated with the delayed EBV infection which predominates in developed countries. In most cases of African BL, primary infection with EBV occurs in the first year of life, whereas the peak incidence of infectious mononucleosis occurs in adolescence. It is suggested that the development of African BL occurs in three phases:

- primary EBV infection "immortalises" infected B lymphocytes

- an immortalised B lymphocyte is stimulated to proliferate by some immunological challenge such as malaria infection, resulting in the formation of an immortalised B cell clone

- in the process of cell division, a single cell in the immortalised clone develops one of the three chromosomal translocations which induce malignant transformation, leading to a clonal B cell malignancy

Hodgkin's disease is a heterogeneous condition which has been suspected of having an infectious aetiology since it was first described in 1832. It seems likely that a number of different mechanisms are involved in the aetiology of the different forms of HD and in different age groups. Recent evidence has shown that EBV is implicated in the pathogenesis of HD in a large proportion of cases in children and adults over the age of 50 years. A multi-step aetiology similar to that for African BL is also proposed for HD.

Host Factors

The concept of "built-in susceptibility" to haemopoietic malignancy remains unproven, except in particular, well-defined circumstances. Numerous case reports exist of families with several cases of leukaemia or lymphoma, but it is difficult to discern whether these are the result of genetic predisposition or shared exposure to a leukaemogen. Many reports do not specify the subtypes of disease involved and, in some cases, misdiagnosis is suspected.

There is a clearly increased risk of acute leukaemia in certain inherited and congenital conditions such as Down's syndrome, Bloom's syndrome and Fanconi's anaemia. Lymphoid malignancy is more common in inherited immunodeficiency states such as Bruton's agammaglobulinaemia and ataxia telangiectasia.

Whether, in the absence of inherited states such as these, the blood relations of an individual with a haemopoietic malignancy are at increased risk of developing the same condition is highly contentious. Epidemiological studies have revealed a slight excess of CLL, ALL and ANLL, but no increased risk of CML in blood relations of confirmed leukaemics. Again, this finding could be explained equally well by a genetic predisposition or by shared exposure to some leukaemogenic factor. Interestingly, an increased incidence of immunological dysfunction was noted in the siblings of individuals with CLL. It is unknown whether this represents a possible preleukaemic state or a state which predisposes to the development of CLL.

SAQ 3

What is the mode of inheritance of the immunodeficiencies Bruton's agammaglobulinaemia and ataxia telangiectasia?

The greatly increased risk of ALL in an identical twin of a confirmed case is well established. The risk of coincident development of ALL is highest in infancy. The most likely explanation for this phenomenon is the transmission of malignant cells from one twin, in whom the disease arose, to the other via the shared placental circulation *in utero*. In a minority of cases, a true constitutional predisposition may be present.

The Role of Oncogenes in Haemopoietic Malignancy

Cellular proto-oncogenes are highly conserved constituents of the normal human genome. They encode proteins which act as growth factors, growth factor receptors, signal transducers or controllers of nuclear function. In short, proto-oncogene products play a major role in the control of cellular growth, differentiation and division within the body. It is hardly surprising, then, that disruption of proto-oncogene function can lead to malignant transformation.

Four types of chromosomal aberration which can lead to oncogene activation commonly are found in haemopoietic malignancies:

- **translocations and inversions** which involve sections of chromosome breaking off and relocating either elsewhere on the same chromosome or onto another chromosome altogether. Translocation of a proto-oncogene can disrupt its function by bringing it under the influence of its new neighbours, by removing it from the influence of its old neighbours or by altering the biochemical action of the gene product. Several examples of oncogene activation by these mechanisms have been discovered and are discussed in detail below.

- **deletions and numerical changes** which involve the loss or gain of part or all of a chromosome. Chromosomal trisomy can lead to increased expression of proto-oncogene products and may contribute to the early stages of malignant transformation. Equally, certain deletions remove proto-oncogenes, leading to the production of cells which are impervious to normal growth control mechanisms.

- **point mutations** in proto-oncogenes can cause the function of the gene product to be altered. For example, the products of the c-*ras* oncogenes are involved in cellular signal transduction pathways. Substitution of glycine by valine or aspartic acid at positions 12 or 13 in RAS proteins greatly diminishes their GTPase activity, thereby weakening signal transduction and leading to deranged cell growth. Such mutations are found in at least 50% of cases of ANLL.

- **gene amplification** which involves the repeated replication of short segments of DNA to produce as many as 100 copies and leading to a gene dosage effect. Amplification of DNA is manifest as homogeneously staining regions and double minute chromosomes which lack centromeres. Both anomalies are found in haemopoietic malignancies. Examples of proto-oncogenes which have been shown to be amplified in certain types of haemopoietic malignancy include the c-*myc* proto-oncogene in M3 ANLL and the *ets*-1 proto-oncogene in M4 ANLL.

The names, chromosomal location and normal function of some important oncogenes are shown in Table 15.1.

Proto-oncogene	Chromosomal Location	Function of Protein Product
N-*ras*	1p11-13	Threonine kinase
src-2	1p34-36	Membrane tyrosine kinase
fms	5q32	M-CSF membrane receptor
pim	6p23	
myb	6q21-22	Regulator of transcription
K-*ras*-1	6p11-12	Membrane threonine kinase
erb-B	7p11-13	Epidermal growth factor membrane receptor
mos	8q22	Cytoplasmic threonine kinase
myc	8q24	Regulator of transcription
abl	9q34	Cytoplasmic membrane tyrosine kinase
tcl-2	11p13	
bcl-1	11q13	
ets-1	11q23-24	
K-*ras*-2	12p12	Membrane threonine kinase
tcl-1	14q	
fos	14q21-31	Nuclear transcrption factor
erb-A	17q21-22	Thyroid hormone receptor
bcl-2	18q21	
src-1	20q12-13	Membrane tyrosine kinase
ets-2	21q22	
sis	22q13	Platelet derived growth factor β chain

Table 15.1 *The chromosomal location of some important oncogenes and the function of their respective protein products*

Cytogenetics and Haemopoietic Malignancy

Normal human cells, other than gametes, contain a total of 46 chromosomes which are composed of 22 pairs of **autosomes**, numbered 1-22 and two chromosomes which determine sex. In males, the **sex chromosomes** are dissimilar and are designated X and Y (46XY) whereas in females the sex chromosomes are both X chromosomes (46XX).

Normal chromosomes are divided into a long and a short arm by a central constriction known as the **centromere**. The long arm of a chromosome is known as the **q arm** whereas the short arm is known as the **p arm**. Preparation of chromosomes for examination by light microscopy involves staining with Giemsa or Quinacrine dyes which reveals a pattern of light and dark bands characteristic of each chromosome type. These bands can be used to describe quite small areas of the chromosome. For example, 8q22 refers to sub-band number 2 on region 2 on the long arm of chromosome number 8 (Figure 15.8).

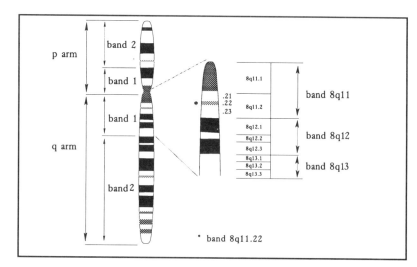

Figure 15.8 *Description of location on chromosome 8 using the banding pattern*

Cytogenetic abnormalities are expressed according to the International System for Human Cytogenetic Nomenclature. Briefly, this system uses the following rules:

- the total number of chromosomes is indicated first, followed by the sex chromosome constitution and then by the gains, losses or rearrangements of the autosomes.

- a (+) before a number eg +21 indicates a gain or tri-somy of that chromosome. A (-) before a number eg -7 indicates a loss or monosomy of that chromo-some.

- a (+) or a (-) after a number eg 5q- indicates a loss of the named part of that chromosome.

- chromosomal rearrangements are indicated by an abbreviation which denotes the type of rearrange-ment, followed by the chromosome(s) involved in parenthesis and then the bands in which the chro-mosomal breaks occurred in a second parenthesis. For example, t(8;21)(q22;q22) indicates a transloca-tion of material between chromosomes 8 and 21 with both breakpoints occurring in band 2 of region 2 of the q arm of the respective chromo-somes. The abbreviations used to denote different types of chromosomal rearrangement are shown in Table 15.2.

SAQ 4

What iatrogenic condition is associated with monosomy 7?

Abbreviation	Meaning	Example
i	isochromosome	i(17)q
del	deletion	5q-
t	translocation	t(8;21)(q22;q22)
inv	inversion	inv (16)(p13;q32)

Table 15.2 *Abbreviations used to denote chromosomal aberrations*

Extensive studies of the cytogenetic constitution of individuals with haemopoietic malignancy have revealed that at least 70% have an abnormal karyotype. Some workers believe that, with modern tech-niques, this figure eventually will be revised upwards to 100%. Although the types of chromosomal abnormality seen in this group of diseases are diverse, the distribution is non-random, both in terms of the chromosomal regions affected and in their association with particular conditions.

Acute Non-lymphoblastic Leukaemia

The most common types of chromosomal abnormality in ANLL are translocations and deletions, most commonly affecting chromo-somes 8, 15, 17 and 21. These are summarised in Table 15.3 and are

Chromosome Abnormality	Variants	Disease Association	Prominent Features
t(8;21)(q22;q22)		M2	eosinophilia/dysplasia-younger patients higher rate of CHR -X, -Y
t(15;17)(q22;q21)	t(15;17)(q22;q11.2)	M3	good prognosis
inv (16)(p13;q32)	16q- t(16)(p13;q22)	M4Eo	eosinophilia/dysplasia
11q23-q24	11q13-q14 t(2;11) t(6;11) t(9;11)(p22;q23) t(11;17) t(11;19) M5	M5	
t(6;9)(p23;q34)		Various	Basophilia, poor prognosis
inv(3)(q21;q26)	t(3)(q21;q26)	Various	dysthrombopoieisis
-5, -7, 5q-, 7q- t(1;7)(p11;p11)		2° ANLL	history of exposure to mutagens

Table 15.3 *Consistent chromosomal abnormalities in ANLL*

described in more detail below. The positions of these non-random breakpoints bear comparison with the chromosomal locations of known proto-oncogenes shown in Table 15.1.

t(8;21)(q22;q22) and M2 ANLL

This translocation is the most consistent structural chromosomal change in ANLL, being present in at least 12% of cases with an abnormal karyotype. The association is especially strong with M2 ANLL where at least 35% of cases with an abnormal karyotype have this abnormality. It is also seen occasionally in M4 and, rarely, in M1 ANLL. Typical features of cases of ANLL in the presence of t(8;21)(q22;q22) include bone marrow eosinophilia or eosinophilic dysplasia, numerous Auer rods and an improved rate of complete haematological remission but only a marginal improvement in long-term survival.

t(8;21)(q22;q22) appears to be more common in younger patients; it is rarely seen in patients over the age of 50 years. The translocation commonly is accompanied by the loss of a sex chromosome. -Y is present in 85% of the males and -X is present in 73% of the females with this translocation. This observation is especially significant because loss of a sex chromosome otherwise is rare in ANLL. The *ets-2* proto-oncogene is moved from 21q22 to 8q22 in this translocation.

t(15;17)(q22;q21) or (q22;q11-12) and M3 ANLL

The t(15;17) translocation currently appears to be specific for M3 ANLL; it has not been described in any other malignancy except cases of CML which have transformed to M3 ANLL. Almost all patients with M3 ANLL have this translocation which is associated with a good prognosis. This translocation disrupts the *pml* gene on chromosome 15 and the retinoic acid receptor gene (*rarα*) on chromosome 17, resulting in the formation of two novel fusion genes, both of which are functional. Synthesis of the novel *pml/rarα* fusion protein leads to the development of M3 ANLL. The proto-oncogene *c-erb A* and the gene which codes for G-CSF also are located at 17q21-22.

Rearrangements of Chromosome 16 and M4 ANLL

Inv (16)(p13;q32) is the most commonly observed chromosomal abnormality in M4 ANLL, being present in about 20% of cases. It is associated with bone marrow eosinophilia, eosinophilic dysplasia and a relatively good prognosis. Cases of M4 with this phenotype are designated as M4-Eo. Variant rearrangements which also are associated with M4-Eo include 16q- and t(16)(p13;q22). The metallothionein gene cluster is split by the breakpoint at 16q22 but the significance of this observation is unknown.

Rearrangements of 11q and M5 ANLL

Deletions and rearrangements of the long arm of chromosome 11 are associated with M5 ANLL. The diversity of rearrangements involving 11q is greater than that seen in M2 and M3 but the most common breakpoints are 11q23-q24 and 11q13-q14, together accounting for more than 90% of cases. Other reported rearrangements include t(2;11), t(6;11), t(9;11), t(11;17) and t(11;19).

t(6;9)(p23;q34) and Bone Marrow Basophilia

Most individuals with t(6;9)(p23;q34) have been shown to have a variable increase in basophil numbers in the bone marrow. It does not appear to be associated with any FAB subtype but is seen most commonly in younger patients with a median age of 38 years. Typically, patients with this translocation have a history of a severe myelodysplastic phase prior to the development of frank leukaemia. This translocation is associated with a poor prognosis.

Interestingly, this translocation involves a breakpoint on chromosome 9 close to that in the Philadelphia chromosome, although the *c-abl* oncogene is not translocated. Basophilia associated with a poor prognosis is also a feature of some cases of CML.

Rearrangements of 3q and Dysthrombopoiesis

Rearrangements of the long arm of chromosome 3 have been reported in a wide range of haemopoietic malignancies, including ANLL, MDS, Philadelphia-negative CML and transformed CML. The single consistent finding in all of these reported cases has been the presence of normal or raised platelet counts and, often severe, dysthrombopoiesis. In particular, the presence of an increased number of hypolobulated micromegakaryocytes in the bone marrow is a common finding. The most commonly described rearrangements involved are inv(3)(q21;q26) and t(3;3)(q21;q26). This implies that the gene(s) which control megakaryocyte differentiation are located on chromosome 3q but the identity and function of these gene(s) remain to be determined.

Numerical Changes and ANLL

Hyper- or hypodiploidy, involving gain or loss of any of the autosomes or sex chromosomes, is relatively common in ANLL. This is the only chromosomal aberration in about 20% of cases of ANLL at presentation. None of the numerical changes is associated with a particular FAB subtype. The most common changes are +8, +11, +19, +21, +22, -5, -7, -12, -17, -20 and -Y.

Secondary ANLL

As described earlier, abnormalities of chromosomes 5 and 7 are the most consistent chromosomal changes seen in ANLL secondary to treatment for a pre-existing malignant condition. About 50% of cases show monosomy 7 (-7) while about 25% show monosomy 5 (-5). 5q- and 7q- also are common.

The translocation t(1;7)(p11;p11) has been reported in a variety of haemopoietic malignancies including secondary ANLL. Interestingly, the presence of this translocation appears to be associated strongly with a history of exposure to mutagenic chemicals or radiation, even in apparently *de novo* cases.

The genes for the haemopoietic growth factors GM-CSF, IL-3, IL-5 and M-CSF and the receptors for M-CSF (*c-fms*) and platelet derived growth factor are all located on 5q while the gene for erythropoietin is located on 7q11-22. It seems likely that deletion of these genes contributes to the myelodysplasia which foreshadows the development of secondary ANLL.

Acute Lymphoblastic Leukaemia

Chromosomal abnormalities are discernible in at least 70% of cases of ALL. For a number of reasons, identification of chromosomal abnormalities in lymphoid malignancy often is technically challenging. Cytogenetic analysis provides useful information to aid disease classification and correlates well with prognosis, and so forms a vital component of the diagnostic work-up in ALL. The most commonly observed chromosomal rearrangements are summarised in Table 15.4 and are described in detail below. Again, the consistent breakpoints are related to the locations of proto-oncogenes.

The Philadelphia Chromosome t(9;22)(q34;q11) in ALL

The Philadelphia chromosome is present in about 15-20% of cases of ALL in adults. It is much less common in ALL of childhood where about 2-3% of cases are Philadelphia positive. Typical fea-

Chromosome Abnormality	Variants	Disease Association	Prominent Features
t(9;22)(q34;q11)		L2	High WBC, immature B cell differentiation
t(4;11)(q21;q23)		mainly L2	WBC > 100x10^9/l, organomegaly, lymphadenopathy, early B precursor differentiation, poor prognosis
t(8;14)(q24;q32)	t(2;8)(p12;q24) t(8;22)(q24;q11)	L3	CNS disease, very poor prognosis
del(6)(q21-23)		cALL	
del(12)(p12)		L1	good prognosis
t(1;19)(q23;p13)		L1	poor prognosis
t(11;14)(p13;q11)	t(8;14)(q24;q11) t(10;14)(q24;q11) inv(14)(q11;q32)	TALL	poor prognosis

Table 15.4 *Consistent chromosomal rearrangements in ALL*

tures of Philadelphia positive ALL include a high white cell count at presentation, L2 morphology and an immunophenotype indicative of immature B cell differentiation. *De novo* Philadelphia positive ALL differs from CML which has transformed into ALL in three ways:

- *de novo* cases are more responsive to cytotoxic chemotherapy and have longer median survival times.

- *de novo* cases rarely have an i(17q) which is a common finding in transformed CML.

- the exact position of the breakpoint within the *bcr* gene on chromosome 22 is more diverse in *de novo* cases as shown in Figure 15.9. The molecular

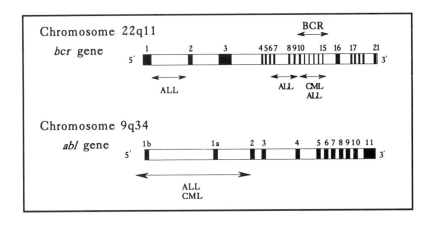

Figure 15.9 *The different Philadelphia chromosome breakpoints on chromosomes 9 and 22 in ALL and CML*

events in the formation of the Philadelphia chromosome are described in more detail later in this chapter.

t(4;11)(q21;q23) and Poor Prognosis ALL

The t(4;11)(q21;q23) translocation is found in about 5% of cases of ALL. It is associated with white cell counts at presentation in excess of 100 x 10^9/l, hepatosplenomegaly, lymphadenopathy, mainly L2 morphology, early pre-B immunophenotype and a very poor prognosis. It is most common in infants and in adults. As described in the next chapter, most of these features are indicators of a poor prognosis. The median survival from diagnosis for bearers of this translocation is about 7 months.

t(8;14)(q24;q32) and L3 ALL

This translocation is associated with B ALL of L3 morphology, an increased incidence of CNS disease and a uniformly poor prognosis. The median survival from diagnosis is 5 months. An identical translocation is seen in Burkitt's lymphoma. The variant translocations t(2;8)(p12;q24) and t(8;22)(q24;q11) also are found, although less commonly, in both conditions. No other translocations have consistently been found in either L3 B ALL or Burkitt's lymphoma.

The proto-oncogene c-*myc* is located at 8q24 and in t(8;14)(q24;q32) is translocated close to the immunoglobulin heavy chain genes at 14q32. In this new position, c-*myc* comes under the influence of the transcription-promoting sequences of the immunoglobulin heavy chain genes, thereby enhancing expression of the oncogene c-*myc*. The protein product of c-*myc* appears to be involved in DNA binding and transcriptional activation. The ultimate consequence of increased production of this protein is neoplastic growth of B lymphoid cells. In the variant translocations, c-*myc* is juxtaposed with either the immunoglobulin light chain κ genes at 2p12 or the immunoglobulin light chain λ genes at 22q11 with the same result. The t(8;14)(q24;q32) translocation is depicted in Figure 15.10.

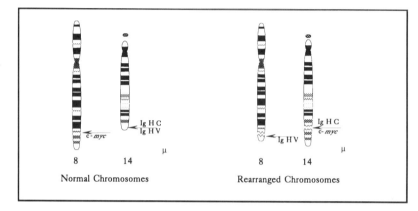

Figure 15.10 *Molecular events in the t(8;14)(q24;q32) translocation IgHC μ - immunoglobulin heavy chain constant region genes IgHV - immunoglobulin heavy chain variable region genes*

del(6)(q21-23) and cALL

Deletions of the long arm of chromosome 6 are relatively common in childhood cALL but have also been seen in adult ALL.

del(12)(p12) and cALL

Deletions of the short arm of chromosome 12 are relatively common in secondary ANLL. About 10% of cases of ALL also carry such deletions. Most cases have been cALL with L1 morphology and have shown a good prognosis.

t(1;19)(q23;p13) and pre-B ALL

The translocation t(1;19)(q23;p13) is associated with pre-B ALL and L1 morphology and a poor prognosis.

Rearrangements of 14q and T ALL

Several rearrangements of the long arm of chromosome 14 are associated with T ALL and other T lymphoid malignancies. These include the translocations t(11;14)(p13;q11), t(8;14)(q24;q11) and t(10;14)(q24;q11) and the inversion inv(14)(q11;q32). None of these rearrangements are particularly common or are associated with particular clinical features. Their only common feature is that they involve rearrangement at 14q11 which splits the Ti_α gene locus.

Numerical Changes and ALL

Changes in total chromosome numbers are relatively common in ALL, affecting about 60% of cases. High hyperdiploidy, with between 50 and 60 chromosomes, is most common in children and is associated with a good prognosis unless accompanied by a rearrangement which confers poor prognosis. The most common extra chromosomes are +21, +6, +18, +14, +10 and +4.

Hypodiploidy typically is associated with a poor prognosis, especially in those rare cases in which the chromosomal complement approaches the haploid number.

Myelodysplastic Syndromes

About 60% of patients with primary myelodysplastic syndromes display one or more chromosomal abnormality. In secondary myelodysplasia, this figure rises to at least 90%. A variety of cytogenetic abnormalities have been described in patients with myelodysplastic syndromes but none are markers of a specific syndrome or associated with particular clinical or prognostic features. The most common changes include +8, +19, +21, -7, 20q- and 5q-. Possession of a single chromosomal abnormality does not appear to affect prognosis significantly but the acquisition of new chromosomal abnormalities or possession of multiple abnormalities at presentation often foreshadows the development of frank leukaemia in patients with MDS.

Non-leukaemic Myeloproliferative Disorders

A variety of chromosomal abnormalities have been reported in patients with myeloproliferative disorders. The most consistent abnormalities are 20q-, +8, +9, 13q- and -7. Single chromosomal abnormalities do not appear to worsen prognosis which generally is rather better than for MDS. Possession of multiple chromosomal abnormalities or -7, however, typically are indicators of poor prognosis and an increased risk of progression to frank leukaemia.

Chronic Lymphoid Leukaemias

The most common chromosomal abnormalities in B CLL are +12 and rearrangements involving 14q32, the site of the immunoglobulin heavy chain genes. Both abnormalities are associated with progressive or refractory disease and frequently also are found in BPLL. The gene(s) on chromosome 12 which are implicated in the induction of malignancy have not been identified. The t(11;14)(q13;q32) translocation brings the *B cell lymphoma 1* or *bcl-1* gene on chromosome 11 into juxtaposition with the immunoglobulin heavy chain gene locus. The nature of the protein product of the *bcl-1* gene and how it might contribute to the induction of CLL is unknown.

T cell variants of the chronic lymphoid leukaemias often display chromosomal rearrangements involving 14q11, 7q35 and 7p13. The Ti_α and Ti_δ genes loci are located at 14q11 while the Ti_β gene locus is located at 7q35 and the Ti_γ gene locus is located at 7p13. The inversion inv(14)(q11;q32) involves breakpoints at the Ti_α gene locus and the *T cell lymphoma-1 (tcl-1)* gene locus which is slightly proximal to the immunoglobulin heavy chain gene locus.

Non-leukaemic Lymphoproliferative Disorders

t(11;14)(q13;q32) and MM

Only two consistent chromosomal rearrangements are found in MM, t(11;14)(q13;q32) and t(14;18)(q32;q21). Both are relatively common in other B cell malignancies as well. The t(11;14)(q13;q32) translocation has been described above. This translocation also is found in small cell lymphocytic lymphoma.

t(14;18)(q32;q21) and MM

In the t(14;18)(q32;q21) translocation, the chromosome 18 breakpoint lies within a region designated the *B cell lymphoma-2 locus (bcl-2)*. The *bcl-2* gene has been shown to encode a 24kd integral membrane protein which is highly transcribed when brought into close juxtaposition with the immunoglobulin heavy chain gene locus on chromosome 14q32. This translocation also is found in follicular small cleaved-cell lymphoma.

Numerical Changes and NHL

Trisomy of chromosomes 2, 3, 7, 12 or 18 is a common finding in NHL, affecting almost two thirds of cases in some studies. However, there appears to be little correlation between a particular trisomy and NHL subtype.

Chronic Myeloid Leukaemia

t(9;22)(q34;q11) and CML

At least 90% of cases of CML display a minute chromosome 22 which results from the reciprocal translocation t(9;22)(q34;q11). This abnormal chromosome 22 is known as the Philadelphia chromosome after the city of its discovery. Molecular analysis of many apparently Philadelphia negative cases of CML reveal similar but variant chromosomal rearrangements. The Philadelphia chromosome is observed also in a minority of cases of ALL and ANLL.

The chromosome 9 breakpoint (9q34) involves the *abl* gene. As shown in Figure 15.9, this gene is unusual in that it contains two alternative first exons (1a and 1b) and therefore is capable of producing two distinct mature mRNA transcripts. This requires that the splice acceptor site of exon 2 is capable of binding to a variety of splice donor sites. This promiscuity is crucial to the malignant potential of the *abl* gene because it also permits the binding of non-*abl* sequences. The precise location of the breakpoint varies from case to case, but always lies within a 200 kb region 5′ to exon 2 of the *abl* gene. Thus, the *abl* gene is translocated to chromosome 22, complete with exons 2-11. The function of the normal ABL protein (p145^{abl}) is poorly understood but it is known to have tyrosine kinase activity and to be important in the regulation of myelopoiesis.

The chromosome 22 breakpoint (22q11) in CML always lies within a 5.8 kb region of the *bcr* gene called the **breakpoint cluster region**. As shown in Figure 15.9, the location of the breakpoint frequently

Recent work at the Children's Cancer Research Institute in Vienna has uncovered an unexpected consistency in the constitution of the Philadelphia chromosome. Detailed family studies have shown that the fragment of the aberrant chromosome which is derived from chromosome 22 always is derived from the maternal chromosome while the chromosome 9 fragment always is paternal in origin. The reason for and significance of this finding remain obscure.

differs in cases of ALL. The normal BCR protein (p160^{bcr}) is known to have serine/threonine kinase activity and is thought to be involved in the activation of GTP-binding proteins within cells.

In the Philadelphia chromosome, the severed end of the *bcr* gene is brought into apposition with the translocated *abl* gene, forming a novel *bcr-abl* fusion gene. The unique product of this fusion gene, p210$^{bcr-abl}$ has a much more powerful tyrosine kinase activity than p145^{abl} and has been shown to interact with its substrates in an altered manner. Although the way in which p210$^{bcr-abl}$ brings about malignant change is unknown, there is little doubt that this protein is implicated in the causation of CML.

Principles of Treatment of Haematological Malignancy

Theoretically ideal treatment for the haematological malignancies requires the selective and total destruction of malignant cells in the absence of significant toxicity to normal cells. As will be seen, this ideal is not attainable in practice. The widespread dissemination of malignant cells in most types of haematological malignancy coupled with the extreme sensitivity of normal haemopoietic and other rapidly dividing tissue make severe toxicity unavoidable. For example, a typical tumour load at diagnosis for ANLL is about 5×10^{11} - 5×10^{12} cells: this compares to a total normal haemopoietic stem cell load of less than 1×10^9. Any treatment which is sufficiently toxic to destroy the leukaemic cells would completely ablate the normal haemopoietic tissue with which it is associated. To overcome this problem, cytoreductive therapy needs to be "pulsed", allowing recovery of normal tissue between treatments. Because the doubling time of leukaemic tissue is much longer than that of normal tissue, this permits the progressive reduction and eventual eradication of the tumour mass as shown schematically in Figure 15.11.

The two modes of treatment which are most widely employed in haematological malignancy are cytotoxic chemotherapy and radiotherapy.

Cytotoxic Chemotherapy

Cytotoxic chemotherapy involves the administration of highly toxic drugs in an attempt to poison the malignant cells. The main advantage of this approach over radiotherapy is that it is effective against

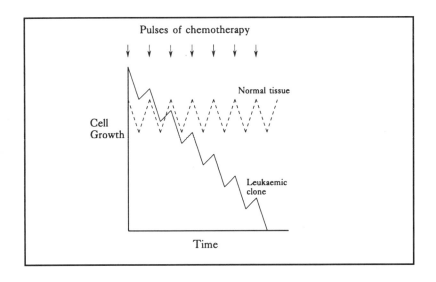

Figure 15.11 *Simplified schematic diagram showing the steady replacement of malignant clone by normal haemopoietic tissue following several cycles of cytoreductive therapy*

disseminated tumours like leukaemia. However, because the drugs are delivered via the bloodstream, poorly vascularised areas are not effectively treated. In particular, destruction of malignant cells in the cerebrospinal fluid requires additional intrathecal therapy. The main disadvantage of cytotoxic chemotherapy is that it is not selective for malignant cells: both normal and malignant cells are poisoned by cytotoxic drugs.

The Cell Cycle

The concept of the cell cycle is central to an understanding of the strategy of cytotoxic chemotherapy. Actively dividing cells are said to be "in-cycle". The length of the cell cycle describes the time between consecutive mitoses for a given cell. As shown in Figure 15.12, the cell cycle consists of four phases, each associated with particular cellular activities:

- the first phase of the cell cycle is designated G_1 (Gap 1). During this period, the cell is diploid (2n, 46 chromosomes). Cellular activity during G_1 is concentrated on preparation for the growth demands of S phase. Variations in the length of the cell cycle of different cell types usually involve variations in the length of G_1.

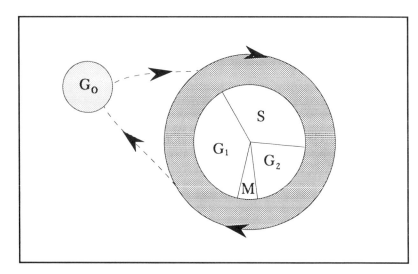

Figure 15.12 *The cell cycle*

- S phase or synthetic phase involves the duplication of the DNA content of the cell such that each chromosome develops an identical twin called a sister chromatid. At the completion of S phase, the cell is tetraploid (4n).

- G_2 phase is associated with the repair of imperfections in the duplicated DNA and final preparations for division.

- M phase describes the period in which cell division, or mitosis, takes place. The two daughter cells which result are diploid and either re-enter the cell cycle if the required growth factors are present or temporarily enter a resting state known as G_0.

The drugs commonly employed as cytotoxic agents can be categorised according to their activity relative to the cell cycle as described in Tables 15.5 and 15.6.

Table 15.5 *Modes of action of cytotoxic drugs relative to the cell cycle*

Class	Action	Comment
I	Phase non-specific	kill dividing and resting cells equally
II	Phase-specific	kill cells in particular phase of cell cycle
III	Cycle-specific	kill dividing cells

Drug	Group	Action	Uses
Class I			
BCNU	nitrosourea	carbamoylation of proteins & alkylation of nucleic acids	HD NHL
Class II			
Cytosine arabinoside	antimetabolite	inhibits DNA synthesis	ANLL NHL
Etoposide	plant alkaloid	inhibits topoisomerase	ANLL NHL
Hydroxyurea	antimetabolite	blocks ribonucleotide reductase	CML
6-Mercaptopurine	antimetabolite	inhibits purine synthesis at PRPP interconversion	ALL
Vinblastine	plant alkaloid	inhibits microtubule assembly	ALL HD NHL
Methotrexate	antimetabolite	inhibits folate-dependent reactions	ALL NHL
Class III			
Actinomycin D	antibiotic	inhibits DNA/RNA synthesis by intercalation between bases	ALL
Adriamycin	antibiotic	as actinomycin D	ALL ANLL NHL
Busulfan	alkylator	forms inter- & intra-strand crosslinks in DNA	CML
Chlorambucil	alkylator	as busulfan	CLL
Cyclophosphamide	alkylator	as busulfan	NHL
Melphalan	alkylator	as busulfan	MM
Miscellaneous			
L-Asparaginase	enzyme	inhibits protein synthesis by depleting L-asparagine	ALL
Prednisolone	steroid hormone	unknown	ALL HD NHL

Table 15.6 *Classification and modes of action of selected cytotoxic drugs*

Class I cytotoxic drugs show no selectivity for malignant cells, they are equally toxic to all cells. Class II and III drugs, because of their selectivity for dividing cells, are more toxic to malignant tissue which has a greater number of cells in cycle. However, this selectivity is lost with prolonged exposure.

Mode of Action of Cytotoxic Drugs

The precise mode of action of many cytotoxic drugs remains obscure. Some drugs have been shown to exert particular toxic effects by *in vitro* experiments, and are classified according to this activity. It is likely, however, that their activities *in vivo* are more complex. Cytotoxic drugs can be broadly classified according to their mode of action or other similarities in their properties:

- alkylating agents
- anti-metabolites
- anthracyclines
- steroid hormones
- plant alkaloids
- enzymes
- miscellaneous agents

Alkylating Agents

Alkylating agents are polyfunctional molecules with highly reactive alkyl groups which form crosslinks between the side chains of proteins and nucleic acids. These crosslinks interfere with the function of cellular enzymes and the replicative function of DNA. Attempts to repair the damage to DNA caused by these drugs results in their mutagenic potential.

The alkylating agents are class III cytotoxic drugs, affecting only dividing cells. Toxic side effects therefore are manifest most severely in rapidly dividing tissue, leading to pancytopaenia, alopecia and ulceration of mucous membranes.

SAQ 5

For which enzyme is the antimetabolite methotrexate a competitive inhibitor?

Commonly prescribed alkylating agents include **cyclophos-phamide, chlorambucil, busulfan, procarbazine** and **cisplatin**. Cyclophosphamide differs from the other members of this group in that it is administered in an inactive form and is activated *in vivo* by hepatic microsomal enzymes. **Acrolein**, the toxic derivative of cyclophosphamide, is excreted via the urinary system leading to side effects such as haemorrhagic cystitis and even bladder cancer.

Anti-metabolites

Anti-metabolites are analogues of compounds involved in essential biosynthetic pathways. As described in Chapter 4, **methotrexate** is a close structural analogue of folic acid and therefore acts as a competitive inhibitor of the enzyme dihydrofolate reductase leading to failure of thymidine and purine nucleotide synthesis. Other commonly prescribed examples of this group of drugs include **5-fluorouracil** which prevents the methylation of deoxyuridylate to form deoxythymidylate, **6-azauridine** which acts by inhibiting orotidylate decarboxylase, **cytosine arabinoside** which inhibits DNA polymerase and **6-mercaptopurine** which is activated intracellularly by hypoxanthine guanine phosphoribosyltransferase (HGPRT) to thioinosinic acid and thereafter interferes with *de novo* purine synthesis by phosphoribosyl pyrophosphate and other interconversions.

The anti-metabolites are class II agents, acting primarily on cells in S phase. The side effects of treatment with anti-metabolites generally are similar to those for alkylating agents.

Anthracyclines

The anthracycline antibiotics include **daunorubicin, actinomycin D** and **adriamycin**. They act by binding directly to GC rich regions of DNA and inhibiting DNA and RNA synthesis. There is also some evidence that they may inflict cellular damage by the generation of toxic oxygen radicals. The anthracyclines are class III cytotoxic agents.

Side effects of anthracycline therapy include cardiotoxicity, myelo-suppression, mucositis and severe tissue necrosis following accidental extravasation.

Steroid Hormones

The glucocorticosteroids **prednisone** and **prednisolone** are widely used in the treatment of lymphoid malignancy. These drugs have been shown to bind to specific cytoplasmic receptors in target cells and to be translocated into the nucleus. However, the precise mode of action of these drugs remains obscure. Because of their strong lympholytic activity and their relative lack of myelosuppressive activity, glucocorticosteroids are widely used in the treatment of lymphoid malignancy. They are also used to induce immunosuppression in autoimmune disorders.

Side effects of glucocorticosteroid therapy include water and salt retention, hypokalaemia, osteoporosis, muscle wasting and neutrophilia secondary to inhibition of neutrophil function.

Plant Alkaloids

The two main groups of plant alkaloids are the **vinca alkaloids** such as **vincristine** and **vinblastine** which are derived from the periwinkle and the **epipodophyllotoxins** such as **etoposide** which is a semi-synthetic derivative of podophyllotoxin, an extract of mangrove root.

Vincristine and vinblastine act by binding to tubulin, thereby preventing microtubule and mitotic spindle formation. Both substances are metabolised in the liver and excreted via the bile. Side effects of vincristine therapy include neurotoxicity, alopecia and severe tissue necrosis following accidental extravasation. The vinca alkaloids are class II cytotoxic agents, primarily affecting cells in S phase.

Etoposide is thought to act by inhibiting the enzyme topoisomerase II and inducing strand breaks in double-stranded DNA. Side effects of etoposide therapy include vomiting, alopecia peripheral neuropathy and myelosuppression. Etoposide is a class II agent.

Enzymes

Normal blood cells meet their requirement for the amino acid asparagine by endogenous synthesis. In contrast to normal lymphoid tissue, however, the leukaemic blast cells in ALL have a relative deficiency of the enzyme L-asparagine synthetase, and so have a requirement for the uptake of asparagine from the extracellular fluid. Intravenous infusion of the bacterial enzyme **L-asparaginase** rapidly destroys the extracellular pool of asparagine, thereby selectively depriving the tumour cells and destroying their capacity to synthesise proteins which incorporate this amino acid. L-asparaginase is most active against cells in G_1. L-asparaginase is derived from *Escherichia coli* and *Erwinia carotova*.

Side effects of L-asparaginase therapy include sensitisation to a bacterial product, disturbances of pancreatic and hepatic function and inhibition of protein synthesis leading to a deficiency of albumin, fibrinogen, antithrombin III, insulin and lipoproteins. In some cases, antithrombin III deficiency has been associated with thrombosis.

Miscellaneous Agents

Using the imperfect classification system described above leaves a number of cytotoxic drugs which do not fit happily into any category. These include the antibiotic **bleomycin** which is a mixture of sulphur-containing polypeptides and has been shown to cause DNA strand breaks. Its principal use is in the treatment of lymphoid malignancy. Side effects of bleomycin therapy include sensitisation to, a bacterial product, cutaneous reactions and cardiotoxicity.

2'-deoxycoformycin is widely used in the treatment of HCL and acts by inhibiting the enzyme adenosine deaminase. Side effects include renal, ocular and neurotoxicity.

Combination Chemotherapy

It is now standard practice to prescribe cytotoxic drugs in combinations with the intention of inducing an additive or, ideally, a synergistic effect on the tumour cells. This approach has been shown to improve significantly the results obtained. Combinations of drugs are selected according to the following principles:

- each drug employed must be effective when used as a single agent

- drugs with different modes of action should be used

- the major toxicity of each drug should differ from others in the combination

- there should be no synergistic toxicity

- each drug must be used in its optimum dose and treatment schedule.

In practice, compromises often are required, but each combination should be as close to this ideal as possible. Some widely used combinations are shown in Table 15.7.

Combination	Components	Use
CHOP	Cyclophosphamide Hydroxydaunomycin (Adriamycin) Oncovin (Vincristine) Prednisolone	NHL
MOPP	Mustine Oncovin (Vincristine) Procarbazine Prednisolone	HD
DAT	Daunorubicin Ara-C (Cytosine arabinoside) 6-Thioguanine	ANLL
VP	Vincristine Prednisolone	ALL
MAZE	M-Amsa (amsacrine) aZacytidine Etoposide	ANLL
MACE	M-Amsa (amsacrine) Cytosine arabinoside Etoposide	ANLL

Table 15.7 *Commonly used combination chemotherapy regimes*

Multi-drug Resistance

Apart from the severe side effects, one of the most important limitations to the successful use of cytotoxic chemotherapy is the development of multi-drug resistance (MDR). As its name suggests, MDR is characterised by the development of tumour resistance to treatment with a range of structurally and functionally unrelated cytotoxic drugs. It is a common finding in relapsed leukaemias and also in secondary ANLL. MDR is associated with failure of remission induction and poor prognosis.

The development of the MDR phenotype has been shown to be associated with the expression of a 170kD transmembrane protein (P-glycoprotein). This protein is coded for by a gene located at 7q21-23 called *mdr-1*. A structurally related gene, *mdr-2*, is located nearby. P-glycoprotein acts as an energy-dependent efflux pump for a wide range of cytotoxic drugs, thereby reducing their toxic effects. The function of the *mdr-2* gene product is unknown, but it does not act as an efflux pump.

Atypical patterns of MDR have also been described, associated with alterations in topoisomerase activity, glutathione-S-transferase activity or CTP synthetase activity.

Attempts to reverse MDR with calcium-channel blocking agents such as verapamil or the anti-oestrogen tamoxifen have had mixed results. Reversal of MDR is readily achievable *in vitro* but at concentrations of drug which would be toxic *in vivo*. The use of a monoclonal antibody to block P-glycoprotein activity is an approach which shows early promise.

Radiotherapy

Ionising radiation frequently is used in the treatment of haematological malignancy, with one of three broad aims:

- in localised tumours such as stage I HD or localised NHL, radiotherapy may be **curative.**

- in disseminated tumours such as the leukaemias and MM, radiotherapy is used as a component of therapy (eg eradication of CNS disease) or for alleviation of symptoms ie **palliation.**

- total body irradiation can be used to destroy haemopoietic tissue as a precursor to bone marrow transplantation. This process, known as **conditioning**, is described in more detail in the next chapter.

Radiotherapy is designed to exploit the biological damage inflicted by ionising radiation upon both normal and malignant tissue. Radiation damage to biological tissue is mediated in two different ways: direct damage involves the disruption of chemical bonds in DNA and proteins while indirect damage is caused by the free radicals which are generated by the ionisation of water and dissolved oxygen. Direct radiation damage is greatest where heavy particles such as protons, neutrons, π mesons or α particles are used.

Modern radiotherapy and imaging equipment permits the accurate targeting of localised tumours while minimising damage to surrounding normal tissue. High-energy electromagnetic radiation such as γ-rays or X-rays can penetrate deep into the body without causing significant damage to superficial tissues while low energy X-rays can be used to treat surface tumours such as leukaemic skin deposits with minimal deep tissue damage.

Different tissues vary in their susceptibility to radiation damage but, broadly, once a given threshold dose is exceeded the number of cells killed increases exponentially with increasing radiation dose. The size of the threshold dose below which radiation is ineffective and the rate of cell kill once the threshold is exceeded is determined by three factors:

- the type of radiation used. As outlined above heavy particles exert the greatest destructive effect while high energy electromagnetic radiation is the most penetrating.

- the characteristics of the irradiated tissue. Broadly, cellular damage is greatest in rapidly dividing tissue which has a relatively long mitotic phase and in undifferentiated cells.

- the oxygen tension of the irradiated tissue. Indirect damage by free oxygen radicals is maximal when the tissue oxygen tension is high. For this reason, poorly vascularised or massive tumours are relatively resistant to radiotherapy.

The limiting factor in the use of radiotherapy remains the non-specific nature of the tissue damage produced. Even with the highly sophisticated techniques and equipment available today, some degree of toxicity is unavoidable. In general, the degree of toxicity is indirectly proportional to the volume of normal tissue exposed. Relatively large doses of radiation can be tolerated where the tumour is small and discrete so that the radiation beam can be accurately focused and exposure of surrounding normal tissue minimised. In these circumstances, radiotherapy may be curative. Disseminated tumours can only be subjected to relatively low doses of ionising radiation if extreme toxicity is to be avoided. In these circumstances, radiotherapy is limited to palliation. The short-term toxic effects of radiotherapy include bone marrow hypoplasia, gastrointestinal haemorrhage, diarrhoea, pulmonary and cardiac fibrosis and renal damage. In the longer term, exposure to ionising radiation is carcinogenic, particularly where alkylating agents and radiotherapy are used concurrently.

The tumouricidal effect of radiotherapy can be maximised relative to the toxic effects by **fractionation** of the total dose into several smaller doses with time for recovery of normal tissue between cycles as described earlier in this chapter. Experimental approaches to the induction of radiosensitivity include the use of hyperbaric oxygen chambers or sensitising drugs such as metronidazole.

Suggested Further Reading

Cartwright, R.A., Alexander, F.E., McKinney, P.A. et al. (1990). *Leukaemia and Lymphoma: an Atlas of Distribution with Areas of England and Wales 1984-88*. London: Leukaemia Research Fund.

Wiernik, P.H., Canellos, G.P., Kyle, R.A. and Schiffer, C.A. (1991). *Neoplastic Diseases of the Blood. (2nd ed.)*. Edinburgh: Churchill Livingstone.

Lee, R.G., Bithell, T.C., Foerster, J., Athens, J.W. and Lukens, J.N. (1993). *Wintrobe's Clinical Hematology*. London: Lea and Febiger.

Hoffbrand, A.V. and Pettit, J.E. (1993). *Essential Haematology*. Oxford: Blackwell Scientific Publications.

Answers to Self-Assessment Questions

1. The genes for GM-CSF, M-CSF, IL-3 and IL-5 are all located on chromosome 5. The gene for erythropoietin is ocated on chromosome 7.

2. EBV infection causes infectious mononucleosis in the developed world.

3. Bruton's agammaglobulinaemia is an X-linked recessive condition. Ataxia telangiectasia is an autosomal recessive condition.

4. Treatment with alkylating agents is a common cause of secondary MDS and ANLL which commonly is associated with monosomy 7 or 7q-.

5. Methotrexate is a competitive inhibitor of the enzyme dihydro folate reductase.

The Acute Leukaemias

The acute leukaemias are a heterogeneous group of malignant disorders which are characterised by the uncontrolled clonal proliferation and accumulation of poorly differentiated blast cells in the bone marrow and other body tissues. Since the first description of leukaemia in 1845, these disorders have been the subject of intense study; they have been classified and re-classified many times and fought over by experts. In recent years the vast amount of effort expended on the study of the acute leukaemias has begun to bear fruit. For some affected individuals at least, acute leukaemia has been transformed from a uniformly fatal condition to one with a significant chance of a cure. However, despite all of the efforts of committed "leukaemologists" over the years, the cause and underlying haemopoietic abnormality of the leukaemias remain to be clearly established. In this chapter the acute leukaemias are considered under the following headings:

- leukaemogenesis

- recognition and classification of acute leukaemia

- pathophysiology

- important clinical and laboratory characteristics

- treatment and management

Acute Leukaemogenesis

The acute leukaemias are thought to develop as a result of a genetic alteration within a single stem cell in the bone marrow. Mitotic division in the progeny of the cell produces a clonal population which, once sufficient clonal mass has been achieved, gives rise to the clinical manifestations of the disease. Clonality of acute leukaemia has been clearly established by techniques such as analysis of glucose 6 phosphate dehydrogenase (G-6-PD) isoenzymes, X-linked restriction fragment length polymorphisms (RFLP),

Rudolf Virchow (1821-1902)

The name leukaemia was coined by Virchow in 1847. He described the disease some two years earlier, the year before he lost his first university appointment in Berlin, apparently a victim of his "uncompromisingly radical political attitudes!" His seminal observation was made at the autopsy table when he noted massive splenomegaly and a peculiar appearance of the blood in a recently deceased patient. The normal ratio of pigmented (red) cells and colourless (white) cells seemed to be reversed in the blood of the deceased. He described this condition as "weisses blut" or "white blood" which, when translated into Greek two years later, became "leukaemia".

John Bennett (1812-1875)

It is generally believed that John Bennett in Edinburgh simultaneously discovered leukaemia with Virchow. Bennett was described as "a man of brilliance but short temper, certain of his own virtues, pugnacious, and unable to suffer fools"! Bennett also made his orginal observation at the autopsy table in a patient with a very similar case history. Bennett felt the blood had pus in it because microscopic examination revealed the presence of a huge number of cells usually associated with the presence of pus. He described the condition as "pyaemia".

A major disagreement between Virchow and Bennett was conducted in the journals for several years. During the decades that followed, Virchow now reinstated to his position but still maintaining his enlightened social and political views, made some seminal observations about leukaemia. These were all made without the ability to stain and count blood cells and it is remarkable how close his guesses were to the truth as it is known today.

immunoglobulin and T lymphocyte receptor gene rearrangements, cytogenetics, chromosomal translocation breakpoints and DNA point mutations.

Cumulative evidence, presented by epidemiologists and others, suggests that acute leukaemia is one of the several potential expressions of aberrant stem cell physiology whose range includes aplastic anaemia and myelodysplasia. The exact nature of the aberrant stem cell physiology is the subject of research.

Epidemiological Evidence

Hereditary Factors

Several hereditary disorders are associated with an increased risk of developing acute leukaemia. These include Fanconi's anaemia, Bloom's syndrome, ataxia telangiectasia and Down's syndrome. Defects in these disorders include chromosome instability secondary to defective DNA repair or some form of immune deficiency. Acute lymphoblastic leukaemia is particularly prevalent in those disorders associated with immune deficiency and in "exaggerated" infection with the Epstein-Barr virus (EBV). In Down's syndrome (+21) a 20- to 30-fold increased frequency of acute leukaemia has been reported. While there is an increased risk with these disorders it is equally true that only a minority of cases develop acute leukaemia.

Radiation, Chemicals and Drugs

Exposure to ionising radiation, chemicals and drugs is a known cause of leukaemia. As described in the previous chapter, the most studied of these is ionising radiation-related leukaemogenesis. In particular, persons exposed to nuclear fall-out from atomic bombs, persons receiving radiation therapy for malignant disease and children exposed to diagnostic X-rays *in utero* have all been shown to suffer from an increased probability of developing leukaemia. Descriptive population studies have shown an increased incidence of leukaemia in families living close to electrical pylons or who are exposed to high levels of radon gas, and in children of fathers who work in nuclear reprocessing plants. Such studies are highly controversial. The mechanisms involved in radiation-induced leukaemogenesis are described in the previous chapter.

The evidence that chemicals and drugs cause leukaemia mostly comes from an increased incidence of leukaemia in patients who have received cytotoxic drugs for the treatment of cancers, or who have been chronically exposed to benzene. Exposure to chloramphenicol and phenylbutazone has also been reported to increase the risk of developing bone marrow aplasia or myelodysplasia which may progress to leukaemia.

Virus-related Leukaemias

Viruses are a common cause of leukaemia in animals, including primates. However, viruses have not been implicated in most human leukaemias. Data from epidemiological studies suggest that ALL in children reflects an unusual response to common infection(s) but no causative virus has yet been isolated. Adult T lymphoblastic leukaemia/lymphoma (ATLL) and Burkitt's lymphoma are related to viral infection with human T-cell lymphotropic virus I (HTLV I) and Epstein-Barr virus (EBV) respectively. However, not all persons infected with HTLV I develop leukaemia and EBV is also the cause of infectious mononucleosis, a non-malignant disorder. EBV has been shown to immortalise human B lymphoblasts *in vitro* and also is implicated in the aetiology of malignant lymphoproliferative diseases in immunodeficient individuals. It is suggested that EBV infection precedes and possibly causes a clonal expansion in Burkitt's lymphoma. However, whether the clonal expansion occurs before or after translocation of the *myc* oncogene is not yet clearly established.

Molecular Evidence

Oncogenes and Tumour-suppressor Genes

Oncogenes are highly conserved genes that are widely distributed among human chromosomes. The exact chromosomal locations of many oncogenes have now been identified and several are involved in the chromosomal abnormalities documented in ALL and ANLL. Oncogenes originally were isolated as the discrete genetic elements of tumour viruses which were responsible for the oncogenic potential of the virus. Oncogenes are classified according to the function of the protein which they encode as shown in Table 16.1.

Oncogene Classification	How isolated	Protein Location	Function
Class 1 (Growth factors)			
sis	Retrovirus	Secreted	Platelet-derived growth factor
Class 2 & 3 (Growth factor receptors)			
erb B	Retrovirus	Membrane	Epidermal growth factor receptor
fms	Retrovirus	Membrane	Receptor for MCSF
trk	Tumour	Membrane	Receptor for nerve growth factor
src	Retrovirus	Cytoplasm	Protein-tyrosine kinase
abl	Retrovirus	Cytoplasm	Protein-tyrosine kinase
Class 4, 5 & 6 (Intracellular transducers)			
raf	Retrovirus	Cytoplasm	Protein-serine kinase
gsp	Tumour	Cytoplasm	G protein a subunit
ras	Retrovirus, tumour	Cytoplasm	GTP/GDP-binding domain
Class 7 (Nuclear transcription factors)			
jun	Retrovirus	Nucleus	Transcription factor
fos	Retrovirus	Nucleus	Transcription factor
myc	Retrovirus, tumour	Nucleus	DNA-binding protein
erb A	Retrovirus	Nucleus	Member of steroid receptor family

Table 16.1 *A selection of characterised oncogenes and the proteins that they encode*

The proteins encoded by oncogenes have been shown to act at different stages of the pathways by which growth signals are transduced through the cell to the nucleus. The signal may trigger the cell into cycle, activate a particular cellular function, or trigger differentiation. Oncogenes have been demonstrated to drive immortalised cell lines to undergo malignant transformation and to cause tumours in transgenic mice. However, in both these situations the oncogenes were not the sole cause of the malignancy. In the immortalised cell lines, the insertion of the oncogene is a secondary event subsequent to the transformation events which occur as part of the immortalisation process. In the transgenic mice, tumours did not occur in all tissues, but as discrete clonal proliferations. This suggests that the mere presence of an activated oncogene is insufficient to induce malignant change. A secondary event subsequent to oncogene activation is required for tumour induction.

The insertion of an oncogene to cells *in vitro* accelerates their growth rate and allows growth under conditions prohibitive for normal cells. This growth effect is dominant: it occurs in the presence of normal cells. However, research using somatic cell genetics has shown that malignant transformation is recessive to normal growth. These findings suggest the presence of genes that can overpower the effect of oncogenes. A number of such genes have been identified and they are known as **anti-oncogenes** or **tumour-suppressor genes**. The exact nature of the function of tumour-suppressor genes such as *p53* and *rb*, remains to be established but they appear to regulate aspects of cell cycle and mitosis. Their protein products frequently are located within the cell nucleus. The loss of function of a tumour-suppressor gene may therefore be one step in a multi-step process of malignant transformation. Compelling evidence for this theory has emerged from studies of the role of the *rb* tumour suppressor gene in the induction of retinoblastoma, a tumour of the eye.

There is an apparent link between the activation of oncogenes or the loss of function of tumour-suppressor genes and the perturbation between cell proliferation and differentiation which is the motif of malignancy. A single event is insufficient to cause malignant transformation. Several changes within one oncogene, or changes in two or more oncogenes or tumour-suppressor genes, are necessary to cause malignant transformation. The mechanisms by which oncogenes can be activated include the following:

- chromosome translocations and rearrangements

- point mutations

- inactivation

- promoter insertion

- amplification

The molecular basis of the numerous chromosome translocations and rearrangements in acute leukaemia is under intense study. The most studied translocations, particularly *myc* and the immunoglobulin genes and *pml* and *rarα*, have been described in the previous chapter and are implicated in leukaemogenesis. Point mutations are best illustrated by studies of the *ras* and *fms* oncogenes in acute

The study of haematological morphology parallels developments in microscopy and chemistry. The simple microscope of Van Leeuwenhoek (c 1700) revealed the red blood cells, whereas the colourless white blood cells were not reliably identified until about 1830 by Addison and Gulliver. The major breakthrough occurred with the work of Paul Ehrlich (1854-1915) who is regarded as one of the founding fathers of cytochemistry. It was his interest and enthusiasm, including the testing of thousands of new stains, which led to the reliable identification of the subtypes of white blood cells. The early stains developed detected lipids, carbohydrates and assessed the acidic or basic nature of the cell. Enzyme detection did not really progress until the 1940's with the development of the azo dyes which can be used to detect intracellular enzymes such as esterases, phosphatases and dehydrogenases. By the mid 1970's cytochemistry was the best diagnostic tool available for acute leukaemia. The next advance came with the use of monoclonal antibodies and immunocytochemistry which resulted in improvements in diagnosis and reclassification of some types of leukaemia.

leukaemia where evidence is accumulating to implicate these as a step in the multi-step process of leukaemogenesis. The other mechanisms of oncogene activation are the subject of active research.

The continuing search for the causes of leukaemia is following two distinct lines of enquiry. The "circumstantial" evidence is being compiled by the epidemiologists who have clearly identified some of the factors or agents that contribute to leukaemia. The "factual" evidence is being compiled by molecular biologists who have identified a multitude of ways to damage a gene and cause the progeny to behave like a tumour. There are early signs that these two apparently divergent approaches are beginning to converge and that coherent theories describing the mechanisms of leukaemogenesis will emerge in the near future.

Recognition and Classification of the Acute Leukaemias

Recognition of acute leukaemia requires the examination of appropriately stained blood and bone marrow smears. The presence of more than 30% blast cells in the bone marrow at clinical presentation is an objective criterion for defining acute leukaemia. Frequently, in cases of grossly elevated white cell counts at presentation, the diagnosis is self-evident from the peripheral blood. However, a bone marrow aspirate, and often a biopsy, are still necessary for confirmation purposes and accurate classification.

Accurate classification has become increasingly important as therapeutic advances have been made both in the treatment and the management of the disorder. Phenotypic characterisation of the leukaemic cells at presentation is essential to enable the selection of appropriate treatment and the monitoring of the progress of the disease during treatment. More recently, the genotypic characterisation of leukaemic cells has been added to the vast armamentarium of technologies available to the leukaemologist. These technologies, including cytomorphology, electron microscopy, cytochemistry, immunocytochemistry, cytogenetics, and molecular techniques involving the manipulation of DNA and RNA, are utilised to define cellular characteristics or markers and the precise nature of the leukaemic proliferation or clone as shown in Table 16.2.

Full Blood Count (FBC)

Requested because of clinical symptoms such as bruising, organomegaly or bone pain.
Occasionally a chance finding on routine medical screening.
FBC usually shows anaemia, thrombocytopaenia and variable WBC

Morphology

Peripheral blood may contain blast cells
Bone marrow has greater than 30% blast cells.

Immunophenotyping

Flow cytometry or immunocytochemistry using panels of monoclonal antibodies
Classification into ALL, with T or B characteristics
Classification into ANLL, M0 to M7 subtypes
Bi-phenotypic if evidence of both lymphoid and non-lymphoid markers

95% of cases are diagnosed by this point

Cytochemistry

To confirm or supplement immunophenotyping results
Particularly for monocytic lineage leukaemias

99% of cases are diagnosed by this point

Cytogenetics

For clonality and prognostic information

DNA analysis

Needed for rare cases

99.9% of cases are diagnosed by this point

Table 16.2 *The diagnosis of acute leukaemia*

The Morphological and Cytochemical Approach to Classification

This approach to the classification of acute leukaemia relies on the examination of the morphology of the leukaemic cells using light microscopy. The information gleaned in this way is supplemented using a battery of cytochemical stains to detect subcellular components as shown in Table 16.3. Electron microscopy also is required in some cases. Using this approach, it is possible to identify two main types of acute leukaemia namely lymphoblastic (ALL) and myeloblastic (AML) or non-lymphoblastic (ANLL), and to subdivide each into a number of subtypes. The term ANLL is preferred to AML because it better encapsulates the extreme complexity of these forms of leukaemia.

Method	Substances stained	Main uses
Sudan Black	Neutral fats, phospholipids lipoproteins	Identification of granulocyte precursors
Peroxidase	Myeloperoxidase	Identification of neutrophil and eosinophil precursors
PAS	1,2-glycol groups of glycogen etc	Block positive in M6
Chloroacetate esterase	Esterase isoenzymes 1, 2, 7 and 8	Differentiation of granulocytic and monocytic maturation (M4 & M5)
Non-specific esterase	Esterase isoenzymes 3, 4, 5 and 6	Differentiation of granulocytic and monocytic maturation (M4 & M5)
Acid phosphatase	Acid phosphatase	Useful in TALL and HCL
TdT	Terminal deoxynucleotidyl transferase	Differentiation of ALL and ANLL*

Table 16.3 *The substances stained by and applications of basic cytochemistry tests*
* rarely positive in ANLL

Classification of individual cases is far from straightforward, however. The disordered growth and differentiation which characterises the leukaemic process increases the likelihood of aberrant expression of cell markers and can make recognition of the different subtypes difficult. Interpretation of the results obtained requires significant skill and, ultimately, relies upon the experience and judgement of a trained haematologist.

In an attempt to improve the reproducibility and comparability of the classification process, a group of expert haematologists from France, America and Britain (FAB) collaborated to define a more objective set of criteria for the classification of the acute leukaemias. The initial FAB collaborative study, which took place in 1976, was based on the examination of more than 200 different cases of acute leukaemia by expert morphologists. The FAB group recommended that the acute lymphoblastic leukaemias should be coded into three variants, which are designated L1-L3 according to the predominant morphology of the leukaemic lymphoblasts, and that the non-lymphoblastic leukaemias should similarly be coded into six subtypes, which are designated M1-M6. The classification should only be made after the examination of both peripheral blood and bone marrow films, including the performance of a 500 cell differential count. In addition, a myeloperoxidase or Sudan black stain should be used to facilitate the recognition of myeloblasts.

In 1985, two further entities, viz acute megakaryoblastic leukaemia (AMegL) and a type of myeloblastic leukaemia with virtually no evidence of differentiation, were recognised and incorporated into the FAB classification scheme as M7 and M0 respectively. These two subtypes were identified using an electron microscope to examine peroxidase cytochemistry at an ultrastructural level. The FAB classification scheme is summarised in Table 16.4.

In extremely rare circumstances it is impossible to classify the acute leukaemia into either ALL or ANLL with any technology. This unusual entity, not included in the FAB scheme, is therefore termed acute undifferentiated leukaemia (AUL). In cases of AUL it is important to confirm that the disease is of haemopoietic origin and to exclude other non-haemopoietic malignancies that have spread to the bone marrow.

The Immunological and Genetic Approach to Classification

With advances in diagnostic technology, further classification schemes have emerged. For example, the application of immuno-cytochemistry techniques which employ monoclonal antibodies to recognise lineage and differentiation markers on leukaemic cells has enabled the subdivision of ALL into at least four separate entities viz early pre-B ALL, pre-B ALL, B ALL and T ALL. The most important of these subdivisions is between T ALL and B ALL. Prognostic and therapeutic significance has been attached to these subtypes but, unfortunately, little correlation exists between the immunological subtypes and the morphological subtypes of ALL according to the FAB scheme.

Acute Lymphoblastic Leukaemia

Designation	Alternative	Bone Marrow Appearances
L1		Homogeneous population of small lymphoblasts with scanty cytoplasm and scanty nucleoli. Nucleus occasionally cleft
L2		Heterogeneous population of large lymphoblasts with moderately abundant cytoplasm and one or more nucleoli. Nucleus commonly indented or cleft
L3	Burkitt's type	Homogeneous population of large lymphoblasts with prominent nucleoli and deeply basophilic, vacuolated cytoplasm

Acute Non-lymphoblastic Leukaemia

Designation	Alternative	Bone Marrow Appearances
M0		Identified by ultrastructural myeloperoxidase activity or immunophenotyping
M1	AML without maturation	Monomorphic with one or more distinct nucleoli, occasional Auer rod and at least 3% myeloperoxidase positivity
M2	AML with maturation	50% or more myeloblasts and promyelocytes and common single Auer rods. Dysplastic myeloid differentiation may also be present
M3	APL	Dominant cell type is promyelocyte with heavy azurophilic granulation. Bundles of Auer rods confirm diagnosis. Microgranular variant exists (M3v)
M4	AMMoL	As M2 but >20% promonocytes and monocytes.
M5	AMoL	>80% monoblasts is poorly differentiated (M5a) >80% monoblasts, promonocytes or monocytes is well differentiated (M5b)
M6	AEL	>50% bizarre, dysplastic nucleated red cells with multinucleate forms and cytoplasmic bridging. Myeloblasts usually >30%
M7	AMegL	Fibrosis, heterogeneous blast population with cytoplasmic blebs. Platelet peroxidase positive

Table 16.4 *Summary of the FAB classification scheme for the acute leukaemias*

The advent of techniques enabling the manipulation of DNA has allowed lymphoid ontogeny to be studied at a genetic level. The hierarchical rearrangement of the immunoglobulin and T lymphocyte receptor genes is well defined and DNA probes are available to study these processes in the diagnostic laboratory using techniques such as Southern blotting and the Polymerase Chain Reaction (PCR). The results of these studies can be incorporated in the classification of ALL but due to either the aberrant biology of leukaemic cells, or the existence of bi-phenotypic leukaemias they have not clarified the classification scheme much further. These techniques have a more significant role to play in the monitoring of the disease and in the understanding of its biology.

A summary of blast cell markers in ALL subtypes, using the technologies of morphology, cytochemistry, immunocytochemistry and recombinant DNA, is shown in Table 16.5.

	Early Pre-B	Pre-B	B	T
Morphology				
FAB L1	90%	90%	10%	95%
FAB L2	10%	10%	15%	5%
FAB L3	0%	0%	75%	0%
Cytochemistry				
Acid phosphatase	–	–	–	+
5'-Nucleotidase	+	+	–	–
Nuclear TdT	+	+	–	+
Immunocytochemistry				
Cytoplasmic μ	–	+	–	–
Membrane Ig	–	–	+	–
CD 10	+++	+	+/–	–
HLA-DR	+++	++	++	+/–
CD19,cyt CD22	+	+	+	–
CD7,cyt CD3	–	–	–	+++
Gene rearrangement				
Heavy chain	+	+	+	–
Light chain	+/–	+/–	+	–
T cell receptor	–/+	–/+	–/+	+

Flow cytometry involves the detection of particles such as cells, bacteria or chromosomes as they move in a liquid stream through a laser-controlled "sensing" zone. The particles of interest are often rare "events" in a mixture of normal or contaminating particles. As each particle passes through the laser beam, it scatters some of the light in all directions. If the particle has been marked with a fluorescent dye, the laser will cause it to fluoresce. The pattern of scattered and fluorescent light produced reveals much about the particle. For example, forward angle light scatter (FALS) gives an indication of cell size, while right angle light scatter (RALS) gives an indication of cell granularity. Modern flow cytometers can make several separate measurements on each particle, at the rate of several thousands of particles per second. The results can be displayed using single histograms or more complex multiparametric diagrams. Some flow cytometers are even capable of sorting out of the main particle stream particles of special interest which can then be used in further experiments.

Table 16.5 *Blast cell markers of the acute lymphoblastic leukaemias*

The immunological classification of ANLL is not as clear-cut as that of ALL. The specificity of myeloid-associated markers is not as strong and the correlation with the widely accepted FAB subgroups of ANLL is poor. The exceptions to this generalisation are AMegL (FAB code M7), AEL (FAB code M6) and acute undifferentiated myeloblastic leukaemia (FAB code M0). These are now identified with immunocytochemistry using anti-glycophorin A to detect the erythroid component in AEL; anti-platelet glycoproteins (CD41,42 and 61) to detect the megakaryoblastic component in AMegL; and a stem cell-associated antibody CD34 combined with a myeloid-associated antibody CD33 to detect the only evidence of myeloid differentiation in the M0 FAB subgroup.

A major advantage with the immunocytochemistry techniques, when compared to the traditional morphology and cytochemistry methods, is that they can be automated in a flow cytometry analytical system using lasers and fluorescence detection. A summary of blast cell markers in ANLL subtypes using the technologies of morphology, cytochemistry and immunocytochemistry is shown in Table 16.6.

	M0	M1	M2	M3	M4	M5	M6	M7
Cytochemistry								
Myeloperoxidase	−	+	++	+++	+	+/-	−	−
Chloroacetate esterase	−	+/-	+	++	+	−	−	−
Non-specific esterase	−	−	−	−	+	++	−	−
Immunocytochemistry								
CD34	+	+/-	−	−	−	−	−	−
CD33	+	+	+	+	+	+	−	−
CD13	−	+	+	+	+	+	−	−
CD14	−	−	−	−	+	++	−	−
HLA-DR	+	+	+	−	+	+	−	−
Glycophorin A	−	−	−	−	−	−	+	−
CD41,42,61	−	−	−	−	−	−	−	+

Table 16.6 *Blast cell markers of the acute non-lymphoblastic leukaemias*

A major shortcoming of the markers described to date is that they are markers of normal haemopoietic differentiation and can therefore only be described as leukaemia-associated markers. Unfortunately, no leukaemia-specific antigenic marker currently is routinely available for classification purposes.

Cytogenetics, the study of chromosomes, has been applied to the acute leukaemias for many years. Numerous non-random patterns of chromosomal alterations have been demonstrated in bone marrow cells from the majority of patients with acute leukaemia. Routinely prepared metaphase preparations have shown clonal karyotypic abnormalities in about 50% of patients with ANLL and 60% of patients with ALL. Whereas high-resolution chromosome banding techniques have shown clonal cytogenetic abnormalities in virtually all patients with either ANLL or ALL. Cytogenetic abnormalities of leukaemic cells can be characterised as changes involving chromosome number (ploidy) or chromosome structure, for example translocation (t), inversion (inv), deletion (del).

The demonstration and typing of chromosomal abnormalities is becoming increasingly important as an aid to the diagnosis and classification and as a prognostic indicator in the leukaemias. As described in the previous chapter, many of the chromosomal rearrangements commonly found in the leukaemias involve disruption or translocation of the loci of oncogenes, the immunoglobulin genes, the T lymphocyte receptor genes or genes encoding growth factors. As our knowledge of the chromosomal locations of oncogenes and of the role they play in leukaemogenesis has expanded, the need to integrate cytogenetic data within a classification scheme for acute leukaemia has become obvious.

With the increasing sophistication of techniques employed by cytogeneticists, it seems likely that new, leukaemia-specific markers will be discovered in the near future. Fluorescent *in situ* hybridisation (FISH) is an example of a highly sensitive and specific technique currently being applied to the study of chromosomal rearrangements in acute leukaemia (see sidebox). A summary of some of the most important chromosomal abnormalities associated with acute leukaemia is shown in Table 16.7. A large number of other chromosomal abnormalities have been reported in association with acute leukaemia. However, these do not show the same strong correlation with a particular leukaemic subtype as those shown in Table 16.7 and so are less useful in the classification of the disease. Hyperdiploidy and hypodiploidy are very important numerical observations, particularly in early pre-B cell ALL.

The most recent classification scheme for the acute leukaemias attempts to combine the most important facets of the above schemes. The MIC (**M**orphology, **I**mmunology and **C**ytogenetics) is likely to prove to be of great biological and clinical significance,

---

In situ hybridisation is a technique by which specific portions of chromosomes can be marked by hybridisation with a labelled nucleic acid probe. The label used can be a radio-isotope, an enzyme or a fluorochrome. Fluorescent *in situ* hybridisation (FISH) is revolutionising molecular cytogenetics. It is now possible to detect structural and numerical aberrations in disorders where conventional karyotyping is very difficult or impossible. The important feature of FISH is that the nucleic acid is retained *in situ*, and not degraded during processing. FISH techniques can be applied to most biological tissues, including whole cells, tissue sections, chromosomes and bare nuclei. The probes used are usually between 10 to 25 kilobases in length. Longer probes give weaker signals, probably because they penetrate less efficiently into cross-linked tissue and smaller probes may be difficult to visualise. Chromosome "paints" which label complete chromosomes are useful in the detection of numerical abnormalities.

Type of leukaemia	Chromosome abnormality	Genes involved	FAB type
ALL	t(9;22)(q34;q11)	*abl, bcr*	L1,L2
Pre-B ALL	t(1;19)(q23;p13	*prl, e2a*	L1
	t(4;11)(q21;q23)		L1,L2
B ALL	t(8;14)(q24;q32)	*myc*, IgH	L3
	t(2;8)(p12;q24)	Igκ, *myc*	L3
	t(8;22)(q24;q11)	*myc*, Igλ	L3
T ALL	t(11;14)(p13;q11)	*tcl2, Ti*$_\alpha$	L1,L2
	t(8;14)(q24;q11)	*myc, Ti*$_\alpha$	L1,L2
AML	t(8;21)(q22;q22)	*ets2*	M2
APL	t(15;17)(q22;q12)	*pml, rar*α	M3
	t(15;17)(q22;q21)		
AMoL	del/t (11)(q23)	*ets1*	M5
AMMoL	inv16,16q- and t(16;16)		M4
AEL	t(8;16)(p11;p13)		M6

Table 16.7 *Non-random structural chromosome abnormalities in the acute leukaemias*

Morphologic, Immunologic, and Cytogenetic (MIC) Working Classification of Acute Lymphoblastic Leukaemias (1986). First MIC Cooperative Study Group. *Cancer Genetics and Cytogenetics*, **23**: 189-197.

Morphologic, Immunologic and Cytogenetic (MIC) Working Classification of the Acute Myeloid Leukaemias (1988). Second MIC Cooperative Study Group. *British Journal of Haematology*, **68**: 487-494.

possibly the "holy grail" for leukaemologists! The MIC classification schemes for ALL and ANLL were the result of collaborative workshops in 1985 and 1986 respectively and recognised the recent advances by immunologists and cytogeneticists in leukaemia diagnosis. Where possible, immunological and cytogenetic data were correlated with the FAB codification scheme. As techniques advance and new data continues to accumulate, the MIC scheme is adapted accordingly: this scheme is in a state of continual evolution. The most consistent correlates are shown in Table 16.7 but as the diagnostic technology in non-cytomorphological methods develops, the linkage of new findings to FAB subgroups will be more difficult.

Pathophysiology of the Acute Leukaemias

Acute leukaemia causes morbidity and mortality through three general mechanisms:

- deficiency in normal blood cell number or function

- invasion of vital organs with impairment of organ function

- systemic disturbances shown by metabolic imbalance

The treatment of leukaemia with cytotoxic chemotherapy also is associated with significant morbidity. In fact, it is often difficult to distinguish between the effects of treatment and the pathophysiology of the disease itself.

Infection

Infection is one of the most common causes of death and a significant cause of morbidity in patients with acute leukaemia. The natural course of acute leukaemia eventually includes a phase of impaired host defence. This is manifest as impairment of phagocytic defences most often due to neutropaenia but also, occasionally, due to qualitative abnormalities of phagocytic cells. Neutropaenia may be secondary to the "crowding out" of normal neutrophil production by leukaemic tissue in the bone marrow or may be secondary to cytoreductive therapy. Numerous qualitative defects of neutrophil function have been reported in acute leukaemia but the pathological significance of these is uncertain. For example, defective phagocytosis and deficiency of the lysosomal enzymes involved in intracellular microbial killing, lysozyme, lactoferrin and myeloperoxidase commonly are present. The clinical effects of neutropaenia and neutrophil dysfunction and the pattern of infecting organisms are discussed in more detail in Chapter 14.

The usual hallmark of infection is fever. Unfortunately, the leukaemic process itself can cause fever, leading to complications in the recognition of infection. Differentiation between fever caused by infection and fever caused by the leukaemia process itself often is difficult. Typically, humoral and cell-mediated immunity are normal in acute leukaemia but, as the disease progresses, immune function deteriorates and the frequency and severity of infection increases.

The prevention of infection is a vital part of the treatment of acute leukaemia, and the subject of intensive haematological and microbiological monitoring. Antibiotic regimes are implemented at the first sign of fever because of the association of infection with mortality. In some leukaemia treatment centres severely neutropaenic patients are treated with prophylactic antibiotics, regardless of signs of infection.

Haemorrhage

Haemorrhage is a common problem in acute leukaemia both at pre-sentation and during treatment. Usually it is the direct result of thrombocytopaenia, but may be secondary to qualitative defects of platelets, disseminated intravascular coagulation (DIC), liver dis-ease, or more rarely, hyperviscosity syndrome. **Petechiae** (tiny pin-point haemorrhages in the skin) and **ecchymoses** (bruises) are the most frequent clinical manifestations. Haemorrhage into the gut, subarachnoid space, or lungs frequently is life-threatening. The risk of severe haemorrhage is inversely related to the circulating platelet count: life-threatening haemorrhage is unlikely until the platelet count falls below $20 \times 10^9/l$. Occasionally, platelet dysfunction can result in bleeding problems at higher platelet counts. In either case, the most effective form of treatment is platelet transfusion. Some treatment centres aim to prevent haemorrhage by a regime of pro-phylactic platelet transfusion.

Disseminated intravascular coagulation is particularly troublesome in APL due to the presence of thromboplastin-like substances in the abnormal granules of the leukaemic promyelocytes, but it may be seen in any form of acute leukaemia. As described in Chapter 23, gram-negative septicaemia is associated with intractable DIC, which commonly results in death.

Anaemia

Normocytic, normochromic anaemia is extremely common in acute leukaemia and is responsible for the symptoms associated with fatigue and a sense of ill health. The severity of the anaemia typi-cally reflects the severity of the disease. The unregulated prolifera-tion of leukaemic tissue results in the physical "crowding out" of normal haemopoietic elements, leading to a reduction in erythro-poiesis, thrombopoiesis and leucopoiesis. In some cases, the anaemia may be exacerbated by ineffective erythropoiesis or, more rarely, haemolysis. In most anaemic individuals, erythropoietin lev-els are raised in proportion to the degree of anaemia but the normal erythroid precursors show diminished responsiveness to this hor-mone. It is thought that leukaemic cells elaborate one or more inhibitors of normal haemopoiesis.

Infiltration of Vital Organs

The organs infiltrated at presentation and during the course of acute leukaemia vary according to the subtype involved, but may include liver, spleen, lymph nodes, meninges, brain, skin, eyes and testes. In contrast to the solid tumours, the frequency of organ infiltration by acute leukaemia far exceeds the frequency of symptomatic complications associated with such infiltration. Broadly, there are three types of complication associated with organ infiltration in acute leukaemia:

- **hyperleucocytosis**. The extremely high white cell counts sometimes encountered at presentation in acute leukaemia are associated with markedly increased whole blood viscosity because leukaemic blast cells are poorly deformable. This leads to a "sludging" effect in the microcirculation, and predisposes to the formation of microthrombi or acute haemorrhage. The organs most commonly involved are the brain, lungs and eyes. The increase in whole blood viscosity usually is partially offset by the presence of anaemia. Injudicious attempts to correct anaemia by transfusion of packed red cells may precipitate problems due to hyperviscosity.

- **leucostatic tumours**. Rarely, leukaemic blast cells may lodge in the vascular system of infiltrated organs and proliferate, forming macroscopic pseudotumours which eventually erode the vessel wall, resulting in, often severe, secondary haemorrhage associated with the site of infiltration. Leucostatic tumours are associated with hyperleucocytosis, particularly where expansion of the leukaemic cell load occurs rapidly. Such tumours were a relatively common cause of death in the days before effective cytoreductive therapy was available. The organs most commonly affected are the brain, liver and lungs

- **sanctuary site relapse**. Leukaemic infiltration of the testes and meninges is observed in all forms of acute leukaemia but is most common in ALL. These organs provide an effective sanctuary for resident leukaemic blasts because they are poorly penetrated by cytotoxic drugs. In the absence of specific additional prophylactic therapy to these organs, they may provide a source for the resurgence of leukaemic proliferation, leading to relapse. Meningeal and testicular relapse are most commonly seen in childhood ALL.

Metabolic Disturbances

Metabolic disturbances are common in acute leukaemia and may be caused by the disease process or by its treatment. For example, a reduction in plasma sodium ion concentration, or **hyponatraemia** is relatively common in ANLL secondary to the production of a vasopressin-like substance by myeloblasts. A reduction in potassium ion concentration, or **hypokalaemia** is also common, especially in AMMoL and AMoL secondary to the renal damage caused by the release of lysozyme by the leukaemic blast cells. Spontaneous lysis of leukaemic blast cells causes the release of abnormally large amounts of purines into the plasma. The increased rate of purine catabolism which results leads to an increased concentration of uric acid, the major breakdown product of purines, or **hyperuricaemia**. Untreated, hyperuricaemia causes gouty arthritis and renal damage. Some degree of hepatic dysfunction is common in the course of acute leukaemia and may result in deranged plasma concentrations of liver enzymes and lactic acidosis.

Several of the drugs used in the treatment of leukaemia are nephrotoxic and therefore may increase the severity of minor metabolic disturbances. When the presenting leukaemic cell load is high, successful cytoreductive therapy can induce severe metabolic disturbances secondary to massive cell lysis. An increase in the plasma concentrations of potassium ions, **hyperkalaemia**, phosphates, **hyperphosphataemia**, hyperuricaemia and a decrease in the plasma concentration of calcium ions, **hypocalcaemia**, are all common sequelae of massive tumour lysis. These abnormalities may be severe enough to require dialysis, particularly where renal damage is present.

Important Characteristics of the Acute Leukaemias

Acute Lymphoblastic Leukaemia

Acute lymphoblastic leukaemia is the most common malignant disease affecting children, accounting for approximately 30% of childhood cancers. The age distribution of the disease is skewed with 75% of cases occurring in children under the age of 15 years. Beyond childhood, the age distribution is uniform with a median between 30 and 40 years. Before the 1960s ALL was almost always fatal whereas now at least 50% of childhood cases are considered curable. Unfortunately, this is not the case with adult ALL which is much more refractory to treatment.

A number of prognostic indicators have been identified which can be used to stratify individual cases into different risk groups and to tailor treatment accordingly. Broadly, those individuals who are judged to have a relatively poor prognosis by these criteria are treated more aggressively than those judged to have a good prognosis. There is considerable controversy and confusion about the relative merits of different prognostic indicators because, ultimately, the form of treatment adopted is the most important factor in determining survival. For this reason, the relative prognostic power of various disease characteristics varies from study to study. The most widely accepted prognostic indicators are summarised in Table 16.8.

These prognostic indicators are most useful at presentation and have greater predictive power in children. The most important prognostic feature at presentation is the white cell count because this provides an indication of the size of the tumour load and the likelihood of successful remission induction. The next most important factor in terms of its predictive power is age at presentation. Infants have a poor prognosis because of the high tumour load relative to their body mass and a greater incidence of extramedullary involvement. Adults have a poorer prognosis than children because of differences in the biology of ALL in adults. Males have a slightly poorer prognosis than females because of the possibility of testicular relapse. Extramedullary involvement typically only occurs in the presence of a high tumour load and so is an indicator of a poor prognosis. The presence of a mediastinal mass on chest X-ray is indicative of the presence of a hypertrophic thymus and is associated with T ALL. The presence of anaemia at presentation indicates a slowly progressing tumour: there is no time for anaemia to develop before the onset of symptoms in more aggressive tumours.

The majority of cases of ALL present with clinical symptoms of bone marrow failure and organ infiltration. Bone pain is common in childhood ALL. Superficial lymphadenopathy and moderate enlargement of the spleen and liver occur at some time in the

Prognostic Indicator	Favourable	Unfavourable
White cell count	$<10 \times 10^9/l$	$>50 \times 10^9/l$
Age	3 to 7 years	<1 year or >10 years
Sex	Female	Male
Race	White	Black
Time to remission	<14 days	>28 days
Lymphadenopathy	Absent	Massive
Organomegaly	Absent	Massive
Mediastinal mass	Absent	Present
CNS leukaemia	Absent	Present
FAB classification	L1	L2 and L3
Haemoglobin	<7 g/dl	>10g/dl
Platelet count	$>100 \times 10^9/l$	$<30 \times 10^9/l$
Serum immunoglobulin	Normal	Decreased
Immunological markers	Early pre-B ALL	T ALL
		B ALL
		Mixed lineage
Cytogenetic markers	Hyperdiploidy	Pseudodiploidy
	6q-	t(9;22)
		t(8;14)
		t(4;11)
		t(14q+)

Table 16.8 *Prognostic indicators in acute lymphoblastic leukaemia*

course of the disease in most cases of ALL. Leucocytosis (predominantly leukaemic blast cells) and thrombocytopaenia are common at presentation. Occasionally, many of the characteristic signs of ALL are absent at presentation.

Immunocytochemistry largely has superseded other methods used in the identification and classification of ALL. The Philadelphia chromosome t(9;22)(q34;q11), usually associated with chronic myeloid leukaemia, is also seen in some cases of ALL. It is documented more frequently in adults than children, often in association with other chromosomal abnormalities and indicates a poor prognosis. As described in the previous chapter, the breakpoint in the t(9;22) of ALL, within the *bcr* gene on chromosome 22, differs from that documented in chronic myeloid leukaemia.

Early Pre-B Acute Lymphoblastic Leukaemia

More than 70% of cases of ALL in children and about 50% of cases in adults type as early pre-B ALL. This form of ALL is characterised by a lack of immunoglobulin markers on the cell surface or within the cytoplasm and, in about 90% of cases, by the presence on the cell surface of CD10 and typically is associated with a good prognosis. Because of its frequency, this form of ALL has been called "common ALL" in earlier classification systems. Very occasionally, the phenotype of early pre-B cell ALL is observed with no expression of CD10. This may be referred to as "null ALL". Hyperdiploidy is most frequently documented in early pre-B cell ALL. Chromosomal translocations are associated more often with the other subtypes of ALL.

Pre-B Acute Lymphoblastic Leukaemia

The leukaemic blast cells in pre-B ALL are characterised by the presence of cytoplasmic immunoglobulin heavy (μ) chains in the absence of light chains or surface immunoglobulin. Most cases are coded as FAB subtype L1 and 90% of cases are CD10 positive. Approximately 30% of cases exhibit the karyotype characterised by t(1;19)(q23;p13) which has been reported to convey a risk of early relapse during standard therapy.

B Acute Lymphoblastic Leukaemia

B ALL is a relatively rare condition, representing less than 2% of cases of ALL. The leukaemic blasts in this subtype of ALL show signs of greater maturity than those in the other subtypes: CD10 expression is weak; immunoglobulins are expressed on the cell surface and molecular genetic analysis reveals a clonal rearrangement of both heavy and light chain immunoglobulin genes. The blast cells in the majority of cases of B ALL are morphologically coded as FAB subtype L3. B ALL is associated with chromosomal translocations involving the c-*myc* oncogene and the immunoglobulin genes ie (t(8;14)(q24;q32), t(8;22)(q24;q11), t(2;8)(p12;q24)). These are the same translocations which characterise Burkitt's lymphoma. For this reason, B ALL is sometimes known as Burkitt's type ALL. This form of ALL is associated with a uniformly poor prognosis.

The discovery of Common ALL Antigen (CALLA) by Dr M Greaves in 1975 caused a great deal of excitement among leukaemologists because it appeared to be the first leukaemia-specific marker to be identified. He produced a polyclonal antibody that reacted with up to 80% of cases of childhood ALL by immunisation of a rabbit with ALL blast cells. However, as the use of monoclonal antibodies to type ALL progressed, it became apparent that there was no specific antibody to detect leukaemic cells: all antibodies produced to date detect a normal cell at some stage of differentiation.

The structure and function of CALLA has been established, and it has been renamed CD10. It is a zinc metalloprotease of mwt 100,000 that hydrolyses peptide bonds, thereby reducing cellular responses to peptide hormones. Among the many biologically active peptides it cleaves are bradykinin, endothelin, angiotensin and oxytocin. CD10 is encoded by a gene on chromosome 3q21-q27. CD10 positivity is widely distributed in normal tissue: it is found in precursor T and B lymphocytes, granulocytes, brain, kidney and muscle, but its main diagnostic utility is as a marker of ALL.

T Acute Lymphoblastic Leukaemia

T ALL accounts for between 10 and 15% of ALL in both children and adults. This subtype of ALL is rarely seen in children under the age of 1 year or in adults over the age of 50 years. T ALL occurs more frequently in males and usually is associated with a high white cell count and mediastinal mass at diagnosis. The incidence of central nervous system involvement is higher than in other types of ALL. T ALL is associated with a poor prognosis. The diagnosis of T ALL frequently is complicated by aberrant expression of immunological markers of differentiation. The most sensitive marker of T ALL is the finding of a clonal rearrangement of the Ti_β gene. Chromosomal translocations are relatively common in T ALL with the genes encoding Ti_α, Ti_β and Ti_γ frequently involved. The genes which code for Ti_β and Ti_γ chains are located on chromosome 7, while those for Ti_α and Ti_δ are located on chromosome 14.

Acute Non-lymphoblastic Leukaemia

Acute non-lymphoblastic leukaemia can occur at any age but is more common in adults, showing an increasing frequency with advancing age. ANLL accounts for 12% of cases of acute leukaemia in children under the age of 10 years and 28% between ages 10 to 15 years. In adults, ANLL accounts for 80 to 90% of cases of acute leukaemia. ANLL often occurs as a secondary event, particularly following a period of myelodysplasia or treatment for other neoplasms. ANLL diagnosed as a primary disorder is known as *de novo* ANLL.

The clinical features of ANLL are similar at all ages and are the consequence of the replacement of normal marrow elements by malignant blasts, often resulting in impaired haemopoiesis and organomegaly. The most common presenting symptoms are pallor and fatigue secondary to anaemia, bleeding problems secondary to thrombocytopaenia, infection secondary to neutropaenia and unexplained weight loss. Infiltration of the skin and gums occurs in approximately 10% of patients with ANLL and is particularly associated with AMoL and AMMoL. Disseminated intravascular coagulation occurs more commonly in ANLL than ALL and is most closely associated with APL. About 1 in 4 individuals with ANLL present with white cell counts in excess of $100 \times 10^9/l$, leading to problems associated with leucostasis, particularly within the pulmonary, CNS and genitourinary systems.

The recognition of prognostic indicators in ALL stimulated the search for similar indicators in ANLL. Consistent findings have been difficult to obtain, partly because of the heterogeneity of ANLL and partly because of the wide variety of therapeutic regimes used worldwide. The most widely accepted prognostic indicators are summarised in Table 16.9.

Prognostic Indicator	Favourable	Unfavourable
Age	<45 years	<2 years or > 60 years
Leukaemia diagnosed	*De novo*	Prior myelodysplasia
White cell count	$<25 \times 10^9/l$	$>100 \times 10^9/l$
CNS disease	Absent	Present
Cytoreduction	Rapid	Delayed
Auer rods	Present	Absent
Eosinophils	Present	Absent
Megaloblastic RBC	Absent	Present
FAB type	M3 or M4	M5, M6 or M7
Immunochemistry		
Myeloid	CD14 -, CD13 -	CD14 +, CD13 + & CD34 +
HLA DR	Negative	Positive
TdT	Absent	Present
Lymphoid	CD2 +, CD19 +	Biphenotypic
Cytogenetics	t(15;17)	-7, del(7q)
	t(8;21)	-5, del(5q)
	inv(16)/del(16q)	11q23 abnormalities
		3q21/3q26 abnormalities

Table 16.9 *Prognostic indicators in acute non-lymphoblastic leukaemia*

The cell of origin in ANLL most often shows myeloid or monocytic differentiation. Approximately 5 to 10% of cases have erythroid or megakaryocytic differentiation. Morphology and cytochemistry usually are sufficient to permit the recognition and classification of the majority of cases of ANLL. The presence of Auer rods, crystalline structures derived from primary granules by coalescence of the granules within autophagic vacuoles, is a characteristic of myeloblasts in ANLL often regarded as pathognomonic. Electron microscopy and immunocytochemistry are necessary to diagnose the remaining cases of ANLL. Cytogenetic abnormalities are common in ANLL and frequently are associated with a particular morphological subtype and clinical presentation.

Acute Myeloblastic Leukaemia

This subgroup includes the three FAB subtypes M0, M1 and M2 and is characterised by the presence of myeloblasts with increasing cytochemical and morphological evidence of myeloid differentiation. The most differentiated, M2, is associated with the cytogenetic abnormality t(8;21). This entity occurs mostly in children or young adults and is associated with anaemia, thrombocytopaenia and splenomegaly at diagnosis. The myeloblasts usually contain Auer rods and the mature myeloid cells are dysplastic. The biological significance of the t(8;21) is unknown. However, the translocation of the *ets*-2 oncogene from 21q to 8q in this syndrome and the association of trisomy 21 (Down's syndrome) with an increased incidence of acute leukaemia may be of significance.

Acute Promyelocytic Leukaemia (APL)

Approximately 6% of patients with ANLL present with APL (FAB subtype M3) which is characterised by the predominance of promyelocytes in the bone marrow. The leukaemic promyelocytes frequently are abnormal in their granulation pattern and possess multiple Auer rods. APL is most common in young adults and is characterised by a low white cell count and thrombocytopaenia at presentation, coupled with disseminated intravascular coagulation (DIC). The recognition and intensive treatment of the associated DIC in APL has improved its prognosis. The chromosomal translocations t(15;17)(q22;q21) and (q22;q11-12) are considered pathognomonic of APL. The chromosome breakpoints involved in this translocation have recently been isolated. They are localised on a previously unknown gene, *pml* on chromosome 15 and in the gene that encodes the α retinoic acid receptor (*rarα*) on chromosome 17. The balanced and reciprocal translocation leads to the formation of two expressed fusion genes. The *pml/rarα* fusion protein is thought to be responsible for the APL phenotype and the differentiation block of the leukaemic blasts. Retinoic acid has the ability to induce differentiation of the leukaemic clone in APL and is currently under investigation for clinical use in this disorder.

Acute Myelomonoblastic Leukaemia (AMMoL)

The AMMoL subtype (FAB subtype M4) is characterised morphologically by the presence of both myeloid and monocytic differentiation. The latter is best demonstrated by the use of non-specific esterase cytochemistry, in particular α naphthyl butyrate esterase, and positive reactions with the CD14 monocyte-associated surface marker. Abnormalities of chromosome 16 are associated with a variant of AMMol with abnormal eosinophil morphology which is associated with a good prognosis.

Acute Monoblastic Leukaemia (AMoL)

AMoL accounts for between 2 and 10% of cases of ANLL and is characterised by the presence of monoblasts that are either poorly differentiated (FAB subtype M5a) or well differentiated (FAB subtype M5b). Cytogenetic abnormalities in AMoL often involve translocations between chromosome 11 and chromosomes 9, 10 or 17. The t(9;11) abnormality involves the translocation of the *ets-1* oncogene to the α interferon gene on chromosome 9. AMoL, and to a lesser extent AMMoL, are associated with a risk of DIC and CNS disease.

Acute Erythroleukaemia (AEL)

AEL (FAB subtype M6) most commonly affects those over the age of 50 years and is more common in men than in women. This subtype is regarded as ANLL with predominant erythroid differentiation and accounts for approximately 3% of cases of ANLL. The morphology of the erythroid cells typically is severely dysplastic with multinucleated erythroblasts and cytoplasmic bridging. AEL frequently represents an erythroleukaemic transformation of myelodysplasia. Aneuploidy has been reported in 63% of patients and abnormalities often involve either chromosome 5 or 7.

Acute Megakaryoblastic Leukaemia (AMegL)

AMegL (FAB subtype M7) represents between 3 and 12% of adult cases of ANLL and occurs as *de novo* leukaemia, secondary leukaemia following cytotoxic chemotherapy and as transformed myeloproliferative and myelodysplastic syndromes. Cytogenetic abnormalities are variable but have included abnormalities of chromosomes 8 and 21. A subset of AMegL occurs in infants and is characterised by extensive organomegaly and the chromosomal translocation t(1;22)(p13;q13). The *N-ras* and platelet-derived growth factor β (*PDGF*-β) genes are located near the breakpoints on chromosomes 1 and 22 respectively. Activation of the PDGF-β gene may be important in the pathobiology of this subtype.

Treatment and Management of Acute Leukaemia

The treatment of acute leukaemia can be divided into two categories; cytotoxic drug therapy to eradicate the leukaemic cells and general supportive therapy for bone marrow failure. There are significant differences between ALL and ANLL in age incidence, drug sensitivity, treatment approach and overall prognosis which justify a different therapeutic strategy in each case. Bone marrow transplantation has become another therapeutic option to be considered in the treatment of acute leukaemia. A further development, the use of haemopoietic growth factors, is being assessed in clinical trials in conjunction with cytotoxic drug therapy and bone marrow transplantation.

Cytotoxic Chemotherapy

The aim of cytotoxic drug therapy is to induce a remission (an absence of any clinical or conventional laboratory evidence of disease) and then progressively to eradicate the residual leukaemic cells by courses of consolidation, intensification and maintenance therapy. The principles of cytotoxic chemotherapy and the modes of action of commonly prescribed drugs are described in the previous chapter. Several cytotoxic drugs are combined to increase the cytotoxic effect, improve remission rates and the length of remission, and to reduce the frequency of drug resistance. Drug combinations are given in cycles with treatment free intervals to allow the recovery of normal haemopoietic tissue. Standard treatment regimes specific for ALL and ANLL have been devised from multicentre trials of cytotoxic drug combinations. These may be varied to take into account the prognostic factors of each case at diagnosis and classification. A summary of typical treatment protocols for ALL and ANLL is shown in Table 16.10.

Maintenance cytotoxic drug therapy has been found to be effective in treating ALL but not ANLL. A feature of treatment regimes for ANLL is prolonged and severe bone marrow failure due to the lack of selectivity of the myelotoxic drugs used. Intensive supportive care is necessary during this period of treatment. Treatment of relapsed acute leukaemia is more successful in ALL than ANLL.

Acute Lymphoblastic Leukaemia	Acute Non-Lymphoblastic Leukaemia
Remission Induction	
eg vincristine, prednisolone, daunorubicin, asparaginase	eg cytosine arabinoside, daunorubicin, thioguanine, etoposide
Consolidation	
1-3 cycles of consolidation eg vincristine, daunorubicin, prednisolone, thioguanine etoposide, cytosine arabinoside	3 cycles of consolidation eg cytosine arabinoside, daunorubicin, thioguanine, mitozantrone, m-amasacrine
Cranial prophylaxis	
<2 years of age: multiple intrathecal methotrexate >2 years of age: cranial irradiation and intrathecal methotrexate	
Maintenance (2 years)	
eg methotrexate, mercaptopurine, prednisolone,vincristine	
Bone marrow transplantation (BMT) is another treatment option, particularly for poor prognosis groups who have HLA matched siblings.	

Table 16.10 *Typical treatment schedule for the acute leukaemias*

Leukaemic cells in the CNS are beyond the reach of most cytotoxic drugs. Meningeal leukaemia used to occur in 75% of children and 50% of adults with ALL during the first 4 years of treatment. Consequently prophylactic cranial treatment consisting of intrathecal methotrexate and irradiation is included in most treatment regimes for ALL to prevent CNS relapse of the leukaemia. The general exception to this is the treatment of children less than 2 years of age where cranial irradiation is avoided and higher doses of methotrexate are given. Meningeal relapse occurs less commonly in ANLL overall, but is most closely associated with AMMoL and AMoL. For this reason, cranial therapy often is included in the treatment regime for these conditions. Testicular leukaemia occasionally occurs in ALL, necessitating irradiation with re-induction cytotoxic drug therapy.

In recent years, the phenomenon of relapse of acute leukaemia associated with the emergence of drug-resistant clones has been observed. An important mechanism in this process is the presence of increased levels of expression of the multi-drug resistance gene and its gene product glycoprotein p170 in the leukaemic cells. This membrane glycoprotein acts as an efflux pump, transporting the cytotoxic drugs out of the cell. Other mechanisms of drug resistance, including altered metabolism of cytotoxic drugs due to changes in cellular enzymes, are also known.

Supportive Therapy

The availability of separate blood components (red cells, platelets and fresh frozen plasma) has radically improved the general supportive therapy of patients with acute leukaemia. Packed red cells are used to treat anaemia; platelets to treat the haemorrhagic complications associated with thrombocytopaenia which can be particularly severe during cytotoxic drug therapy; and fresh frozen plasma, usually combined with platelets, is used to treat the DIC which often is troublesome in APL.

As already described, patients with acute leukaemia are highly susceptible to infection. The prompt and effective treatment of established infection and attempts to prevent infection are vitally important components of leukaemia treatment. The infections usually are bacterial but viral, fungal and protozoal infections also occur with increased frequency. Measures taken to reduce the risk of infection include nursing in isolation facilities, antibiotic therapy to reduce gut and other commensal flora, and vigorous microbiological surveillance. Anti-endotoxin and anti-tumour necrosis factor are more recent immunotherapy approaches to the severe complications of certain infections.

Patients receiving cytotoxic drug therapy are very prone to severe and prolonged nausea and vomiting which may have serious metabolic consequences. Various drug regimes are employed to counteract this particular problem. These and other side effects of the cytotoxic drugs need to be taken into account in the design of appropriate supportive care protocols.

Bone Marrow Transplantation

Bone marrow transplantation (BMT) involves the elimination of host haemopoietic stem cells using large doses of cytotoxic drugs and total body irradiation and the subsequent infusion of replacement bone marrow cells. The transplanted marrow may be from an HLA-matched donor (**allogeneic transplant**) or may be from a sample of stored patient bone marrow "harvested" during disease remission (**autologous transplant**). BMT is used in some centres to treat ANLL in first remission in patients under 45 years of age, and to treat ALL in successful second remission. It is also considered for other cases of acute leukaemia with particularly poor prognostic indicators.

The rigours of bone marrow transplantation are such that it is only offered to those under the age of 45 years who are physically in good condition. The conditioning process involves the administration of large doses of cyclophosphamide as a cytotoxic and immunosuppressive agent followed by either total body irradiation (TBI) or total lymphoid irradiation (TLI) to induce marrow ablation. The dose of radiation employed needs to be as high as possible but is limited by the damage it causes to the lungs, gastrointestinal tract and central nervous system. The conditioning process is associated with a range of severe toxic effects such as nausea, vomiting, diarrhoea, abdominal pain, haemorrhagic cystitis, interstitial pneumonitis, cardiomyopathy, hair loss, reddening of the skin, sterility, thyroid dysfunction and, in children, impairment of growth and intellectual ability. TLI is associated with lower pulmonary toxicity than TBI.

A major cause of failure in any form of organ transplantation is the possibility of rejection of the graft by the host immune system. Graft rejection can be minimised by only using HLA-matched tissue and by the use of immunosuppressive agents such as cyclosporin. However, because bone marrow transplantation involves the engraftment of immunocompetent tissue, an additional complication exists, viz the possibility of rejection of the host by the graft. This phenomenon is known as **graft versus host disease (GVHD)**, and is an important cause of morbidity and mortality in bone marrow transplant recipients. The incidence of GVHD can be reduced by post-transplant immunosuppressive therapy or by pre-transplant purging of T lymphocytes from the donor marrow. Unfortunately, the reduction in the incidence of GVHD achieved using T lymphocyte-depleted bone marrow is offset by a concomitant increase in the rate of graft rejection. Acute GVHD is associated with T-lymphocyte mediated attack of skin, liver and lung tissue. There is some evidence that a minor degree of chronic GVHD may contribute to a reduction in the risk of leukaemic relapse following bone marrow transplantation. This is thought to be mediated by a "**graft versus leukaemia effect**".

In the absence of a suitable donor, transplantation of autologous bone marrow harvested during disease remission may be used. This form of treatment is associated with a higher rate of engraftment and the absence of GVHD. However, these advantages are balanced by a greater risk of leukaemic relapse and the absence of the graft versus leukaemia effect. The risk of leukaemic relapse following autologous bone marrow transplantation can be reduced by pre-transplant purging of the leukaemic cells from the marrow sample using monoclonal antibodies.

Haemopoietic Growth Factors

A further development in the treatment of acute leukaemia, the use of recombinant human haemopoietic growth factors, is being assessed by clinical trials. Haemopoietic growth factors are administered in conjunction with cytotoxic drug therapy to improve the eradication of leukaemic cells and to accelerate the recovery of normal haemopoiesis. An important consideration in the trials is the potentially adverse effect of the growth factors in accelerating the proliferation of the leukaemic cells. The utility of haemopoietic growth factors is also being assessed in BMT where it is envisaged that they will accelerate the haemopoietic reconstitution process.

Suggested Further Reading

Lee, R.G., Bithell, T.C., Foerster, J., Athens, J.W. and Lukens, J.N (1993). *Wintrobe's Clinical Hematology.* London: Lea and Febiger.

Hoffbrand, A.V. and Pettit, J.E. (1993). *Essential Haematology.* Oxford: Blackwell Scientific Publications.

Bain, B.J. (1990). *Leukaemia Diagnosis: A Guide to the FAB Classification.* London: Gower Medical Publishing.

Catovsky, D. (1991). *The Leukaemic Cell.* Edinburgh: Churchill Livingstone.

The Chronic Leukaemias

The leukaemias are malignant disorders which are characterised by the unbridled clonal proliferation of abnormal blood cells in the bone marrow and other body tissues. As described in the previous chapter, the malignant clone in acute leukaemia is poorly differentiated. In contrast, the malignant clone in the chronic leukaemias is relatively well differentiated and usually is readily identifiable on morphological grounds. The chronic leukaemias can be divided on the basis of the lineage of the malignant clone into chronic myeloid leukaemias and chronic lymphoid leukaemias. Each of these groups is capable of further division as described below. In this chapter the chronic leukaemias are considered under the following headings:

- leukaemogenesis

- recognition and classification

- pathophysiology

- treatment and management

Chronic Myeloid Leukaemia

The term chronic myeloid leukaemia (CML) originally was used to distinguish chronic leukaemias involving marrow-derived cells from those arising in lymphoid tissue. Nowadays, CML is defined as a clonal myeloproliferative disorder of the totipotential haemopoietic stem cell and almost invariably is characterised by the presence of a chromosomal marker, the **Philadelphia chromosome** t(9;22)(q34;q11), in the leukaemic cells. The presence of the Philadelphia chromosome in erythrocyte, granulocyte, platelet, B lymphocyte precursors and the proof of clonality using polymorphic genetic markers such as G-6-PD confirm that CML is derived from a single totipotential stem cell.

CML occurs with an annual incidence of about 1 per 100,000 of the population with no apparent geographic variation. There is a slight excess incidence of CML in males. There was a significant increase

SAQ 1

What is the chromosomal location of the G-6-PD gene?

in the incidence of CML in survivors of the atomic explosions in Hiroshima and Nagasaki. No other universally accepted predisposing factors have been identified.

CML is characterised by an insidious onset of ill-health and is associated with a massive increase in the circulating granulocyte count and splenomegaly. CML affects all age groups but is seen most frequently in middle age. Until recently, the prognosis of patients with CML was poor with a median survival of three years. However, recent reports have indicated an improved prognosis due to earlier detection, improved anti-CML therapy and better supportive care. CML is a haematological disorder of considerable historical significance and has provided a model for the study of the acquired genomic changes that occur in malignant disease.

Leukaemogenesis of CML

Much of the research into the causation of CML has centred on the role of the Philadelphia chromosome. As described in Chapter 15, the typical reciprocal translocation t(9;22)(q34;q11) involves the translocation of the c-abl oncogene which is located at 9q34 to a point within the breakpoint cluster region of the *bcr* gene at 22q11, forming a chimeric *bcr-abl* gene.

The function of the normal *abl* gene product (p145^{abl}) is incompletely understood but it is known to have tyrosine kinase activity and may play a role in the regulation of several different growth factor receptors, including those for epidermal growth factor, platelet derived growth factor, and colony stimulating factor receptors. The normal *bcr* gene product (p160^{bcr}) is known to have serine/threonine kinase activity and shows considerable homology to a number of cell cycle proteins. It is thought to play an important role in cellular signal transduction. Both *bcr* and *abl* genes are expressed in virtually all types of normal cells.

The chimeric *bcr-abl* fusion gene produces a novel 8 kb mRNA transcript which encodes a chimeric protein of molecular weight 210,000 (p210$^{bcr-abl}$). This protein contains 1104 amino acids encoded by the translocated *abl* gene and either 927 or 902 amino acids encoded by the disrupted *bcr* gene. The size of the *bcr*-derived portion of the mRNA transcript is determined by the presence or absence of *bcr* exon 3 in the chimeric fusion gene. P210$^{bcr-abl}$ has a much more powerful tyrosine kinase activity than p145^{abl} and has

In 1960, an abnormally small group G chromosome, the Philadelphia chromosome (Ph), named after the city of its discovery was identified in the bone marrow cells of patients with CML. Subsequently, up to 90% of CML patients were shown to be Philadelphia-positive using conventional cytogenetic techniques. With the introduction of Giemsa banding techniques in 1973, the Ph chromosome was shown to result from a reciprocal translocation of genetic material between chromosomes 9 and 22, t(9;22)(q34;q11). The molecular genetics of the Ph chromosome have now been elucidated as described in the main text.

been shown to interact with its substrates in an altered manner. Although the way in which p210$^{bcr-abl}$ brings about malignant change is unknown, there is little doubt that it plays a pivotal role in CML, particularly in the chronic phase.

As described in Chapter 15, up to 80% of Ph-positive acute leukaemia patients have a chromosomal breakpoint which is proximal to the breakpoint cluster region. This results in the production of a smaller 7.5 kb mRNA transcript which encodes a novel 190kD protein (p190). This type of chromosomal rearrangement is most closely associated with ALL but has rarely been seen in CML and ANLL. These latter cases are distinguished by the presence of a pronounced monocytic component. The clinical features and prognoses of p210$^{bcr-abl}$ and p190 Ph-positive acute leukaemias are similar.

As described later in this chapter, CML typically is a triphasic disease. It can be separated on the basis of various clinical and laboratory characteristics into a **chronic phase**, an **accelerated phase** and a terminal **blastic phase**. During the chronic phase of CML the t(9;22)(q34;q11) typically is the only chromosomal abnormality present. However, progression into the accelerated phase is accompanied by the acquisition of additional chromosomal abnormalities in about 80% of cases. The most common additional abnormalities are the acquisition of an extra Philadelphia chromosome (+Ph), trisomy 8 (+8) and i(17q).

It seems likely that disease progression occurs as a consequence of the activation of additional oncogenes within one or more leukaemic stem cells, thereby favouring the establishment and expansion of new malignant clones which have the characteristics of acute leukaemia. A number of oncogenes have been shown to be altered in blastic phase leukaemic cells, including the recessive tumour suppressor gene *p53* which is located on chromosome 17 and *myc* which is located on chromosome 8. There is, as yet, no direct evidence that any of these oncogene abnormalities is implicated in the induction of the blastic phase of CML.

Current evidence suggests that the genesis of CML is a multi-step process:

Recent work has implicated the novel chimeric protein p210$^{bcr-abl}$ in the pathogenesis of CML. The human *bcr-abl* gene has been successfully expressed in murine bone marrow cells. When these transfected cells were reinfused into lethally irradiated mice, the majority developed chronic phase CML and a further group developed acute leukaemia. Further, experiments using human CML cells in *in vitro* culture, have shown that blocking the expression of the chimeric p210$^{bcr-abl}$ protein by anti-sense oligonucleotides abolishes the leukaemic phenotype.

These observations suggest that cure of CML requires complete elimination or suppression of the Ph-positive clone and have led to the evaluation of novel treatment strategies such as the use of anti-sense oligonucleotides or synthetic peptides which are directed against p210$^{bcr-abl}$ mRNA or its protein product.

SAQ 2

What is the defining feature of an isochromosome?

- The first step towards the induction of CML is thought to involve the clonal proliferation of a genetically unstable, Philadelphia chromosome-negative totipotential stem cell. The abnormal clone which results has a proliferative advantage over normal haemopoietic stem cells. The cause and nature of the stimulus for this clonal proliferation is unknown.

- Chronic phase CML is thought to be triggered by the acquisition of a Philadelphia chromosome and the expression of $p210^{bcr-abl}$ in a single member of the expanded totipotential stem cell clone.

- Progression of the disease to the accelerated and blastic phases is thought to be prompted by the acquisition of further chromosomal abnormalities which may involve the loss of tumour suppressor genes or the activation of proto-oncogenes. The processes involved in the evolution of the malignant clone towards the blastic phase are poorly understood, at present.

Recognition and Classification of CML

Recognition of CML requires the examination of appropriately stained blood and bone marrow smears and cytogenetic studies. Frequently, in cases of grossly elevated white cell counts at presentation, the diagnosis is self-evident from the peripheral blood. However, a bone marrow aspirate is still required to provide material for cytogenetic evaluation and to assess the degree of fibrosis.

The classification of CML and its variants is based on the presence or absence of the Philadelphia chromosome and the morphology of the leukaemic clone as shown in Table 17.1. Up to 90% of cases of CML have clear cytogenetic evidence for the presence of the Philadelphia chromosome. The application of molecular genetic techniques to cases of atypical CML in which the Philadelphia chromosome cannot be identified by conventional means has revealed evidence for the rearrangement of the *bcr* and *abl* genes in at least 35% of cases. As described below, the division of CML into typical and atypical forms is clinically relevant: atypical CML has a relatively poor prognosis. The morphological variants of typical CML are rare.

Subtype	Philadelphia Chromosome	Frequency
Typical CML	Present	>90%
Atypical CML	Absent	<10%
Juvenile CML	Absent	Uncommon
Chronic neutrophilic leukaemia	Absent	Rare
Chronic basophilic leukaemia	Varies	Rare
Chronic eosinophilic leukaemia	Varies	Uncommon

Table 17.1 *Classification of chronic myeloid leukaemia*

Pathophysiology of CML

Typical CML

In the majority of patients, typical CML is a triphasic disease: most cases present in the **chronic phase** of the disease but progression to the **accelerated phase** and, ultimately, to the **blastic phase** is inexorable and is neither delayed nor prevented by current conventional treatment.

Chronic Phase CML

The three defining features of typical chronic phase CML are a raised granulocyte count, the presence of the Philadelphia chromosome and splenomegaly. The total WBC at presentation often exceeds 100×10^9/l and may be as high as 1000×10^9/l although, with increasing access to health care in the developed world, it is becoming increasingly frequent for CML to be discovered when the total WBC is as low as $20\text{-}40 \times 10^9$/l. Typically, all stages of granulocyte differentiation are present in the peripheral blood but a rise in the level of circulating myelocytes and mature neutrophils is especially prominent. Typically, the proportion of myeloblasts and promyelocytes is low during chronic phase. The absolute basophil, eosinophil and monocyte count may all be increased. The cells of the leukaemic clone have been shown to have an increased rate of cytoplasmic maturation relative to nuclear maturation. This is most obviously manifest as an increased number of cytoplasmic granules in CML promyelocytes. A variety of functional abnormalities have also been noted in the leukaemic clone including defects of chemotaxis and phagocytosis and deficiency of granule contents such as

The earliest known cases of leukaemia involved a 28 year old slater called John Mentieth, who was admitted to the Edinburgh Royal Infirmary on 27 February 1845 and a 50 year old cook called Marie Straide who was admitted two days later to the Charite Hospital in Berlin. Both succumbed shortly after admission and were examined *post mortem* by Drs Bennet and Virchow respectively. With the benefit of hindsight, it seems likely that both of these unfortunates were suffering from CML. Both complained of progressive lethargy and a painful, swollen abdomen, probably reflecting anaemia and massive splenomegaly. Straide also had a severe cough and Mentieth had numerous solid tumours scattered about his body, a classical feature of end-stage untreated CML rarely seen these days.

lactoferrin, myeloperoxidase and alkaline phosphatase. This last observation is exploited in the differentiation of early CML from other causes of leucocytosis where the level of alkaline phosphatase is normal or increased.

Other peripheral blood cell abnormalities which are common in chronic phase CML include normocytic, normochromic anaemia and thrombocytosis. Broadly, the severity of both abnormalities increases with increasing total WBC count. As described below, bleeding is not an uncommon complication of CML, despite the raised platelet count. In such cases, investigation usually reveals an acquired defect of platelet function.

A range of other abnormalities have been noted in chronic phase CML, although these do not contribute to the recognition of the disease. The circulating levels of myeloid progenitor cells such as CFU-GEMM, CFU-GM, BFU-E and CFU-Meg are greatly increased in CML. These cells all carry the Philadelphia chromosome and thus reflect expansion of the leukaemic clone. The serum vitamin B_{12} level typically is massively increased, reflecting synthesis of transcobalamins I and III by the leukaemic granulocytes. Hyperuricaemia is also common and reflects the increased white cell turnover.

Expansion of the leukaemic clone is associated with extreme hypercellularity of the bone marrow with progressive loss of fat spaces, extension of haemopoietically active marrow into the long bones and extramedullary haemopoiesis, resulting in splenomegaly and, less commonly, hepatomegaly. An increase in marrow reticulin fibres is common at presentation, progressing in most cases to outright fibrosis.

The typical physical features of chronic phase CML include pallor, lethargy and fatigue which are secondary to the anaemia; abdominal distension or discomfort secondary to splenomegaly; sternal tenderness or more generalised bone pain secondary to expansion of haemopoietically active marrow and, occasionally, purpura or bleeding secondary to platelet dysfunction.

Accelerated Phase CML

The accurate recognition of disease progression from chronic to accelerated phase is becoming increasingly important for the treatment of CML. However, as described below, attempts to define

It has very recently become possible to assay and study the most primitive haemopoietic progenitor cells, the long term culture-initiating cells (LTC-IC), in normal subjects and in patients with CML. Initial studies have shown that, in cases of CML, the concentration of Ph-positive LTC-IC is raised in the peripheral blood but decreased in the bone marrow relative to normal and that these cells appear to have a defect of self-maintenance in long term culture. It is hoped that future studies in this area will lead to the characterisation of the molecular changes which promote clonal expansion in CML.

prognosis in terms of features existing at presentation or which develop in the course of chronic phase have met with little success. Accordingly, there are no universally agreed objective criteria for defining the point at which CML enters the accelerated phase. Broadly, most workers accept that the transition to accelerated phase is accompanied by increasing refractoriness to treatment which may be reflected in one or more of the changes listed in Table 17.2.

Laboratory Features

>15% blasts in bone marrow or peripheral blood
>30% blasts + promyelocytes in peripheral blood
>20% basophils in peripheral blood
<100 x 10^9/l platelets (not treatment-related)
Acquisition of additional cytogenetic abnormalities
Increasing collagen fibrosis of bone marrow

Clinical Features

Increasing splenomegaly which is refractory to treatment
Increasing chemotherapy requirement

Table 17.2 *Objective criteria for the recognition of transition to accelerated phase CML*

The median duration of the chronic phase from presentation is 3 years. Transition to the accelerated phase usually is a gradual process, with minimal physical sequelae. Once the accelerated phase is clearly established, however, progression to the blastic phase is inexorable and usually occurs within a few months.

Blastic Phase CML

In most cases, establishment of the accelerated phase of CML is followed by a sustained downward spiral in which the disease becomes progressively more refractory to treatment, the blast cell count rises inexorably and physical symptoms steadily worsen. In such cases, definition of the point at which transition to the blastic phase is established is somewhat arbitrary. One widely accepted criterion for the establishment of blast crisis is that the circulating blast cell count should exceed 30% of the total leucocyte count. Occasionally, blast transformation is identifiable in an extramedullary site such as the spleen prior to the appearance of frank signs of blastic phase in the bone marrow or peripheral blood. In some cases, the transition to the blastic phase of CML occurs abruptly, with no apparent warning and no clearly defined accelerated phase.

Progression of chronic phase to blastic phase CML has been likened to the evolution of a chronic leukaemia into an acute leukaemia. The accumulation of blast cells which results is accompanied by the development of progressive anaemia, neutropaenia and thrombocytopaenia. Most cases of blastic phase CML show features of M1 or M2 ANLL, but monoblastic, erythroblastic, megakaryoblastic and lymphoblastic transformation also occur. The treatment for blastic phase CML is the same as that for the acute leukaemia which it most closely resembles but usually is much less successful. Haematological remissions are harder to obtain and typically are of shorter duration than in *de novo* acute leukaemia. The most common causes of death in blastic phase CML are infection secondary to neutropaenia and haemorrhage secondary to thrombocytopaenia.

Atypical CML

The absence of the Philadelphia chromosome in an individual with an otherwise CML-like picture is the defining feature of atypical CML. Using traditional cytogenetic techniques, about 10% of cases fall into this group. However, the application of modern molecular genetic techniques to cases of atypical CML has uncovered evidence for the expression of $p210^{bcr-abl}$ in about one third of such cases. The prognosis for these "cryptic" typical CMLs appears to be similar to those with clear cytogenetic evidence of a Philadelphia chromosome.

The 6% of cases of CML which show no evidence of $p210^{bcr-abl}$ expression have a much poorer prognosis with a median duration of survival from presentation of about 18 months.

Juvenile CML

As described in Chapter 15, the most common form of leukaemia in infants and children is ALL. Typical CML is rare in this age group but, where present, is clinically indistinguishable from the adult disease.

A distinct form of CML occurs in infants with a peak incidence between 1 and 5 years of age. Juvenile CML, as this form is known, is characterised by a CML-like blood picture with a prominent monocytic component, thrombocytopaenia, and a raised foetal haemoglobin concentration which may exceed 50% of the total. Typical clinical features at presentation include anaemia, hepato-splenomegaly, respiratory tract infection and eczematoid rash. JCML is associated with a uniformly poor prognosis: most affected infants die within 18 months of presentation.

Treatment and Management of CML

The mainstays of conventional cytotoxic chemotherapy of CML are busulphan and hydroxyurea. Rapid and prolonged haematological remission with resolution of physical symptoms can be achieved using either of these drugs. Busulphan, an alkylating agent, is preferred in older patients who are not candidates for bone marrow transplantation, or who cannot attend hospital regularly. Its use is associated with unpredictable, prolonged myelosuppression, pulmonary fibrosis, skin pigmentation, amenorrhoea and infertility. Hydroxyurea acts by inhibiting the enzyme ribonucleotide reductase, and currently is the drug of choice in the developed world because its use is associated with fewer and less severe side effects. In particular, lack of pulmonary toxicity makes this drug more appropriate as a "conditioning" agent prior to bone marrow transplantation.

Haematological remissions are obtainable in at least 80% of cases of CML with the use of busulphan or hydroxyurea. However, disease progression is not significantly altered by such treatment: the median duration of the chronic phase of CML is much the same in treated and untreated individuals. In addition, cytogenetic studies have revealed the persistence of the Philadelphia chromosome-containing clone, even during apparently complete remission. For these reasons, conventional cytotoxic chemotherapy of CML must be considered to be palliative rather than curative.

Numerous attempts have been made to pinpoint features of chronic phase CML which may be useful as indicators of prognosis and therefore could aid treatment selection. Unfortunately, these efforts have met with little success: the only widely accepted indicators of prognosis are the absence of the Philadelphia chromosome and extreme basophilia, both of which confer a poor prognosis. Other

The earliest agent which could clearly be shown to be effective in the treatment of leukaemia and lymphoma was a 1% aqueous solution of AsO_3, known as Fowler's solution. This highly toxic substance had been in use for centuries as an effective poison and, in more dilute form, for almost a hundred years as a general tonic and cure-all when, in 1865, it was administered to a woman with CML by a German physician called Lissauer. The temporary remission which resulted prompted others to repeat the experiment with similar success. Unfortunately, the remissions were short-lived and arsenic fell into disuse when, at the turn of the century, radiotherapy became available.

proposed prognostic indicators are shown in Table 17.3. As new and improved treatment options for CML become available, the need to find some means of stratifying cases with respect to prognosis increases.

Clinical Indicators at Presentation Increasing age Clinically high grade disease Significant weight loss Hepatomegaly Splenomegaly **Laboratory-associated Indicators** Absence of Philadelphia chromosome Anaemia Thrombocytosis, thrombocytopaenia Megakaryocytopaenia High blast + promyelocyte count in blood or bone marrow High basophil count in blood or bone marrow Increased collagen fibrosis in bone marrow **Treatment-associated Indicators** Delayed induction of remission Short duration of remission Impaired response to busulphan or hydroxyurea Failure of suppression of Ph-positive clone Poor initial response to α-interferon therapy

Table 17.3 *Proposed indicators of poor prognosis in CML*

An alternative agent which has been used with some success in the treatment of chronic phase CML is α-interferon. Using this agent alone, haematological remission has been obtained in up to 70% of newly diagnosed cases of chronic phase CML. Perhaps of even greater importance is the observation that this drug appears selectively to suppress the leukaemic clone, leading to a significant reduction in the proportion of Philadelphia chromosome-positive progenitor cells in the bone marrow and peripheral blood. The introduction of recombinant human α-interferon has enabled the performance of clinical trials of this drug, both alone and in combination with conventional cytotoxic agents. Early results from these trials suggest that improved survival and durable cytogenetic remission is obtainable in about 20% of patients. The toxicity of α-interferon is relatively mild, consisting of fever, chills and flu-like symptoms. More serious side effects occur in a minority of patients with prolonged treatment, including anorexia, weight loss and neurotoxicity.

The only form of treatment for CML which currently offers the chance of a cure is bone marrow transplantation. Allogeneic transplantation has been shown to offer significantly improved disease-free survival times, particularly when transplantation is performed early in the chronic phase. The use of T lymphocyte-depleted bone marrow, reduces the incidence of graft-versus-host disease but is associated with an increased incidence of graft failure and relapse because of the reduction in the "graft-versus-leukaemia" effect. When an HLA-matched donor is unavailable, autologous marrow transplantation may be attempted using bone marrow harvested during the chronic phase or following successful treatment with α-interferon. The application and difficulties associated with bone marrow transplantation are considered in more detail in the previous chapter.

Chronic Lymphoid Leukaemias

As described in Chapter 15, chronic lymphoid leukaemia can be subdivided into three main subtypes viz chronic lymphocytic leukaemia (CLL), prolymphocytic leukaemia (PLL) and hairy cell leukaemia (HCL). Each of these subtypes can be further subdivided on the basis of immunological phenotype as described below. Minor subtypes of chronic lymphoid leukaemia exist and will be described briefly. The distinction between the chronic lymphoid leukaemias and other lymphoproliferative disorders such as lymphoma frequently is unclear, particularly when the latter presents or relapses in a "leukaemic phase" caused by overspill of the lymphoma cells from the tissue into the circulation. The lymphomas are described in Chapter 19.

Recognition and Classification of Chronic Lymphoid Leukaemias

The chronic lymphoid leukaemias traditionally have been classified according to the morphological appearances of the predominant leukaemic cell type as shown in Table 17.4.

It was Virchow who first proposed that there was more than one form of leukaemia. He suggested that one form was characterised by massive splenomegaly and marked expansion of the numbers of one type of colourless cells in the blood while the other was characterised by swelling of the lymph nodes and an increase in the other main type of colourless blood cells (remember that Romanowsky staining was not yet available and the distinctions between the types of leucocyte were far from clear). Virchow coined the terms splenic leukaemia and lymphatic leukaemia to describe these two types. Several years later, in 1879, it was suggested that the predominant cells in the splenic form of leukaemia emanated from the bone marrow and so the term myeloid leukaemia was coined and gradually came to replace the term splenic leukaemia.

Abbreviation	Name	Morphology
CLL	Chronic lymphocytic leukaemia	Small, round, mature cells. Many "smear" cells.
PLL	Prolymphocytic leukaemia	Large cells, abundant cytoplasm, single prominent nucleolus
HCL	Hairy cell leukaemia	Multiple cytoplasmic projections, "fried egg" appearance
SLVL	Splenic lymphoma with villous lymphocytes	Medium sized cells with short villi in polar distribution
WM	Waldenstrom's macroglobulinaemia	Lymphoplasmacytoid cells abundant pale blue cytoplasm
MM	Multiple myeloma	Plasma cells, some multinucleate forms
LGL	Large granular lymphocyte leukaemia	Large lymphoid cells with prominent azurophilic granules
SS	Sezary cell syndrome	Large lymphoid cells with

Table 17.4 *The morphological classification scheme of the chronic lymphoproliferative disorders*

However, the advent of monoclonal antibodies in 1976, provided a new way of classifying the chronic lymphoid leukaemias, based on the lineage and stage of differentiation of the leukaemic cells. Immunophenotyping, as this process is known, can be performed on lymphoid cells derived from peripheral blood, bone marrow, lymph node biopsy, tissue biopsy or from other body fluids such as a pleural effusion. The primary distinction to be made in each case is between T and B lineage disease. Further subdivision into differentiation or maturation stage can then be performed to provide the classification scheme shown in Tables 17.5 and 17.6.

CD No.	CLL	PLL	HCL	SLVL	FL	NHL	WM	MM
CD2	−	−	−	−	−	−	−	−
CD5	+	−	−	−	−	−	−	−
CD10	−	−	−	−	+	−	−	+/-
CD11	−	−	+	−	−	−	−	−
CD19	+	+	+	+	+	+	+	−
CD22	+/-	+	+	+	+	+	+	−
CD25	−	−	+	+/-	−	−	−	−
CD38	−	−	−	−	−	−	−	+
SIgM	−	+	+	+	+	+	+	−

Table 17.5 *Immunophenotype classification of B cell chronic lymphoid leukaemias*

CD No.	CLL	PLL	SS	LGL	ATLL
CD2	+	+	+	+	+
CD3	+	+	+	+	+
CD4*	−	+/−	+	−	+/−
CD5	+	+	+	+	+
CD7	+	+	−	+	+
CD8*	+	+/−	−	+	+/−
CD10	−	−	−	−	−
CD16	−	−	−	+/−	−
CD19	−	−	−	−	−

Table 17.6 *Immunophenotype classification of chronic T lymphoid leukaemias*
* Chronic T lymphoproliferative leukaemias usually express either CD4 or CD8 but a small number of PLL and ATLL cases may express both markers

HCL, SLVL, WM and MM are exclusively B lymphoid diseases while SS and LGL leukaemia are exclusively T lymphoid diseases and CLL and PLL may involve either lineage. In most studies, TCLL and TPLL represent about 5% and 25% of cases of CLL and PLL respectively.

Identification of a chronic lymphoid leukaemia by immunophenotyping of peripheral blood cells requires the demonstration and typing of the malignant lymphoid clone against a background of normal, polyclonal lymphocytes. Recognition of a B lymphoid clone is relatively simple in such circumstances because the proportion of circulating B lymphocytes normally is low. One reliable way to identify a B lymphoid clone is to demonstrate immunoglobulin light chain restriction. In contrast, recognition of a malignant T lymphoid clone must take place against a dominant background of normal, mature T lymphocytes. Immunophenotyping in such cases often is inconclusive, unless the morphology of the leukaemia is characteristic, for example the cerebriform nuclei of SS are easily spotted. Definitive demonstration of the presence of a clonal T lymphoid disorder frequently relies upon the demonstration of a clonal rearrangement of the T lymphocyte receptor.

Chronic Lymphocytic Leukaemia

Chronic lymphocytic leukaemia (CLL) is by far the most common of the chronic lymphoid leukaemias, comprising about 70% of all cases. CLL most commonly affects the elderly inhabitants of developed countries. This may be partly due to the increased life expectancy in such countries but there also appears to be a genetic

Splenic B cell lymphoma with circulating villous lymphocytes (SLVL) is a non-Hodgkin's lymphoma which primarily affects splenic tissue but with variable overspill into the peripheral blood of villous lymphocytes which superficially resemble the hairy cells of HCL. SLVL affects a slightly older age group than HCL but the main diagnostic difference between these two disorders lies in the histological appearance of the spleen.

Mycosis fungoides is a chronic T helper lymphoma of the skin. Sezary syndrome represents a similar condition which is characterised by lymphomatous skin lesions, exfoliative erythroderma and the presence in the peripheral blood of large lymphoid cells with moderately abundant cytoplasm and irregular, cerebriform nuclei, the so-called Sezary cells.

Large granular lymphocytic leukaemia (LGL) is an alternative designation for the rare T8+ lymphocytic variant of CLL.

component because the disease is rare in expatriate as well as indigenous Japanese. CLL is twice as common in men as in women. There have been rare reports of a familial tendency towards the development of CLL.

Leukaemogenesis of CLL

Research into the molecular and cytogenetic changes which accompany the development of CLL has been hampered by the low mitotic rate of the leukaemic cells. Even following stimulation with mitogenic factors such as tetradecanoylphorbol acetate (TPA), Epstein-Barr virus (EBV) or, in TCLL, phytohaemagglutinin (PHA), metaphase preparations can be obtained in little more than half of cases. Because of these technical difficulties, there is far less agreement about the frequency, nature and significance of non-random chromosomal abnormalities in CLL than for CML or the acute leukaemias. The most widely accepted non-random chromosomal abnormalities in CLL are shown in Table 17.7.

Table 17.7 *Non-random chromosome abnormalities associated with chronic lymphocytic leukaemia. The frequency quoted represents the percentage of cytogenetically abnormal cases*

Lineage	Abnormality	Frequency
B	+12	33%
B, T	14q+	25%
B	13q-	10%

Many other cytogenetic abnormalities have been reported in cases of CLL, but typically represent isolated case reports or small series showing random defects, and therefore are difficult to interpret. Most workers agree however, that as the complexity of any observed chromosomal rearrangement increases, so the individual prognosis deteriorates. The presence of trisomy 12 as an isolated defect does not appear to confer any appreciable worsening of the prognosis. The application of fluorescent *in situ* hybridisation (FISH) and interphase cytogenetic techniques should aid in the search for other non-random chromosomal abnormalities and may implicate novel oncogenes or tumour suppressor genes in the genesis of CLL. To date, the only oncogenes which have been shown to be rearranged in BCLL have been the K-*ras-2* oncogene which is located at 12p11-p12 and the *bcl-1* oncogene which is located at 11q13.

Recognition and Classification of CLL

Recognition of classical CLL is relatively straightforward and is based on the presence of an absolute lymphocytosis and the morphological appearance of the lymphocytes. Lymphocyte counts at presentation may range from 5 to $1000 \times 10^9/l$ but, most commonly, lie between 20 and $50 \times 10^9/l$. The leukaemic cells in BCLL characteristically are small, round, mature cells, with a thin rim of featureless sky blue cytoplasm. The microscopic hallmark of CLL is the presence of a large number of "smear" cells on the blood film. This artefact is caused by damage to unduly fragile BCLL cells during spreading of the blood film and is not associated with other chronic lymphoid disorders.

The bone marrow always is involved in CLL: an infiltrate which occupies 30 to 50% of the available space is common. As the disease progresses, the leukaemic clone progressively squeezes out normal haemopoiesis, resulting in anaemia and thrombocytopaenia. Erythroid hyperplasia in the bone marrow is strongly indicative of the presence of autoimmune haemolysis, a common complication of CLL. Trephine biopsy of the bone marrow shows one of three different patterns of infiltration, diffuse, interstitial or nodular. Diffuse infiltration is associated with bulky disease with concomitant suppression of normal haemopoiesis and a poor prognosis.

Sensitive techniques such as immunophenotyping, flow cytometry and dual-labelling of cells have enabled the reliable recognition of CLL, even in the absence of an absolute lymphocytosis. This extreme laboratory sensitivity is not yet reflected in agreed classification schemes, however; this facility is most useful for the demonstration of minimal residual disease during treatment.

The characteristic immunophenotype of BCLL includes the presence of the membrane markers CD5, CD19, CD20, CD21 (the EBV-C3d receptor), CD22 and HLA DR. Typically, the antigen density on BCLL cell membranes is lower than that on normal lymphocytes. CLL cells also express CD25 (the IL-2 receptor) weakly. Of these markers, CD5 expression is considered to be essential for a diagnosis of CLL. CD5 is a pan T cell marker which is involved in T lymphocyte activation. This marker has also been demonstrated on foetal splenic lymphocytes and on a small subset of adult lymph node germinal centre lymphocytes. These CD5+ B lymphocytes are postulated to be involved in the regulation of autoimmunity, a hypothesis which accords well with the observed excess of auto-

---

The mechanisms underlying the common occurrence of certain non-random genetic rearrangements is becoming clear eg the rearrangement of the immunoglobulin and T lymphocyte receptor genes is mediated by an enzyme called DNA recombinase which recognises specific DNA sequences to signal cleavage and recombination sites. The heptameric DNA sequence CTGACAG followed 12 bases later by the nonameric DNA sequence ACAAGCCT signals a cleavage site while the heptameric DNA sequence CAATGTG followed 23 bases later by the nonameric DNA sequence GGTTTTTGT signals a recombination site. Analysis of the regions flanking the *bcl*-1 and *bcl*-2 oncogenes has revealed the presence of homologous DNA recombinase recognition sequences which makes these sites "hotspots" for recombination events.

immune disease in CLL. The clonal nature of BCLL is easily confirmed by the demonstration of immunoglobulin light chain restriction (the leukaemic cells express either κ or λ light chains, but never both) or the presence of a clonal immunoglobulin gene rearrangement.

Pathophysiology of CLL

CLL is an insidious and slowly progressive disease. Typical presenting features include general malaise and fatigue secondary to anaemia, mild hepatosplenomegaly and painless, symmetrical lymphadenopathy most commonly involving the cervical, supraclavicular, axillary and inguinal lymph nodes. Splenomegaly in CLL typically is minimal; massive enlargement of the spleen is associated with HCL or PLL. In contrast to the acute leukaemias and lymphomas, symptoms such as unexplained fever, severe weight loss and night sweats are uncommon in CLL, although occasionally, a severe chest infection is the presenting feature. However, susceptibility to bacterial or fungal infection tends to increase as the disease advances due to progressive immunodeficiency, neutropaenia and hypogammaglobulinaemia. As many as 25% of cases of CLL are free of physical symptoms at diagnosis.

The most common cause of anaemia in CLL is bone marrow failure but autoimmune haemolytic anaemia (AIHA), haematinic deficiency and pure red cell aplasia are all potential complications. AIHA occurs in about one third of cases but, if recognised early and treated successfully, does not confer a poor prognosis. Several triggers of pure red cell aplasia have been documented including parvovirus infection, T lymphocyte suppression of erythropoiesis and the development of autoantibodies directed against erythropoietin.

Clinical Staging of CLL

As a rule, disease progression in CLL occurs in an orderly fashion: the leukaemic cells slowly saturate the peripheral blood, bone marrow and then gradually infiltrate more and more lymph nodes. The most important determinants of survival are the total tumour load and the tumour doubling time. In more than half of cases, the tumour doubling time is in excess of 5 years. In the remainder of cases, the typical tumour doubling time is less than 1 year. Clinical staging is an attempt to define the prognosis in individual cases by providing objective criteria to measure disease bulk and progression, thereby facilitating the selection of treatment strategy. There are two main staging schemes in use for CLL; the Rai scheme (Table 17.8) and the more recent International Working Party scheme (Table 17.9).

Stage	Areas involved	Haemoglobin	Platelet Count	Survival (months)
0	Blood and bone marrow	>11	>100	>150
I	0 + lymph nodes	>11	>100	101
II	0 or I + hepato-splenomegaly	>11	>100	71
III	0 or I or II	<11	>100	30
IV	0 or I or II or III	< or >11	<100	30

Table 17.8 *The Rai clinical staging scheme for chronic lymphocytic leukaemia*

The Rai clinical staging scheme assumes that the peripheral blood lymphocyte count is greater than 15.0×10^9/L and that anaemia and thrombocytopaenia are secondary to bone marrow failure rather than to autoimmune disease or haematinic deficiency.

Stage	Areas involved	Haemoglobin	Platelet Count	Survival (months)
A	< 3 areas	>10	>100	>120
B	3, 4 or 5 areas	>10	>100	84
C	Not considered	<10	<100	24

Table 17.9 *The International Working Party clinical staging scheme for chronic lymphocytic leukaemia*

The International Working Party (IWP) clinical staging scheme also assumes that anaemia and thrombocytopaenia are secondary to bone marrow failure. For the purposes of staging, an area is defined as palpable lymph nodes in the neck, axillae or groin, or an enlarged liver or spleen. The IWP clinical staging system is simpler than the Rai scheme and also has the advantage that it allows a diagnosis of CLL to be made on lymphocyte counts as low as 5.0×10^9/l. The IWP scheme largely has superseded the Rai scheme although Rai stage 0 is retained as it identifies the earliest possible stage of CLL to be defined.

In about 30% of cases, CLL gradually transforms to the more aggressive disease PLL. This is manifest as a gradual increase in the numbers of prolymphocytes in the peripheral blood and is accompanied by progressive splenomegaly and increasing resistance to treatment. The morphology and immunophenotype of the prolymphocytes in transformed CLL are identical to those of *de novo* PLL. Further, once the circulating prolymphocyte count reaches 50% of the total, transformed CLL is clinically indistinguishable from *de novo* PLL.

A second form of transformation of CLL exists viz immunoblastic transformation or **Richter's syndrome**. This type of transformation affects about 5% of cases of CLL and is similar in some respects to the blastic phase of CML. Immunoblastic transformation always is associated with a poor prognosis and generally is regarded as a terminal event. In most cases, immunoblastic transformation is confined to the lymph nodes and biopsy is required to confirm its occurrence but, rarely, the peripheral blood and bone marrow are involved and the disease may superficially resemble acute leukaemia. Molecular analysis has shown that the immunoblasts often arise from a different B lymphoid clone to the BCLL cells. Although some short-lived responses to chemotherapy have been reported, transformed CLL typically is refractory to treatment and death usually occurs within a few months of immunoblastic transformation.

Treatment and Management of CLL

A wide selection of treatment options exist for CLL, ranging from minimal supportive care to aggressive cytotoxic chemotherapy and radiotherapy. Which option is selected in an individual case largely is determined by age and clinical stage. For example, an 85 year old man presenting with Rai stage 0 disease is unlikely to require anything more than minimal supportive therapy and regular haematological monitoring to provide early warning of disease progression. In contrast, a much younger patient with more advanced disease requires aggressive treatment which is aimed at induction of a complete haematological remission. Regardless of the treatment group selected, much of the treatment of CLL is palliative rather than curative.

The most intensive cytotoxic chemotherapy for CLL is intended to induce a complete haematological remission which currently is defined as a return to a normal peripheral blood lymphocyte count and a reduction in bone marrow lymphocytes to less than 30% of the total. This definition takes no account of the presence of minimal residual disease: most individuals who meet these criteria still have demonstrable disease. An alternative aim of therapy in some individuals is to induce a partial remission of CLL while causing minimal toxicity. Partial remission of CLL is defined as a measurable reduction in disease bulk, enabling reallocation to a lower clinical stage which carries an improved prognosis.

The drug combinations used in the treatment of CLL consist of alkylating agents such as chlorambucil or cyclophosphamide and the corticosteroid prednisolone. The response to chemotherapy typically is greater in the early stages of the disease: about 50% of individuals with low stage disease achieve a good response, but complete remission is attainable in less than 30% of individuals with high stage disease. Lower doses of these drugs can be used to maintain remission or at least to slow disease progression. However, long-term use of high dose steroids is contra-indicated because of side effects such as osteoporosis and weight gain. Tumour lysis syndrome is a possible complication of successful cytoreductive therapy in CLL, particularly where the circulating lymphocyte count prior to treatment is exceptionally high.

Troublesome splenomegaly which is not alleviated by chemotherapy can be treated by splenic irradiation or splenectomy. Splenic irradiation precipitates a reduction in the circulating lymphocyte count, as well as shrinkage of the spleen and lymph nodes, even those not included in the radiation field. Splenectomy also is indicated for the treatment of refractory autoimmune haemolysis (AIHA) or thrombocytopaenia (AITP).

Because the practical aim of treatment for CLL is to prolong and improve the quality of life, it is important that secondary symptoms such as anaemia, thrombocytopaenia and infections are treated promptly and effectively. The use of prophylactic immunoglobulin and the prompt institution of antimicrobial chemotherapy at the first sign of bacterial or fungal infection have reduced morbidity and mortality in CLL significantly. Long-term prophylactic penicillin therapy is required post-splenectomy to prevent life-threatening pneumococcal infections. Vaccination can also be offered, but frequently fails because of the impaired immune response in CLL. Uncomplicated anaemia and thrombocytopaenia can be treated by transfusion. Autoimmune disease usually responds well to prednisolone, cyclophosphamide or azathioprine.

Newer drug therapies which are still the subject of clinical trials include fludarabine monophosphate, 2'-deoxycoformycin and 2-chlorodeoxyadenosine. Preliminary results show that fludarabine therapy induced some degree of remission in up to 50% of cases, some of whom were refractory to conventional chemotherapy, but was associated with myelosuppression and an increased incidence of bacterial infections. 2'-deoxycoformycin, currently more commonly used in HCL, has induced significant remission in up to 50% of individuals with advanced disease.

Immunotherapy is an alternative form of treatment which has been tried with limited success in some cases of high stage CLL. This form of treatment involves the intravenous administration of a monoclonal antibody such as CDw52 (Campath) which has a lytic effect on the CLL cells. Some remissions have been attained using immunotherapy but the results are inferior to cytotoxic chemotherapy or radiotherapy. In addition, because no leukaemia-specific antigen has yet been found, immunotherapy is lytic to normal cells as well as the target cells.

Bone marrow transplantation is not considered to be a treatment option except in relatively young individuals with a suitable HLA-matched donor. The extreme rigours of the conditioning and transplantation process make this form of treatment unsuitable for anyone over the age of 55 years. Autologous bone marrow transplantation is unsuitable because it requires the induction of complete haematological remission which is difficult to achieve in CLL.

Prolymphocytic Leukaemia

Prolymphocytic leukaemia (PLL) is a relatively uncommon condition. It accounts for less than 10% of the chronic lymphoid leukaemias. Like CLL, PLL most commonly is a B lymphoid malignancy which afflicts the elderly of developed countries and affects men more commonly than women. PLL was, for many years, thought to be an unusual variant of CLL. However, with the advent of immunophenotyping, it became clear that PLL is a separate disease. In contrast to CLL, where the T lymphoid variant is rare, TPLL accounts for about 25% of cases.

Leukaemogenesis of PLL

In contrast to CLL, metaphase preparations are relatively easy to obtain from cases of PLL. Most studies have shown that the incidence of clonal chromosomal rearrangements is very high in PLL and that rearrangements of 14q are particularly common as shown in Table 17.10.

Lineage	Abnormality	Frequency
BPLL	14q32 rearrangements	50 to 75%
	+12	isolated cases
	t/del(12)	isolated cases
TPLL	14q11 rearrangements	>50%
	7q35 rearrangements	isolated cases

Table 17.10 *Non-random chromosome abnormalities associated with prolymphocytic leukaemia*

The most common chromosomal rearrangement in BPLL is t(11;14)(q13;q32) which involves the translocation of the *bcl*-1 oncogene from 11q13 to the site of the immunoglobulin heavy chain gene locus at 14q32, thereby promoting expression of B lymphocyte growth factors. This translocation is relatively common in many B lymphoid malignancies, but it appears to be particularly common in BPLL. Many other cytogenetic abnormalities have been described in BPLL, including +12 and rearrangements of 3p, 11p and 12p.

Rearrangements of 14q are also common in TPLL but, in this case, the breakpoint usually is located at 14q11, the locus of the T lymphocyte receptor α chain gene. The most common abnormality is inv(14)(q11;q32) which involves the Ti_α and *tcl*-1 gene loci. Other cytogenetic abnormalities reported in TPLL involve rearrangement of 7q35, the site of the Ti_β gene.

Recognition and Classification of PLL

Recognition of PLL is relatively straightforward and is based on the presence of a markedly raised white cell count which is composed of more than 55% of prolymphocytes. The white cell count at presentation typically is greater than $100 \times 10^9/l$ and may reach as high as $1000 \times 10^9/l$. TPLL usually is associated with higher white counts than BPLL. Most cases have thrombocytopaenia and anaemia at presentation, which are secondary to bone marrow infiltration and splenomegaly.

The peripheral blood picture seen in BPLL is characteristic: examination of the bone marrow seldom is required for diagnostic pur-

The predominant cell in PLL has the morphological stigmata of immaturity In spite of the morphological name prolymphocyte, which usually implies immaturity, the predominant cell in PLL is, in fact, further along the differentiation pathway than either CLL or HCL cells.

poses although examination of a trephine biopsy can provide useful prognostic information. The prolymphocytes of BPLL are relatively large cells which are characterised by the abundance of their pale blue cytoplasm, which is free of granules and their central nucleus with its prominent, single nucleolus. A number of subtle differences in the morphology of the prolymphocytes of TPLL enable the skilled microscopist to recognise this subtype. Typically, the prolymphocytes in TPLL are slightly smaller than their BPLL counterparts, have an irregular nucleus which often is cleft, and a slightly more basophilic cytoplasm which may include azurophilic granules. As shown in Table 17.11, immunophenotyping provides a much more reliable way of differentiating between the two subtypes of PLL.

CD No.	BPLL	TPLL
CD2	−	+++
CD3	−	+++*
CD4	−	++ **
CD5	+/−	+++
CD7	−	+++
CD8	−	++ **
CD10	−	−
CD19	+++	−
CD20	+++	−
CD22	+++	−
CD25	+/−	−
FMC7	+++	−
SIgM	+++	−
κ/λ	+++	−

Table 17.11 *Differentiation of TPLL and BPLL by immunophenotyping*
* *A proportion of T-PLL patients fail to express surface CD3*
** *60% of T-PLL are CD4+, CD8-; 20% are CD4-, CD8+ and 20% are CD4+, CD8+*

Pathophysiology of PLL

PLL is characterised at presentation by moderate splenomegaly in the absence of lymphadenopathy and typically follows a more aggressive course than CLL. There is no formally accepted clinical staging system for PLL. However, many treatment centres employ a modified Rai scheme, similar to that used for CLL (Table 17.8). The majority of PLL patients present with stage III or IV disease.

Treatment and Management of PLL

PLL is a more aggressive disease than CLL and typically is moderately refractory to treatment. Effective treatment for PLL is hampered by the advanced age of those affected and, because of the hyperleucocytosis, by the need to avoid tumour lysis syndrome. In most cases, the first step of treatment is to reduce the circulating white cell count by leucopheresis or splenic irradiation. The latter option causes a significant reduction in the splenomegaly, appears to lengthen the duration of subsequent remission and generally is well tolerated by elderly patients. Splenectomy may further improve the duration of remission but, in contrast to HCL, does not impede disease progression.

The disease debulking manoeuvres described above are insufficient to induce remission in PLL: in almost every case, supplementary cytotoxic chemotherapy is required. The most commonly used treatment schedule involves the use of **C**yclophosphamide, **H**ydroxydaunomycin (adriamycin), **O**ncovin (vincristine) and **P**rednisolone (CHOP). This schedule is widely used in the treatment of non-Hodgkin's lymphoma, which typically affects a younger age group who are better able to withstand the rigours of cytotoxic chemotherapy. Because of their advanced age, PLL sufferers require energetic supportive care while undergoing chemotherapy. Most individuals will have some, generally short-lived, response to treatment but complete remissions are rare. Several other treatments have been tried in PLL with limited success, including α-interferon, immunotherapy with CDw52 and 2'-deoxycoformycin which has proved to be useful in a few cases of TPLL. Currently, clinical trials are in progress to assess the potential benefit of using 2-chlorodeoxyadenosine and fludarabine in the treatment of PLL.

Hairy Cell Leukaemia

Hairy cell leukaemia (HCL) is a rare B lymphoid disorder, accounting for no more than 10% of cases of chronic lymphoid leukaemia. It has a similar age distribution to CLL, and shows an even greater preponderance in males: the male:female ratio is about 4:1 in HCL.

The name hairy cell leukaemia was coined by Schrek and Donnelly in 1966, but the disease was first described by Bouroncle in 1958 and was then called **leukaemic reticuloendotheliosis**. The lineage and normal counterpart of the hairy cell was been the subject of heated scientific debate for many years. However, recent advances in immunophenotyping and genotyping have finally confirmed the cell as being of B lymphoid origin.

Leukaemogenesis of HCL

All of the technical problems associated with cytogenetic analysis of CLL apply equally well to HCL, but the pancytopaenia which accompanies this condition and the difficulty of obtaining an adequate bone marrow sample impose extra difficulties. A number of small studies have shown that the overall incidence of chromosomal abnormalities is high in HCL. The most common abnormalities involved rearrangement of chromosome 14q, with the breakpoint occurring at 14q32. Abnormalities of chromosome 12 also are commonly seen.

Recognition and Classification of HCL

More than 80% of cases of HCL present with pancytopaenia, with neutropaenia and monocytopaenia being especially prominent. The degree of anaemia at presentation is variable and usually is normochromic and normocytic. The platelet count at presentation typically is less than $100 \times 10^9/l$. Identification of the pathognomonic hairy cells is mandatory for a diagnosis of HCL. However, these usually are evident on careful examination of a well-stained blood film. Hairy cells are almost twice as large as normal lymphocytes and have an eccentric nucleus which rarely contains nucleoli. The abundant, pale blue cytoplasm, which may contain azurophilic cytoplasmic inclusions which superficially resemble Auer rods, characteristically is demarcated by long "hair-like" projections. Electron microscopy reveals the presence of cylindrical structures which contain rows of ribosomes known as ribosome-lamellar complexes in about 50% of cases. These complexes are not unique to HCL, they can, on occasion, be demonstrated in other B lymphoid disorders.

Attempts to aspirate bone marrow often result in a "dry tap" because of increased marrow fibrosis. Trephine biopsy shows a characteristic pattern of diffuse infiltrate which has a "honeycomb" appearance. This appearance, thought to be an artefact of fixation, is caused by each hairy cell being surrounded by an apparently clear rim of cytoplasm.

Hairy cells express a characteristic pattern of cell surface antigens which confirms their mature, functional B lymphocytic origin. In common with the malignant cell of other B lymphoid malignancies, they express CD19, CD20, CD22, HLADR, SIgM, and show immunoglobulin light chain restriction. The distinguishing immunological markers of hairy cells are the absence of CD5 and the presence of CD11c, a monocyte-associated marker, CD25, the IL-2 receptor, and FMC7. The applicability of immunophenotyping to the recognition of HCL is limited by the dearth of cells in the peripheral blood and the difficulty in aspirating bone marrow.

Supplementary evidence for a diagnosis of HCL can be obtained by staining a peripheral blood film for the enzyme acid phosphatase. The addition of tartaric acid to the reaction mixture inhibits all of the common isoenzymes of acid phosphatase, except isoenzyme 5 which is found in hairy cells. Tartrate resistant acid phosphatase (TRAP) activity is located in the Golgi area and in the nuclear membrane of hairy cells, and is characteristic. Although TRAP positivity has rarely been demonstrated in other T and B lymphoid disorders, its presence is highly suggestive of HCL, particularly when accompanied by the other stigmata of this disease.

A variant of HCL exists which is distinguished by the presence of a raised white cell count at presentation of up to $100 \times 10^9/l$ and more rounded hairy cells which have a higher nuclear:cytoplasmic ratio and do not express CD25. Bone marrow aspirates typically are easy to obtain in such cases. In further contrast to typical HCL, these variant cases are refractory to α-interferon and 2′ deoxycoformycin therapy.

Pathophysiology of HCL

Most cases of HCL present with fatigue and general malaise secondary to anaemia, severe infections secondary to leucopaenia or bleeding or bruising problems secondary to thrombocytopaenia. Mycobacterial and other uncommon opportunistic infections are a particular feature. Infection is the leading cause of death in HCL, closely followed by autoimmune disease. Some degree of splenomegaly is present in virtually all cases and is accompanied by minimal hepatomegaly in about 50% of cases. Hepatomegaly is secondary to infiltration of hepatic sinuses by hairy cells. Lymphadenopathy is rare except in the terminal phase of the disease. Cell kinetic studies have shown that the pancytopaenia results from a combination of suppression of haemopoiesis and splenic sequestration.

The most widely accepted clinical staging scheme for HCL is based on the degree of anaemia and splenic enlargement as shown in Table 17.12.

Stage	Haemoglobin	Spleen Enlargement
I	normal	slight
II	slight anaemia	moderate
III	severe anaemia	massive

Table 17.12 *Clinical staging of hairy cell leukaemia*

This staging scheme can only be applied prior to splenectomy. Stage I patients have the best prognosis while those assigned to stage III have the worst prognosis. Other staging schemes have attempted to incorporate the circulating neutrophil count and the number of circulating hairy cells, but these have proven to be difficult to establish with reliability.

A second staging system is used post-splenectomy to predict the need for supplementary cytotoxic chemotherapy. On the basis of white cell count, haemoglobin concentration and platelet count at about three months post-splenectomy, individual cases can be stratified into three risk groups: the complete responders, between 40 and 60% of cases, have no cytopaenia and good bone marrow function; the intermediate responders have mild anaemia and/or neutropaenia; and the non-responders, up to 40% of cases, have a severe, progressive cytopaenia. In general, cytotoxic chemotherapy is withheld from the good responders until relapse occurs: poor and intermediate responders require treatment straight away.

Treatment and Management of HCL

Most individuals with HCL are symptomatic at presentation and require immediate treatment. The most common first-line treatment for HCL is splenectomy which has been shown to relieve the pancytopaenia and induce remission in most cases. It is possible to predict with some certainty the benefits of splenectomy in HCL. As a general rule, those who present with significant splenomegaly benefit the most, whereas those with minimal splenomegaly at presentation tend not to respond. The 40% of cases who have progressive disease post-splenectomy require second-line chemotherapy to induce and maintain remission. The use of cytotoxic chemotherapy regimens which have been used with success in the other chronic leukaemias or lymphomas has been discouraging: very few complete remissions have been attained by this means. To make matters worse, conventional cytotoxic chemotherapy tends to worsen the pre-existing neutropaenia, thereby increasing the susceptibility to infection in these individuals.

More promising results have been obtained with the use of α-interferon which has recently become available in human recombinant form. Virtually all poor prognosis cases of HCL have been shown to experience some degree of disease remission following α-interferon therapy. The exact mechanism of action of α-interferon is unknown. Although the neutropaenia is not relieved during α-interferon therapy, the susceptibility to bacterial and fungal infections appears to diminish. However, α-interferon therapy is associated with the development of inhibitory antibodies in those treated and a high incidence of side effects which range from flu-like symptoms to nausea, vomiting and chronic fatigue syndrome.

Another novel treatment for HCL which shows early promise is 2'-deoxycoformycin (DCF) which acts as an inhibitor of the enzyme adenosine deaminase (ADA). As explained in Chapter 14, ADA catalyses the irreversible deamination of adenosine and deoxyadenosine to form inosine and deoxyinosine. DCF therapy results in the intracellular accumulation of deoxyadenosine triphosphate with consequent inhibition of the enzyme ribonucleotide reductase and a severe impairment of DNA synthesis. Lymphocytes are particularly susceptible to the action of DCF. Early results of DCF therapy suggest that complete haematological remission can be attained in up to 90% of cases within a few weeks of commencing treatment. However, the long-term risks of DCF remain to be established.

Early results of 2-chlorodeoxyadenosine, an ADA-resistant purine analogue, suggest that it may also be effective in the treatment of poor-prognosis HCL and that its use is associated with lower toxicity.

Suggested Further Reading

Lee, R.G., Bithell, T.C., Foerster, J., Athens, J.W. and Lukens, J.N. (1993). *Wintrobe's Clinical Hematology*. London: Lea and Febiger.

Hoffbrand, A.V. and Lewis, S.M. (1989). *Postgraduate Haematology*. Oxford: Butterworth-Heinemann.

Chronic Myeloid Leukaemia: State of the Art Symposia - 24th ISH Congress (1992). *British Journal of Haematology*, **82**: 199-203.

Chronic Myeloid Leukaemia: Second International Conference (1993). *Leukaemia and Lymphoma*, **11**: Supplement 1.

Catovsky, D. and Foa, R. (1990). *The Lymphoid Leukaemias*. Oxford: Butterworth-Heinemann.

Answers to Self Assessment Questions

1. The G-6-PD gene is located on the tip of the q arm of the X chromosome at Xq28.

2. An isochromosome occurs when either the long or the short arm is deleted and the other arm is duplicated about the centromere, forming a "mirror image" chromosome.

The Myelodysplastic Syndromes

The myelodysplastic syndromes (MDS) are a highly heterogeneous group of acquired neoplastic disorders which are characterised by varying degrees of trilineage cytopaenia and dysplasia in the presence of a normocellular or hypercellular bone marrow and, in some cases, by progression to acute leukaemia. The phenotypic manifestations of the myelodysplastic syndromes vary from a mild, refractory anaemia to a condition which closely resembles ANLL. The MDS have been recognised in some form for decades and have, over the years, been associated with a variety of descriptive titles, including acquired refractory sideroblastic anaemia, preleukaemia, oligoblastic leukaemia, smouldering leukaemia, chronic erythraemic myelosis and dysmyelopoietic syndrome. These titles have fallen into disuse since 1982 when the FAB group reclassified the MDS into five types viz **refractory anaemia (RA), refractory anaemia with ring sideroblasts (RAS), refractory anaemia with excess of blasts (RAEB), refractory anaemia with excess of blasts in transformation (RAEB-t)** and **chronic myelomonocytic leukaemia (CMML)**. The FAB classification scheme for the MDS is described later in this chapter.

The myelodysplastic syndromes are diseases of the elderly, although MDS secondary to monosomy 7 is seen in children and some workers suggest that juvenile CML should be reclassified as the juvenile equivalent of CMML. Also, congenital chromosome fragility states such as Fanconi's anaemia are associated with MDS, but these are very rare. The median age at presentation of MDS is 65 years. Fewer than 10% of cases are younger than 50 years of age at presentation. Overall, the incidence of MDS is about 1 per 100,000 persons, with males being affected slightly more often than females.

In this chapter the MDS are considered under the headings:

- aetiology

- recognition and classification

- pathophysiology

- treatment and management

Aetiology of the MDS

The mechanisms which underly the genesis and progression of the MDS remain obscure. In common with other haemopoietic malignancies, cytogenetic abnormalities are common in the MDS but no consistent cytogenetic marker exists. The application of techniques such as G-6-PD isoenzyme analysis, restriction fragment length polymorphism analysis and polymerase chain reaction using X-linked markers has provided definitive evidence for the clonal nature of the MDS. However, the state of knowledge about the nature of the primary stem cell mutation and the molecular mechanisms involved remains relatively rudimentary. The demonstration of clonal cytogenetic rearrangements in the erythroblasts, granulocytes, monocytes, megakaryocytes and, sometimes, in the B and T lymphocytes of affected individuals suggests that the initial mutation occurs at the level of the pluripotent stem cell. Further support for the presence of lymphoid involvement is provided by the observation that a small number of cases of MDS transform to ALL.

One of the confounding factors in the quest for knowledge about the MDS is the extreme heterogeneity of their presentation and progression. For the present, we must content ourselves with the accumulation of evidence from various sources until a pattern becomes clear.

Epidemiological Evidence

The MDS are diseases of the elderly as shown in Figure 18.1. The overall incidence of the MDS in the UK is about 1 case per 100,000 per year but this incidence rises to 1 case per 1,000 per year in those older than 60 years of age. It seems likely that, with the demographic changes taking place in developed countries, that the incidence of MDS is set to rise in the coming years.

As described in Chapter 15, a variety of chemical, biological and physical insults may be associated with the induction of haemopoietic malignancy, including exposure to ionising radiation, chemicals, drugs and viruses.

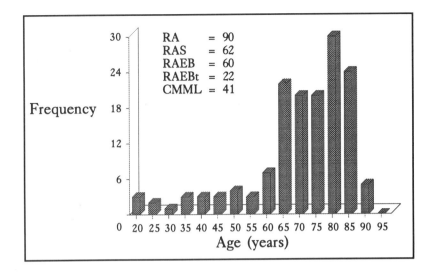

Figure 18.1 *The age-related incidence and distribution of the MDS in Sheffield, UK*

The evidence relating ionising radiation to the MDS is surprisingly weak. Isolated reports exist of RAEB in individuals exposed to thorium dioxide (Thorotrast), an early radioactive X-ray contrast medium. At *post-mortem*, these cases showed histological evidence of residual Thorotrast in the spleen, lymph nodes and bone marrow. It is plausible that chronic exposure of such sensitive sites to ionising radiation may have contributed to the induction of MDS in these cases. Thorotrast has also been associated with the induction of hepatoma.

Epidemiological studies have shown a much higher incidence of the MDS in workers in the petroleum industry and in those exposed to benzene or its derivatives. This is hardly surprising, chronic occupational exposure to benzene has been linked with the induction of bone marrow aplasia and acute leukaemia for many years. Benzene also is present in tobacco smoke, along with a number of other potential mutagens such as nitrosamines and radioactive polonium (^{210}Po). Cigarette smoking has shown a positive association with the development of ANLL but evidence for such a link currently is lacking in the MDS.

As described in Chapter 15, treatment of primary malignancies with alkylating agents such as melphalan, chlorambucil, cyclophosphamide and busulphan is associated with the induction of secondary ANLL. In almost 70% of cases, secondary ANLL is preceded by a myelodysplastic phase. Secondary MDS is even more refractory to treatment than *de novo*, or primary, MDS and is associated with a shorter time course. The majority of cases present as RAEB or RAEB-t, have a greater incidence of cytogenetic abnormalities and at least 60% progress to ANLL. The median delay between the therapeutic exposure and presentation is about 4 years but may be as long as 12 years. The risk of secondary MDS or ANLL following exposure to alkylating agents is substantial. For example, about 10% of cases of Hodgkin's disease treated with alkylating agents develop this complication within 9 years of the start of therapy.

There is no convincing evidence for the role of viruses in the induction of the MDS but several studies have described myelodysplastic features in the bone marrow of patients with HIV and non-A, non-B hepatitis.

Cytogenetic and Molecular Evidence

Chromosomal abnormalities are present in up to 50% of cases of *de novo* MDS and in virtually all cases of secondary MDS. The variety of abnormalities observed is extensive but, as shown in Table 18.1, the most common abnormalities involve chromosomes 5, 7 and 8.

Table 18.1 *Summary of the cytogenetic changes observed in 3000 cases of the MDS*

Abnormality	-7	+7	+8	5q-	7q-	11q-	12q-	13q-	20q-	inv3	i(17q)	t(1;3)	t(1;7)	t(3;3)
Frequency (%)	15	5	19	27	4	7	5	2	5	1	5	1	2	1

None of these chromosomal abnormalities is specific for the MDS and there is no absolute relationship with a particular subtype. However, a number of non-random associations can be discerned:

- Deletion of the long arm of chromosome 5, although seen in all MDS subtypes, is strongly associated with RA: 5q- accounts for up to 70% of cytogenetic abnormalities in this subtype. The most common breakpoints on chromosome 5 are at q13.3 and q31.1 as shown in Figure 18.2. This chromosomal abnormality is associated with a clinical subtype of RA, the **5q- syndrome**, which is characterised by a refractory macrocytic anaemia, thrombocytosis, splenomegaly and a low rate of progression to acute leukaemia. Bone marrow examination reveals the presence of erythroid hypoplasia, dyserythropoiesis and marked dysthrombopoiesis with megakaryocytic hypolobulation. 5q- syndrome is seen most commonly in elderly women. The q arm of chromosome 5 is particularly rich in genes which encode haemopoietic growth factors and their receptors. For example, the genes which encode IL-3, IL-4, IL-5, GM-CSF, M-CSF and the M-CSF receptor (c-*fms*) are all located in this region. As many as 40% of cases of 5q- have been shown to have lost the c-*fms* gene. The potential for the loss of any or all of these genes to contribute to the disruption of ordered haemopoiesis is obvious. Many workers suspect the presence of an as yet undiscovered tumour suppressor gene on 5q. The median survival time for the 5q- syndrome is greater than 5 years.

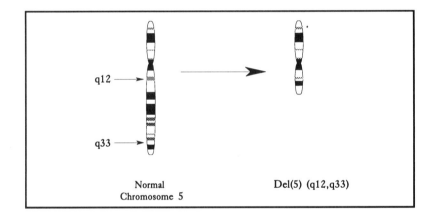

q12

q33

Normal
Chromosome 5

Del(5) (q12,q33)

Figure 18.2 *Schematic representation of the common deletion in 5q- syndrome*

- Monosomy 7 and 7q- also are seen in all MDS subtypes, but are most strongly associated with secondary and paediatric MDS. Deletion of this chromosome is associated with the loss of a major surface glycoprotein (gp130) in neutrophils and a susceptibility to bacterial infections secondary to impaired granulocyte and monocyte chemotactic activity. The genes which encode erythropoietin, plasminogen activator, multi-drug resistance and the proto-oncogenes c-*met* and c-*erb* are all located on chromosome 7. The role, if any, of these genes in the induction of MDS is unknown. Monosomy 7 is associated with a very poor prognosis: the median survival time from presentation is less than 1 year.

- Deletions of the q arm of chromosome 11, with breakpoints in the region q14 to 22, account for 20% of chromosomal abnormalities in RAS. This abnormality is associated with raised iron stores and high ring sideroblast counts. The molecular basis for this association is unknown but the presence of the gene which encodes the H-subunit of ferritin at 11q13 may be significant.

- Deletions of the p arm of chromosome 12 are associated with CMML. The Ki-*ras*-2 oncogene is located on chromosome 12 and is thought to be affected by these deletions.

- Abnormalities of chromosome 17 which involve the loss or disruption of the *p53* tumour suppressor gene are seen in CML in association with transformation to the blastic phase and in up to 5% of cases of primary MDS. Certain dysplastic features such as pseudo-Pelger-Huët and neutrophil vacuolation have also been described in association with abnormalities of the short arm of chromosome 17.

- Dysmegakaryopoiesis and thrombocytosis appear to be associated with abnormalities of chromosome 3.

Despite the variety of cytogenetic abnormalities observed in the MDS, their presence does not, in most cases, provide a useful additional indicator of prognosis. Generally, however, multiple cytogenetic abnormalities are associated with a poorer prognosis than single abnormalities. This is consistent with a multistep hypothesis for the development of the MDS, in which progressive genetic instability and the acquisition of cytogenetic abnormalities are relatively late events as shown in Figure 18.3.

Three patterns of evolution of the MDS have been described:

- a stable group with no increase in bone marrow blasts and a normal karyotype.

- rapid blast transformation with the acquisition of new cytogenetic changes after an initial, stable phase.

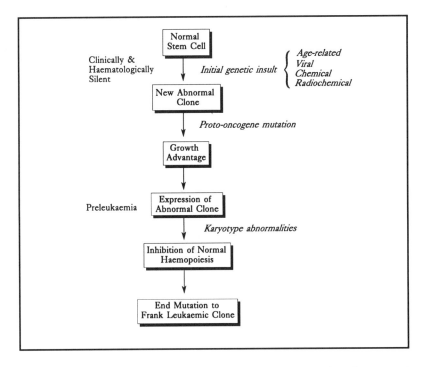

Figure 18.3 *Hypothetical evolution of MDS*

- gradually increasing blasts count in the absence of new cytogenetic changes.

The Role of Oncogenes in the MDS

The role of oncogenes in the development of the MDS and their progression to acute leukaemia remains to be defined. Much of the research to date has centred on the role of the *ras* oncogene family and the M-CSF receptor gene, c-*fms*.

The *ras* group of oncogenes are related to the viral oncogenes of the Harvey murine sarcoma virus and Kirsten murine sarcoma virus. As shown in Table 18.2, and previously in Table 15.1, several *ras* oncogenes exist in humans, scattered throughout the genome. All of these oncogenes encode a p21 protein which is an intermediate of the signal transduction pathways. This protein is located adjacent to the inner aspect of the plasma membrane where it binds to guanosine triphosphate (GTP) in response to incoming cellular signals such as membrane growth factor receptor occupation. Binding of p21 to GTP results in the activation of a variety of cellular enzymes such as phospholipase C, adenyl cyclase, protein A kinases and

ras Oncogene	Chromosome
cKi-*ras*	6
cKi-*ras*-2	12
cHa-*ras*-1	11
cHa-*ras*-2	X
N-*ras*	1

Table 18.2 *The ras oncogene family*

stimulates membrane inositol turnover. Activation of these second messenger pathways normally is terminated by the hydrolysis of GTP to GDP and the release of p21. Analysis of the N-*ras* and Ki-*ras* oncogenes in cases of MDS has shown that point mutations at codons 12, 13 or 61 is present in up to 40% of cases, most commonly in CMML. It is postulated that these mutations encode for an abnormal p21 which is not subject to deactivation following GTP hydrolysis and so stimulates cellular second messenger systems inappropriately. Similar *ras* oncogene mutations have been described in a wide range of malignant conditions, including ANLL and colorectal, stomach, thyroid, bladder, lung and ovarian carcinomas. RAS proteins appear to be involved in terminal differentiation, perhaps partly explaining the presence of ineffective haemopoiesis following their mutation. However, the significance of *ras* mutations in the pathogenesis of MDS is still in doubt. Such mutations have been identified in apparently normal subjects. It seems likely that *ras* mutations are incapable of producing malignant change on their own but that they may contribute to the pathogenesis of disease following malignant change. One study suggested that cases of MDS with *ras* mutations are associated with a significantly poorer prognosis than those which lack this abnormality.

The c-*fms* proto-oncogene epitomises the logic of the MDS-oncogene link. The c-*fms* gene was first isolated from a feline sarcoma virus and specifically encodes the M-CSF growth factor receptor. This receptor has been shown to have tyrosine kinase activity and to play a regulatory role in monocytoid cell division. Analysis of c-*fms* genes in individuals with CMML has revealed point mutations of codons 301 or 969 in up to 20% of cases. Mutations of codon 301 appear to be associated with neoplastic transformation while mutations of codon 969 exert a negative regulatory effect. Similar rates of c-*fms* mutation have been demonstrated in ANLL FAB type M4. As described earlier, loss of c-*fms* may play a role in the 5q-syndrome.

It is hoped that continuing research on the role of oncogenes will help to clarify the aetiology of the MDS and the pathogenesis of their progression to acute leukaemia. The discovery of molecular markers of early disease or indicators of progression to acute leukaemia would represent a major step forward in our understanding of this group of malignant disorders and may facilitate the rational design of new treatment protocols.

Recognition and Classification of the MDS

The presentation of the MDS is highly variable, but about 90% of cases are anaemic and up to 50% are pancytopaenic. In addition, a wide range of dysplastic and dysfunctional states may be present as shown in Tables 18.3 and 18.4. None of these features are, in themselves, diagnostic of the MDS. Rather, it is the pattern of refractory cytopaenia with trilineage dysplastic features in an elderly person which suggest the diagnosis. However, before a diagnosis of MDS can be made, it is important to exclude other potential causes of cytopaenia or dysplasia such as deficiencies of vitamin B_{12}, iron or pyridoxine, drug toxicity, anaemia of chronic disorders, aplastic anaemia, acute leukaemia, chronic myeloproliferative disorders, HIV infection, immune cytopaenias, metabolic disturbances associated with hypothyroidism or renal failure, and non-haematological malignancy.

Red Cells	Granulocytes	Platelets
Ovalomacrocytes	Hypogranularity	Micromegakaryocytes
Dimorphic population	Abnormal granulation	Megakaryocyte fragments
Megaloblastic change	Pseudo-Pelger-Huët	in peripheral blood
Gross poikilocytosis	Nuclear appendages	Platelet dysfunction
Multinuclearity	Gross hypersegmentation	Agranular platelets
Nuclear budding	Decreased myeloperoxidase	Giant platelet granules
Ring sideroblasts	& abnormal esterase activity	
Raised HbF	Neutrophil dysfunction	
Raised HbH	Abnormally localised immature	
Reticulocytopaenia	myeloid precursors in marrow	
Howell Jolly bodies	Monocytosis	
Pappenheimer bodies	Abnormal monocytes	
Basophilic stippling		
Decreased pyruvate		
kinase activity		

Table 18.3 *Commonly observed dysplastic features in the MDS*

Affected Cell Line	Observed Abnormality	Frequency of Observation (%)
Peripheral Blood		
Red cells	Ovalomacrocytosis	100
	Hypochromia	20
	Erythroblastosis	25
White cells	Presence of promyelocytes	25
	Neutrophil nuclear hyposegmentation	15
Platelets	Large, dysplastic forms	75
Bone Marrow		
Red cells	Erythroid hyperplasia	70
	Erythroid hypoplasia	10
	Megaloblastic appearance	85
	Dyserythropoiesis	80
	Excess sideroblasts	20
White cells	Abnormal monocyte maturation	80
	Granulocyte maturation bulge	85
Platelets	Megakaryocytosis	50
	Megakaryocytopaenia	30
	Dysthrombopoiesis	85

Table 18.4 *Frequency of the more commonly observed dysplastic features in the MDS*

When the original FAB classification scheme for acute leukaemia was proposed in 1976, a group of conditions called the dysmyelopoietic syndromes were defined, but were not included in the scheme. At this stage two types of dysmyelopoietic syndrome were recognised, refractory anaemia with excess of blasts (RAEB) and chronic myelomonocytic leukaemia (CMML). In the years that followed, it rapidly became apparent that the range of morphological appearances in the MDS was very wide and that there was some correlation between morphological subtypes and the risk of transformation to ANLL. In 1982, a more detailed FAB classification scheme for the MDS was proposed which took account of these findings. Classification of the MDS according to the FAB scheme requires careful examination of both peripheral blood and bone marrow films. The diagnosis of MDS first requires the exclusion of the acute non-lymphoblastic leukaemias as shown in Figure 18.4. The presence of ring sideroblasts, with their "necklace" of iron-laden mitochondria surrounding the cell nucleus is revealed using the Perl's Prussian blue stain for iron. A number of supplementary

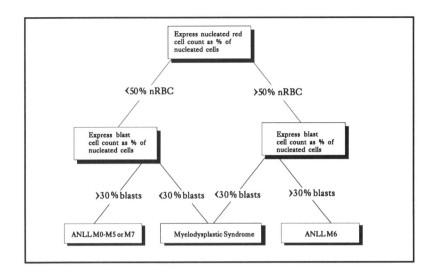

studies may aid the classification of the MDS. For example, the presence of a raised serum lysozyme concentration aids the recognition of CMML.

Following a further refinement in 1985, the FAB classification scheme for the MDS has become widely accepted. The current FAB classification scheme is shown in Table 18.5.

Disorder	Blasts (%) Blood	Marrow	Monocytes (x 10^9/l)	Ring Sideroblasts (%)	Other Features
RA	< 1	< 5	< 1.0	< 15	anaemia
RARS	< 1	< 5	< 1.0	> 15	anaemia, refractory cytopaenia
RAEB	< 5	5-20	< 1.0	< 15	anaemia, refractory cytopaenia
RAEB-t	> 5	20-30	< 1.0	< 15	Auer rods in blast cells
CMML	< 5	< 20	> 1.0	< 15	increased blood granulocyte count and marrow promonocyte count

Table 18.5 *The FAB classification scheme for the MDS*

The classification of the MDS according to the FAB scheme is not simply an exercise in obsessive haematological orderliness: the FAB subtypes carry prognostic significance as shown in Table 18.6.

FAB subtype	Rate of Transformation to Acute Leukaemia (%)	Median Survival (months)
RA	15	32
RAS	10	76
RAEB	30	10
RAEB-t	48	5
CMML	20	18

Table 18.6 *Reported rates of progression of the FAB subtypes of MDS to acute leukaemia*

Refractory Anaemia

Up to 35% of MDS cases are classified as RA. The typical picture includes a macrocytic or, less commonly, normocytic anaemia and reticulocytopaenia which is refractory to haematinic therapy. Basophilic stippling commonly is present. In some cases, dysplastic features are restricted to the red cells but, typically, features such as neutropaenia with hypogranular and hypolobulated neutrophils and thrombocytopaenia with large, agranular platelets also are present. Up to 90% of cases of RA at presentation are pancytopaenic. Bone marrow examination typically reveals hypercellularity with dysplastic, normoblastic or megaloblastic erythropoiesis. Ring sideroblasts are present but do not exceed 15% of the erythroblasts present. The blast cell count always is less than 5% of the total nucleated cells.

Refractory Anaemia with Sideroblasts

As discussed in Chapter 5, RAS is identical to the most common of the sideroblastic anaemias, primary acquired sideroblastic anaemia (PASA), and constitutes up to 20% of cases of MDS. It is characterised at presentation by the presence of anaemia and a dual red cell population: a major population of normochromic macrocytes and a minor population of hypochromic microcytes. Typically, the serum iron, ferritin concentration and transferrin saturation are all raised and Pappenheimer bodies and basophilic stippling are present. Neutropaenia, thrombocytopaenia and trilineage dysplasia are much less common than in RA. The bone marrow typically is hypercellular with prominent normoblastic or megaloblastic erythroid hyperplasia and dysplasia. The *sine qua non* for a diagnosis of RAS is that ring sideroblasts should comprise at least 15% of the erythroblasts present and that blast cells should comprise less than 5% of the total of nucleated cells in the bone marrow.

Refractory Anaemia with Excess of Blasts

RAEB constitutes up to 25% of MDS and is a much more aggressive disease than RA or RAS. It is characterised at presentation by symptomatic anaemia, neutropaenia and thrombocytopaenia. Trilineage dysplasia is more common and tends to be more severe than in the relatively benign forms of the MDS. Blast cells typically are present in the peripheral blood but do not exceed 5% of the total of nucleated cells. Bone marrow examination reveals a variable number of ring sideroblasts and a blast cell count of between 5 and 20% of the total nucleated cell count.

Refractory Anaemia with Excess of Blasts in Transformation

A case of RAEB is said to be in transformation to acute leukaemia (RAEB-t) when any of three markers are present: a peripheral blood blast cell count which exceeds 5% of the total of nucleated cells; the presence of Auer rods in the blast cells in the peripheral blood or the presence of a blast cell population which exceeds 20% of the total of nucleated cells in the bone marrow. If blast cells exceed 30% of the total nucleated cells in the bone marrow, transformation to acute leukaemia is said to be complete. Typically, such cases are profoundly neutropaenic and thrombocytopaenic and trilineage dysplasia is almost universal. Some degree of hepatosplenomegaly commonly is present.

Although both RAEB and ANLL are associated with peripheral blood cytopaenia despite the presence of a hypercellular bone marrow, the mechanisms involved are quite different. In acute leukaemia, the pancytopaenia is directly related to the dominance of leukaemic blast cells in the marrow whereas in RAEB it is the result of ineffective haemopoiesis ie a large proportion of the cells produced are morphologically and functionally defective and are doomed to die in the bone marrow. Further, trilineage dysplasia invariably is present in RAEB while it is infrequent in *de novo* ANLL.

Chronic Myelomonocytic Leukaemia

CMML is characterised at presentation by hepatosplenomegaly, a peripheral blood monocyte count which exceeds $1 \times 10^9/l$ and monocytic dysplasia. Anaemia and thrombocytopaenia are much less common than in other types of the MDS. Where present, the anaemia usually is normocytic and normochromic but macrocytes, microcytes and siderocytes may all be present. Dysplastic features commonly are present but trilineage dysplasia is not as common as in other types of the MDS. Typically, the bone marrow is hypercellular with dysplastic promonocytes being especially prominent. The blast and ring sideroblast counts vary but seldom exceed 20% of the total.

Pathophysiology of the MDS

Erythrodysplasia

Ferrokinetic studies have demonstrated major defects in erythropoiesis in all of the MDS groups, with ineffective erythropoiesis often being evident prior to the development of anaemia and obvious erythrodysplasia. The MDS can be divided into three groups based on plasma iron turnover, marrow iron turnover, red cell iron utilisation and red cell survival. The lowest erythroid output and the poorest red cell survival times are seen in RAEB and RAEB-t. At the other extreme, cases of RAS are marked by profound erythrokinetic abnormalities with greatly increased plasma and marrow iron turnover secondary to ineffective erythropoiesis but longer red cell survival times. One of the major contributors to premature red cell death in RAS is intra-mitochondrial iron accumulation which leads to an increase in the generation of free radicals with concomitant damage to mitochondrial function. The other forms of MDS form a heterogeneous intermediate group.

Other frequently observed changes in the red cells in the MDS include a variety of secondary metabolic abnormalities such as pyruvate kinase deficiency and increased concentration of foetal haemoglobin. Isolated reports exist of an acquired form of HbH disease secondary to defective α globin gene transcription. Changes in red cell antigen expression occasionally are seen, most commonly involving increased i antigen expression and Complement sensitivity.

Leucodysplasia

Leucodysplasia presents as neutropaenia and granulodysplasia in the presence of a normocellular or hypercellular bone marrow. This contrasts with CML where the bone marrow hypercellularity is reflected in the peripheral blood and dysplastic changes are minimal and with the hypoplastic anaemias where peripheral neutropaenia is accompanied by a hypocellular bone marrow and dysplastic features are uncommon. A proportion of Philadelphia chromosome negative CML cases in whom a *bcr-abl* rearrangement cannot be identified show prominent granulodysplastic features. Many workers believe that such cases should be reclassified as MDS.

The morphological abnormalities of granulocytes and monocytes are paralleled by enzyme defects such as myeloperoxidase deficiency, increased monocyte esterase activity and low neutrophil alkaline phosphatase activity and by impaired neutrophil function. Impairment of adhesion, chemotaxis and microbicidal activity in neutrophils have all been described.

In contrast to the granulocyte and monocyte series, lymphocyte morphology typically is normal in the MDS, despite the demonstrable involvement of lymphoid cells in some cases. However, a fall in CD4+ T lymphocytes and NK cells and a lack of Epstein-Barr virus receptors on B lymphocytes are all common. Occasionally, lymphoproliferative disorders such as myeloma, B and T cell lymphomas and hypogammaglobulinaemia have been described in coexistence with the MDS.

Thrombodysplasia

Thrombodysplasia is manifest as the presence of mononuclear and binuclear micromegakaryocytes, mononuclear small megakaryocytes, multi-separated nuclear megakaryocytes and megakaryocytes with bizarre nuclei in the bone marrow and vacuolation, giant granulation and structural abnormalities of microtubules and the surface-connected canalicular system in peripheral blood platelets. In addition, abnormalities of platelet function such as defective adhesion and aggregation responses are common. Acquired platelet glycoprotein defects such as those seen in Bernard-Soulier syndrome have been described in juvenile MDS.

Growth Characteristics

The defective haemopoietic growth characteristics which are the hallmark of the MDS have been extensively investigated using cell culture techniques. Impairment of haemopoietic progenitor cell growth in culture is a consistent feature of all types of MDS. Broadly, the severity of the growth abnormality mirrors the severity of the condition: normal growth of CFU-GM is seen most often in RA and RAS but is unusual in CMML, RAEB and RAEB-t. The *in vitro* growth characteristics of CFU-Meg, BFU-E and CFU-E have all been shown to be defective, but no correlation with FAB subtype exists. Considerable research has been performed to determine the potentially corrective effects of a variety of haemopoietic growth factors and differentiating agents, with mixed results. CD34+ stem cells from MDS patients have been shown to demonstrate diminished responses to M-CSF, G-CSF, GM-CSF, IL-3 and Epo.

The link between the MDS and iron metabolism is again demonstrated by the observation that adherent macrophages derived from MDS patients inhibit the growth of normal CFU-GM in culture but that the inhibition is abolished by the addition of anti-ferritin antibodies to the culture medium. It seems possible that the inhibitory effect of MDS macrophage-derived acidic isoferritins on normal cell growth contributes to the growth advantage of any leukaemic clone which evolves.

Flow cytometric studies have been used to demonstrate the aberrant cell cycle characteristics of the MDS. These studies have shown that those cases with the highest proportion of bone marrow cells in the S and G_2 phases have the best prognosis while those with the highest proportion of cells in the G_1 phase show the greatest propensity for leukaemic transformation. The impaired proliferative capacity of haemopoietic progenitors in the MDS has also been demonstrated using this technique. Some workers believe that determination of the cell cycle characteristics of individual MDS cases may provide useful prognostic information.

Treatment and Management of the MDS

The treatment offered for the MDS is determined by the age of the individual and the severity of the condition. Broadly, the aim of treatment in young patients is curative while in elderly patients with aggressive disease it is palliative. A number of factors have been suggested to have prognostic value in the MDS as shown in Table 18.7.

Poor Prognostic Features

Excess of bone marrow blasts
Abnormal localised immature myeloid precursors (ALIP)
Pancytopaenia
Abnormal chromosome 7
Complex or multiple cytogenetic abnormalities
Increased age at presentation

Table 18.7 *Presenting features which have been suggested to signify poor prognosis in the MDS*

The most widely used grading system, largely because of its ease of application, is the "Bournemouth score", which is summarised in Table 18.8.

Clinical Feature	Score
Hb < 10g/dl	+1
Plt < 100 x 10^9/l	+1
PMN < 2.5 x 10^9/l	+1
PMN > 16.0 x 10^9/l	+1
BM Blasts > 5%	+1

Total Score	Prognosis	Median Survival
0-1	Good	62 months
2-3	Intermediate	22 months
4	Poor	8 months

Table 18.8 *The Bournemouth score for assessing prognosis in the MDS*

Those cases which are identified as having a good prognosis usually are offered supportive treatment such as blood and platelet transfusions to correct the anaemia and thrombocytopaenia and antimicrobial chemotherapy to combat infections. As described above, a proportion of these cases progress to acute leukaemia but it is currently impossible to predict with certainty which will follow this course. Once acute leukaemia is established, treatment follows the protocols described in Chapter 16.

Poor prognosis cases typically are offered some form of treatment but there currently is little agreement about which approach affords the best prospect of cure or prolongation of life. Among the treatment options are:

- allogeneic bone marrow transplantation. This option is only available to those under the age of 50 years.

- the use of differentiating agents such as retinoic acid and low-dose cytosine arabinoside to drive the affected clone to maturity.

- the use of recombinant haemopoietic growth factors such as rhIL-3, rhIL-8, rhGM-CSF and rhG-CSF. This approach has been shown to improve the neutrophil count and partially to restore neutrophil function. It remains to be established whether the use of haemopoietic growth factors accelerates progression of the MDS to ANLL.

- the use of ANLL cytotoxic chemotherapy regimens.

The most common causes of death in the MDS are infectious and haemorrhagic complications secondary to peripheral cytopaenia or leukaemic transformation.

Suggested Further Reading

Mufti, G.J. and Galton, D.A.G. (1992). *The Myelodysplastic Syndromes.* Edinburgh: Churchill Livingstone.

The Non-leukaemic Malignant Disorders

The non-leukaemic malignant disorders are an extremely diverse group of disorders which can be divided according to the origin of the malignant clone into myeloproliferative and lympho-proliferative types. The malignant myeloproliferative disorders include **primary proliferative polycythaemia (PPP)** which is one of many different types of polycythaemia, **primary thrombo-cythaemia** and **myelofibrosis**. The malignant lymphoproliferative disorders include **multiple myeloma (MM)** and related plasma cell disorders, **Hodgkin's disease (HD)** and the various **non-Hodgkin's lymphomas (NHL)**.

The Non-leukaemic Myeloproliferative Disorders

The myeloproliferative disorders, as originally defined, form an amorphous group of malignant disorders which are characterised by the uncontrolled clonal proliferation of bone-marrow derived cells. However, as knowledge of the nature and aetiology of haemopoietic malignant disorders has improved, the use of this term, in its generic sense, has declined. The rather more precise term, non-leukaemic myeloproliferative disorders is retained because it emphasises the interrelatedness of the three remaining members of this hitherto all-embracing group of disorders.

Primary Proliferative Polycythaemia

Primary proliferative polycythaemia is a malignant disorder of haemopoietic stem cells which is characterised by absolute erythro-cytosis and, commonly, a moderately increased granulocyte count and platelet count. It may occur at any age but is predominantly a disease of middle age: the median age at diagnosis is 55 years. Males are affected slightly more commonly than females.

Recognition and Classification of the Polycythaemias

The defining criterion of polycythaemia is a rise in the venous PCV to more than 0.53 in males or more than 0.51 in females, reflecting

The references ranges for venous haematocrit (PCV) are as follows:

Cord blood	0.44-0.62
Child (10 years)	0.37-0.44
Adult male	0.40-0.54
Adult female	0.36-0.47

The venous haematocrit over-estimates the whole body haematocrit (WBPCV) be-cause of normal changes in the ratio of plasma:cells in arterial and venous blood. As a general guide, the WBPCV is about 91% of the venous PCV, but this value varies considerably, for example in pregnancy, splenomegaly and congestive cardiac fail-ure.

an increase, real or apparent, in the circulating red cell count. Under normal physiological conditions, the circulating red cell count is under tight hormonal control and is maintained within remarkably narrow limits. Alterations in the venous PCV can be caused by a reduction in plasma volume or by a true increase in red cell numbers. An absolute increase in the rate of erythropoiesis can be caused by malignant transformation which frees the haemopoietic stem cells from hormonal control or via hypoxic or physiologically inappropriate stimulation of erythropoietin release. Thus, the polycythaemias are a large and diverse group of disorders, only one member of which, PPP, is a malignant disorder. However, an understanding of the aetiology and classification of all types of polycythaemia is essential because recognition of PPP largely is based upon exclusion of the other types. The classification of the polycythaemias is illustrated schematically in Figure 19.1.

SAQ 1

How does chronic, heavy smoking contribute to a secondary polycythaemia?

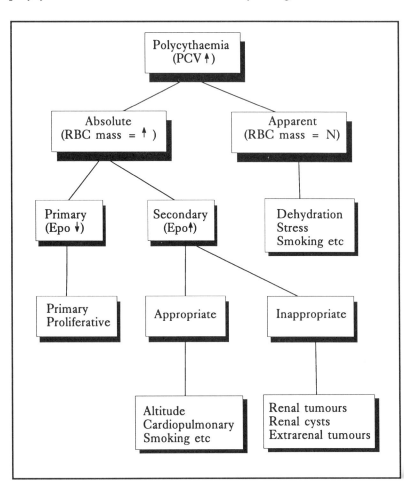

Figure 19.1 *Recognition and classification of the polycythaemias*

Apparent Polycythaemia

Apparent polycythaemia is defined as those cases where an increased venous PCV is not explained by an absolute increase in the red cell mass (RCM) but by a reduction in the plasma volume (PV), or by the combination of an RCM towards the upper limit of normality and a PV towards the lower limit of normality. Apparent polycythaemia is by far the most common finding where the PCV is only minimally increased, accounting for up to 50% of such cases. Alternative names for this condition include relative poly-cythaemia, pseudopolycythaemia, stress polycythaemia, spurious polycythaemia and Gaisböck's syndrome.

Red cell mass and plasma volume are under separate physiological control and so may vary independently of each other. Plasma volume may fall as a result of dehydration secondary to diuretic therapy, severe diarrhoea and vomiting, burns or alcohol ingestion. Prolonged stress, hypertension and smoking have a similar effect. The red cell mass may be increased slightly by hypoxia secondary to minimal degrees of cardiovascular or pulmonary disease or by heavy smoking. Some cases of apparent polycythaemia progress to secondary polycythaemia as their cardiopulmonary insufficiency worsens. Other clinical and laboratory signs which can be used to differentiate between apparent polycythaemia and the other forms are summarised in Table 19.1.

Laboratory Variable	PPP	Apparent Polycythaemia	Secondary Polycythaemia
PCV	Raised	Raised	Raised
RCM	Raised	Normal	Raised
Erythropoietin	Decreased	Normal	Raised
WBC	Raised	Normal	Normal
Plt	Raised	Normal	Normal
Bone marrow	Hyperplastic	Normal	Erythroid hyperplasia
Spleen	Enlarged	Normal	Normal
Arterial pO_2	Normal	Normal	Decreased or normal
Serum ferritin	Decreased	Normal	Normal
Serum B_{12}	Raised	Normal	Normal
LAP	Raised	Normal	Normal
Serum lysozyme	Raised	Normal	Normal

Table 19.1 *Differential diagnosis for the polycythaemias*

Interestingly, animal species which are indigenous to high altitudes such as llama and vicuña, do not normally have high red cell counts. They have adapted to the low oxygen tension of their environment by synthesising a form of haemoglobin with an extraordinarily high oxygen affinity. It is obvious that this helps to maximise the extraction of atmospheric oxygen in the lungs but the mechanisms involved in maintaining optimal oxygen delivery to the tissues in these animals are much less clear.

The heart is a muscular pump with four chambers: the right and left atria which receive blood from the systemic and pulmonary circulations respectively and the right and left ventricles which discharge blood into the aorta and pulmonary artery respectively. Normally, the left and right sides of the heart are separated by a septum. A ventricular septal defect, commonly known as a "hole in the heart", permits shunting of blood from the left to the right ventricle and, unless minor, requires surgical repair. Ventricular septal defects frequently are accompanied by other congenital cardiovascular abnormalities such as persistence of the ductus arteriosus.

Cont

Secondary Polycythaemias

The secondary polycythaemias are the result of increased stimulation of erythropoiesis, either in response to hypoxia or to another, physiologically inappropriate, stimulus. They could be described rather more accurately as the secondary erythrocytoses because leucocytes and platelets are not involved.

Physiologically appropriate release of erythropoietin occurs in response to tissue hypoxia which, broadly, can result from three main defects:

- **a persistently low atmospheric oxygen tension**. This occurs at high altitude and is responsible for the erythrocytosis observed in human mountain dwellers. Other physiological adaptations to high altitude include alveolar enlargement, increased total blood volume and sustained hyperventilation. The physiological cost of this adaptive response is that the scope for further adaptation to cardiopulmonary disease is limited. For this reason, cardiopulmonary disease frequently is more severe in mountain dwellers.

- **inadequate uptake of atmospheric oxygen** results in a reduction in arterial oxygen saturation and so impedes delivery of oxygen to the tissues. Because of the sigmoid shape of the haemoglobin-oxygen dissociation curve, a relatively small drop in alveolar oxygen tension can cause a precipitate fall in arterial oxygen saturation, leading to significant cyanosis and tissue hypoxia. A variety of disorders interfere with oxygen uptake in the lungs. For example, chronic obstructive airways diseases such as chronic bronchitis and emphysema reduce the ventilatory capacity of the lungs. Respiratory failure states such as pulmonary fibrosis, pulmonary oedema and a variety of pulmonary vascular abnormalities result in inadequate perfusion. Cardiovascular abnormalities such as transposition of the great vessels and ventricular septal defects result in significant quantities of venous blood passing directly to the arterial side of the heart without first passing through the lungs.

- **defective transport of absorbed oxygen from the lungs** to the tissues occurs in a variety of inherited and acquired defects of haemoglobin function. High affinity haemoglobins such as haemoglobin Chesapeake and haemoglobins M such as haemoglobin Boston have been described in Chapter 8. Metabolic defects which limit the effectiveness of oxygen transport include methaemoglobin reductase deficiency and 2,3-DPG deficiency. The effects of heavy smoking on haemoglobin are described earlier in this chapter.

> Transposition of the great vessels is another congenital cardiac malformation where the aorta and pulmonary artery are linked to the opposite ventricles, leading to dyspnoea (shortness of breath) and a grey complexion (cyanosis) due to suboptimal oxygenation of the arterial blood.

A variety of disorders are associated with the autonomous synthesis and release of erythropoietin, leading to secondary polycythaemia. This physiologically inappropriate release of erythropoietin occurs as a rare complication of renal disorders such as polycystic kidneys, chronic glomerulonephritis, hydronephrosis and renal tumours, and is occasionally seen in association with a variety of extrarenal tumours such as hepatoma, cerebellar haemangioblastoma and bronchial carcinoma.

Pathophysiology of PPP

The presenting features of PPP are related to the hypervolaemia and hyperviscosity which accompanies the absolute increase in red cell mass. Typical complaints include ruddiness of the complexion, headaches, blurred vision, dizziness, mental impairment and a feeling of congestion in the head. Some degree of splenomegaly is common at presentation and is secondary to vascular engorgement, extramedullary haemopoiesis and fibrosis. Hyperviscosity with impairment of blood flow contributes to the increased incidence of arterial and venous thrombosis seen in this condition. In particular, the incidence of transient ischaemic attacks, intermittent claudication and thrombotic strokes is increased in PPP. Paradoxically, platelet dysfunction with a tendency to bruise and bleed excessively following trauma also are common in all of the non-leukaemic myeloproliferative disorders. An unusual and interesting complaint which is present in up to 25% of cases is severe itching, particularly after a warm bath. This appears to be linked to histamine release from basophils.

> A transient ischaemic attack is manifest as sudden neurological deficit which resolves completely within 24 hours and is thought to be secondary to embolism in the cerebral circulation.
>
> Intermittent claudication is manifest as painful cramping of the legs and feet following exercise and is caused by ischaemia secondary to atheroma of the arteries of the lower limbs.

As shown in Table 19.1, PPP is characterised by an increased haemoglobin concentration, venous packed cell volume and red cell mass in the presence of a normal plasma volume and arterial oxygen saturation. The granulocyte count is raised in about 70% of cases but seldom exceeds $60 \times 10^9/l$. Neutrophil function and morphology typically are normal. The platelet count is moderately increased in about 50% of cases. Bizarre platelet morphology and dysfunction are common. Examination of the bone marrow reveals hypercellularity with prominent granulocytic and megakaryocytic hyperplasia. Erythroid hyperplasia frequently is less obvious. Haemopoiesis is effective. *In vitro* culture of bone marrow results in the growth of erythroid colonies, even in the absence of added erythropoietin. Whether this reflects extreme sensitivity of the malignant clone to the effects of the tiny quantity of erythropoietin present in the culture medium or truly autonomous growth remains to be clearly established. Cytogenetic abnormalities are present in about 15% of cases of PPP at presentation. The most frequently reported abnormalities are aneuploidy, -Y, 20q-, 5q-, +9 and 13q-. These do not appear to influence prognosis significantly. The minimum criteria for a diagnosis of PPP are shown in Table 19.2.

SAQ 2

What is the primary site of synthesis of erythropoietin?

If splenomegaly is present	
	RCM > 36 ml/kg lean body mass in males
	> 32 ml/kg lean body mass in females
and	arterial pO_2 > 92%
and	no evidence for secondary polycythaemia
If splenomegaly is absent	
	RCM > 36 ml/kg lean body mass in males
	> 32 ml/kg lean body mass in females
and	arterial pO_2 > 92%
and	no evidence for secondary polycythaemia
and 2 of the following	
	Plt > $400 \times 10^9/l$
	WBC > $12.0 \times 10^9/l$
	LAP score > 100
	serum vitamin B_{12} > 900 ng/l
	unbound B_{12} binding capacity > 2200 ng/l

Table 19.2 *Minimum criteria for a disgnosis of PPP*

Up to 25% of cases of PPP transform to chronic myelofibrosis and of these up to one third eventually progress to ANLL. The duration of PPP prior to transformation in these cases has varied from less than 2 years to more than 20 years. Treatment with alkylating agents is associated with a higher rate of progression to ANLL.

Treatment of PPP

The primary aim of treatment for PPP is to reduce the risk of thrombosis and to relieve the symptoms caused by hyperviscosity and hypervolaemia. This can be achieved quickly by red cell and platelet apheresis or, where circumstances permit, more slowly by repeated venesection. Removal of up to 500 ml of blood for up to 8 consecutive days greatly relieves symptoms and causes a reduction in the venous PCV to less than 0.45 in most cases. This "remission" may be maintained for several months without the need for further treatment. Venesection does not affect the circulating white cell count or platelet count significantly.

The long-term management of PPP is controversial. Some cases are managed by repeated venesection alone and have a median duration of survival of about 14 years with a low incidence of leukaemic transformation but a relatively high incidence of thrombotic complications. Attempts to minimise thrombotic complications with the use of prophylactic aspirin often increases the incidence of haemorrhagic complications to an unacceptable degree. The addition of myelosuppressive therapy using ^{32}P reduces the platelet count and lessens the risk of thrombosis while lengthening the periods between treatments. Unfortunately, this form of treatment is associated with a higher rate of leukaemic transformation and has a median duration of survival of about 12 years. Attempts also have been made to induce myelosuppression using alkylating agents such as chlorambucil or busulphan, but these are associated with an even higher risk of leukaemic transformation and a median duration of survival of 9 years. The treatment of choice for PPP remains to be clearly established.

Primary Thrombocythaemia

Primary thrombocythaemia is a malignant clonal disorder which is characterised by megakaryocytic hyperplasia and a markedly increased circulating platelet count. Alternative names for this disorder include **essential thrombocythaemia, idiopathic thrombocythaemia** and **primary haemorrhagic thrombocythaemia**. In common with the other myeloproliferative disorders, primary thrombocythaemia is rare in children and young adults. The median age at diagnosis of this disorder is 60 years. Men and women appear to be affected with equal frequency.

SAQ 3

Why is iron deficiency relatively common in primary thrombocythaemia?

Pathophysiology of Thrombocythaemia

The major presenting features of primary thrombocythaemia are thromboembolic complications secondary to the extremely high platelet count and haemorrhagic complications secondary to platelet dysfunction. Thromboembolic manifestations include cerebral transient ischaemic attacks, painful ischaemia of fingers and toes, pulmonary embolism and thrombosis of unusual vessels such as the hepatic veins, the axillary artery and the veins of the penis with resultant priapism. Haemorrhagic manifestations include gastrointestinal bleeding, epistaxis and inappropriately severe bleeding and bruising following trauma. Paradoxically, both thromboembolic and haemorrhagic complications may be present in the same individual. Significant splenomegaly is present in up to 80% of cases. Some degree of hepatomegaly also is common.

Primary thrombocythaemia characteristically presents with a platelet count greater than $1,000 \times 10^9/l$ but platelet counts as high as $10,000 \times 10^9/l$ are not rare. Examination of a blood film reveals the presence of platelet clumping and bizarre morphological abnormalities of the platelets with marked variation in size, shape and granulation. Megakaryocyte fragments may be present in the peripheral blood. Typically, a moderate neutrophilia is present, but the white cell count seldom exceeds $35 \times 10^9/l$. The red cell count and haemoglobin concentration are normal in most cases but some degree of iron deficiency may be present, secondary to chronic blood loss. Examination of the bone marrow reveals hypercellularity with pronounced megakaryocytic hyperplasia, granulocytic hyperplasia and, sometimes, erythroid hyperplasia.

Up to 25% of cases of primary thrombocythaemia transform to myelofibrosis or, rarely, PPP or ANLL. By far the most common cause of death in this disorder is thromboembolic complications.

Treatment of Thrombocythaemia

Many cases of primary thrombocythaemia follow a relatively benign course and do not require treatment. Where thrombotic or haemorrhagic symptoms are troublesome, the usual strategy is to reduce the circulating platelet count by apheresis, by the use of alkylating agents such as melphalan and busulphan or by the administration of ^{32}P. Typically, treatment is only required intermittently and for short periods to maintain the platelet count below $500 \times 10^9/l$. Alternative strategies, including the use of anticoagulant drugs such as heparin and warfarin or the prophylactic use of aspirin to minimise thrombotic complications have shown mixed

results. The median duration of survival with primary thrombocythaemia is about 10 years.

Myelofibrosis

Myelofibrosis predominantly is a disease of the middle-aged and
elderly. It is characterised by progressive collagen fibrosis of the
bone marrow spaces, megakaryocytic hyperplasia and massive
splenomegaly secondary to extramedullary haemopoiesis. An alternative name for this disease is **agnogenic myeloid metaplasia**.
Myelofibrosis affects men and women equally.

Pathophysiology of Myelofibrosis

The onset of myelofibrosis is insidious. Typical complaints at presentation include lethargy and exercise intolerance secondary to
anaemia; weight loss and night sweats secondary to metabolic
derangement; bruising secondary to platelet dysfunction and a feeling of left-sided abdominal fullness secondary to splenomegaly.
Marked splenomegaly is present at diagnosis in at least 50% of
cases and, in about 10% of cases, splenomegaly is massive, extend-
ing down into the pelvic region. In such cases, an inability to eat a
full meal or urinary frequency secondary to compression of the
stomach and bladder by the bulging spleen may be present. The
cause of splenomegaly in myelofibrosis is extramedullary
haemopoiesis. In advanced disease, blood flow to the spleen may
be increased by as much as 10 times, leading to severe portal hypertension, oesophageal varices and ascites. Extramedullary
haemopoiesis in the liver may further exacerbate the portal
hypertension. Radiographic examination sometimes reveals a
greatly increased bone density with narrowing of the medullary
cavity in the long bones and thickening of the trabeculae.

Examination of the blood reveals a leucoerythroblastic anaemia
with prominent polychromasia, anisocytosis and "tear drop" poikilocytosis. The white cell count and platelet count are variable but
frequently are raised. Platelet morphology frequently is grossly
atypical, suggesting overlap with primary thrombocythaemia. As
the disease progresses, the degree of dysplasia increases, the circulating cell counts drop inexorably. and the red cell and white cell
turnover increases leading to a rise in the serum concentrations of
lysozyme, lactate dehydrogenase and uric acid. In advanced cases
with portal hypertension, the serum concentrations of hepatic
enzymes may be abnormal.

Attempts to aspirate bone marrow frequently fail because of the fibrotic overgrowth of the marrow space. Trephine biopsy typically reveals large areas of fibrosis with patchy areas of hypercellularity which contain prominent clusters of dysplastic megakaryocytes. As these ill-fated megakaryocytes die within the marrow space, they release **platelet-derived growth factor (PDGF)** and **platelet factor 4 (PF4)** into the local area. PDGF is encoded by the c-*sis* proto-oncogene which is located on the q arm of chromosome 22 and functions as a fibroblast mitogen. PF4 is a cationic peptide which inhibits neutrophil and fibroblast collagenase enzymes. The combined action of these two substances promotes the inexorable rise in collagenous fibrosis which characterises this condition. Marrow fibrosis thus is a secondary phenomenon in myelofibrosis, the primary defect is thought to lie in a haemopoietic progenitor cell of CFU-Mk and CFU-GM. The increasing hostility of the marrow haemopoietic inductive microenvironment promotes the establishment of extramedullary haemopoiesis in the foetal sites of the spleen and liver.

Treatment of Myelofibrosis

The median survival from diagnosis in myelofibrosis is about 3 years but some cases survive for more than 10 years. About 10% of cases progress to ANLL. Leukaemic transformation appears to be more common in men.

In most cases, the treatment for myelofibrosis is palliative and consists of splenic irradiation to reduce the size of the spleen and to relieve the symptoms of massive splenomegaly such as red cell and platelet sequestration or portal hypertension. Where this measure is ineffective, or where splenomegaly is especially troublesome, splenectomy may be performed. Other supportive measures include the use of blood transfusion to correct the anaemia, allopurinol to correct the hyperuricaemia, haematinic therapy if folate or iron deficiency is present and androgens to correct the ineffective erythropoiesis. Where the disease is advancing rapidly, alkylating agents such as busulphan and chlorambucil or antimetabolites such as 6-thioguanine can be used with limited success. The only prospect of cure in myelofibrosis is offered by bone marrow transplantation which may be attempted in younger cases.

The Non-leukaemic Lymphoproliferative Disorders

The non-leukaemic lymphoproliferative disorders are malignant clonal disorders of the lymphopoietic system.

Multiple Myeloma and Related Plasma Cell Disorders

Multiple myeloma (MM) is a B lymphoid malignancy which is characterised by the proliferation of a malignant clone of plasma cells which synthesise and secrete excessive amounts of monoclonal immunoglobulin. In many respects, MM behaves as a solid tumour with a particular predilection for bone marrow. MM is a disease of the elderly, with the median age at diagnosis being about 62 years. The disease is more common in blacks than in whites and shows a slight excess incidence in men. The aetiology of MM is obscure, although there was a sight excess in survivors of the atomic explosions at Hiroshima and Nagasaki. Experiments in mice suggest that genetic factors and chronic antigenic stimulation may play a role in the induction of plasma cell tumours, but the significance of this observation for the human disease is uncertain.

Pathophysiology of MM

All of the many sequelae of MM are attributable to two causes:

- the uncontrolled growth of a plasma cell tumour which secretes a substance which elicits macrophage-mediated suppression of B lymphocyte function and also osteoclast activating factors such as tumour necrosis factor β (TNFβ) and IL-1β

- the inexorable and pointless synthesis and secretion of large quantities of monoclonal immunoglobulin by the malignant plasma cells

Thus, the most common presenting features in MM are bone pain and hypercalcaemia secondary to osteolysis; anaemia and uraemia secondary to renal impairment caused by deposition of immunoglobulin in the tubules and respiratory tract infection secondary to defective humoral immunity.

Multiple myeloma was first described in 1844, almost a year before the first descriptions of leukaemia by Virchow and Bennett, by S Solly and was known then as mollities ossium.

Skeletal Abnormalities

Osteolytic lesions with a characteristic, "punched-out" appearance occur in about 80% of cases of MM during the course of the disease. At presentation, the bones most commonly affected include the ribs, sternum, pelvis and vertebrae. As the disease progresses, involvement of the skull and the proximal ends of the long bones occurs and pathological fractures of the femur, ribs and sternum become more common. Pathological collapse of the lumbar or dorsal vertebrae with acute lower back pain is one of the classical forms of presentation of MM. Occasionally, the localised plasma cell tumours which cause the osteolysis can break through the bone and invade the surrounding soft tissue. Osteolysis leads to hypercalcaemia which may cause weakness, nausea, polyuria, disorientation and, in severe cases, coma.

Renal Failure

About 25% of cases of MM have significant renal impairment at presentation, but many more enter renal failure during the course of the disease. Immunoglobulin light chains secreted by the malignant plasma cell clone are excreted via the urine at a rate of up to 10 g per day. Precipitation and deposition of these light chains in the renal tubules causes the formation of unyielding, calcified tubular casts which may rupture the tubular basement membrane, stimulating acute and chronic inflammatory responses which eventually result in extensive fibrosis and renal failure. This phenomenon, known as **"myeloma kidney"**, is a common cause of death in this disease.

Amyloidosis

Amyloid deposits consist of partially degraded immunoglobulin light chains arranged in a rigid, pleated fibrillar structure. In about 10% of cases of MM, most commonly involving λ light chains, amyloid deposits accumulate in and inflict damage upon organs such as the kidney, liver, spleen, heart, gastrointestinal tract and tongue. For example, more than 70% of these cases have significant cardiac enlargement and hardening with progressive failure of the pumping action. A particularly distressing manifestation of amyloidosis is macroglossia in which amyloid deposits in the tongue cause extreme swelling and hardening of the tongue with respiratory embarrassment.

SAQ 4

Which chromosomes carry the immunoglobulin light chain (κ and λ) genes?

Neurological Complications

A variety of neurological complications may be troublesome in MM. The most serious such complication, compression of the spinal cord by localised tumour deposits in the vertebrae or epidural space, is manifest as sensory loss, incontinence and paraplegia. These changes may be irreversible in the absence of prompt treatment. Other neurological complications of myeloma include carpal tunnel syndrome, polyneuropathy secondary to amyloidosis, meningeal infiltration and cranial nerve palsies.

The *sine qua non* for a diagnosis of myeloma is the demonstration of a monoclonal immunoglobulin or immunoglobulin light or heavy chain in the serum and, where proteinuria is present, in the urine. However, rare exceptions exist in which all of the other signs of MM are present but the malignant clone does not secrete any form of immunoglobulin or more than one monoclonal immunoglobulin is synthesised. The determination of the immunoglobulin subclass and light chain class of the monoclonal protein provides important prognostic information. The approximate incidence of the different types of myeloma is summarised in Table 19.3.

	IgG		IgA		IgD		IgM			
	κ	λ	κ	λ	κ	λ	κ	λ	κ	λ
Frequency (%)	35	20	15	11	0.2	1.3	0.1	0.1	8	7

Table 19.3 *Distribution of the different types of immunoglobulin heavy and light chains in multiple myeloma*

Analysis of the specificities of the monoclonal immunoglobulins produced in MM has shown that many are directed against ubiquitous antigens such as the Ii blood group family, membrane lipids such as phosphatidylcholine and the glycosaminoglycan heparan sulphate. However, most myelomatous immunoglobulins have no known specificity. Whether this means that they are synthesised aimlessly or that they are directed against as yet unknown antigens remains to be determined.

IgG myeloma is associated with a slower tumour growth rate and a lower incidence of hypercalcaemia and amyloidosis than the other types of myeloma. However, the rate of synthesis of monoclonal immunoglobulin is highest in this form, so the total serum immunoglobulin concentration also is highest in IgG myeloma. The rate of immunoglobulin catabolism is proportional to the

Plasma cell leukaemia is a rare condition which is characterised by a peripheral blood plasma cell count (often greatly) in excess of $2 \times 10^9/l$, anaemia, thrombocytopaenia and many of the clinical features of multiple myeloma. The disease typically occurs *de novo*, but also is seen as a terminal event of pre-existing multiple myeloma. The prognosis for PCL is poor, although a few durable remissions have been reported.

circulating immunoglobulin level. The greatly increased rate of immunoglobulin catabolism in IgG myeloma results in a profound deficiency of normal, polyclonal immunoglobulins and an increased susceptibility to bacterial infection. Because IgG_3 immunoglobulin readily forms large aggregates, this form of myeloma is associated with hyperviscosity.

IgA myeloma also is associated with hyperviscosity because of the tendency of this form of immunoglobulin to polymerise. Hypercalcaemia and amyloidosis are more troublesome in this form of myeloma than in IgG but the incidence of bacterial infection is lower.

IgD myeloma is a particularly malignant form which is associated with a younger age group and is most common in men. The median survival time for this form of myeloma is about a year and sinister findings such as hepatosplenomegaly, lymphadenopathy, extraosseous tumour deposits, renal failure, hypercalcaemia and amyloidosis are much more common than in the other types of myeloma.

IgE myeloma is extremely rare and appears to be associated with the presentation of *de novo* **plasma cell leukaemia** (PCL). This rare disease presents as an acute leukaemia with a circulating plasma cell count greater than $2 \times 10^9/l$, anaemia, thrombocytopaenia, hepatosplenomegaly, osteolysis and renal failure. The white cell count at presentation frequently exceeds $80 \times 10^9/l$ of which more than half are atypical plasma cells.

Bence Jones (BJ) myeloma occurs when immunoglobulin light chains are synthesised in the absence of heavy chains. This form of myeloma is associated with the most rapid tumour growth and the highest incidence of renal failure, hypercalcaemia and amyloidosis. The prognosis is particularly grim for λ chain BJ myeloma.

The presence of a monoclonal immunoglobulin band on serum or urine electrophoresis does not necessarily equate with myeloma; almost 1% of individuals over the age of 25 years and at least 3% over the age of 70 years express such a band. Undoubtedly, some of these cases represent very early myelomas but a significant proportion are completely stable and show no evidence of malignant progression, even after many years. However, myeloma has been shown to have an extremely slow rate of progression and some workers believe that, given enough time, most or even all of these individuals would develop MM or some related condition. These individuals are said to have a **monoclonal gammopathy of unde-termined significance (MGUS)**.

Haematological examination typically reveals a series of changes which reflect the degree of infiltration of the bone marrow by the malignant clone. Typical findings include rouleaux formation secondary to the increased immunoglobulin concentration and a normocytic, normochromic anaemia which is secondary to depression of erythropoiesis although, less commonly, megaloblastic features may be present which are secondary to folate deficiency. The anaemia is accompanied by a variable degree of thrombocytopaenia and leucopaenia which may be severe. In a minority of cases, a leucoerythroblastic blood picture with atypical plasma cells in the peripheral blood is strongly suggestive of the diagnosis. In most cases, the plasma viscosity is raised, occasionally markedly so.

Examination of the bone marrow reveals the presence of an increased number of atypical plasma cells, but the appearance and number of these cells vary greatly between cases and also, because of the patchy nature of the infiltration, between samples. Myeloma plasma cells are large, oval cells with a round, eccentric nucleus and basophilic cytoplasm. Multinucleated and other atypical forms such as **flaming plasma cells** whose bright red cytoplasmic fringes are caused by the accumulation of precipitated immunoglobulin and **Mott cells** which contain grape-like clusters of bluish, spherical inclusion bodies in their cytoplasm known as **Russell bodies** are common. The Russell bodies within Mott cells are located on the outside of the rough endoplasmic reticulum. These inclusion bodies are also commonly seen in smaller numbers as pinkish inclusion bodies, when they represent condensed immunoglobulin within the rough endoplasmic reticulum. However, none of these changes are specific for myeloma. Immunofluorescent staining of the myeloma plasma cells confirms that they are all synthesising a single form of immunoglobulin heavy chain and light chain. Trephine biopsy of marrow exposes the dual nature of infiltration in myeloma. Diffuse infiltration in which myeloma plasma cells coexist with normal haemopoietic tissue is accompanied by a varying number of nodular deposits which consist entirely of myeloma plasma cells. It is these tumour nodules which largely are responsible for the characteristic osteolytic lesions of MM.

It has been suggested that myeloma plasma cells establish a self-supporting autocrine loop by synthesising and secreting IL-5 and

IL-6 which are potent B lymphocyte and plasma cell growth factors. The action of these factors is potentiated by the presence of IL-3 and GM-CSF. Other workers, however, argue that the main source of IL-6 *in vivo* is osteoblasts or bone marrow macrophages.

Because mitotic spreads are difficult to obtain in myeloma, knowledge about the incidence and significance of cytogenetic abnormalities is relatively scanty but, in common with other B lymphoid neoplasms, 14q+ with the breakpoint at 14q32, t(11;14)(q13;q32) and t(8;14)(q24;q32) are frequently observed. The possible significance of these cytogenetic aberrations is discussed in Chapter 15.

A number of other plasma cell tumours exist, including **solitary plasmacytoma of bone** in which an isolated tumour nodule with localised osteolysis occurs and **extramedullary plasmacytoma** in which the tumour affects extraosseous soft tissues. These frequently are associated with a younger age group than MM. Some of these cases, after apparently successful treatment of the primary disorder, go on to develop MM in later years.

Treatment of MM

The assessment of prognosis in MM at presentation involves an evaluation of the extent of tumour infiltration as measured by the haemoglobin concentration and the concentration of the monoclonal immunoglobulin; the degree and rate of osteolysis as measured by the serum calcium concentration and a radiographic survey; the degree of renal impairment as measured by the blood urea concentration and the performance status. A more recently defined prognostic variable is the serum concentration of β_2-microglobulin. The features which are associated with a good or a poor prognosis are summarised in Table 19.4. Almost all cases judged to have a poor prognosis by these criteria die within 2 years of diagnosis whereas more than three quarters of those in the good prognosis category survive for longer than 2 years.

MM is a slowly progressive and insidious disease and by the time it is symptomatic, most workers believe that it has entered a preterminal phase. Certainly, the opportunity for effective curative treatment is limited at the outset in many cases by the presence of irreversible changes such as extensive skeletal damage, renal failure and neurological complications. The severe defect of humoral immunity which accompanies MM seldom is corrected by therapy

---

SAQ 5

What gene complex is located at 14q32 which is involved in many B lymphoid malignancies?

Variable	Good Risk	Poor Risk
Haemoglobin (g/dl)	> 10	< 7.5
Serum calcium (mg/dl)	< 12	> 12
Blood urea (mmol/l)	< 8	> 10
β_2-microglobulin (mg/l)	< 4	> 6
Osteolytic lesions	None, or isolated plasmacytoma	Advanced skeletal destruction
Monoclonal immunoglobulin	IgG < 50 g/l IgA < 30 g/l	IgG > 70 g/l IgA > 50 g/l
Urine Bence Jones excretion	< 4 g/l/24 hours	> 12 g/l/24 hours

Table 19.4 *Risk factors in MM*

and bacterial infections continue to be troublesome. Further, the advanced age of most patients limits their tolerance of aggressive cytoreductive therapy.

Much of the treatment offered is palliative. Local radiotherapy halts the advance of osteolysis and provides pain relief but bone repair seldom occurs. A further improvement in well-being is offered by effective treatment of hypercalcaemia and renal failure. Reduction of the tumour cell load has traditionally been achieved with the use of alkylating agents such as melphalan and cyclophosphamide. Typically, the response to these drugs is slow. Establishment of complete remission may take several months. Once achieved, the duration of remission varies widely from a few months to several years but relapse is inevitable and frequently is refractory to further treatment. The monoclonal immunoglobulin subtype synthesised following relapse frequently differs from that originally present.

A number of more intensive, combination chemotherapy protocols have been proposed as a treatment for MM and are undergoing clinical trials.

Waldenström's Macroglobulinaemia

Waldenström's macroglobulinaemia (WM) is an uncommon B lymphoid malignant disorder which is characterised by hyperviscosity secondary to the excessive secretion of a monoclonal IgM immunoglobulin by the malignant clone. The malignant cells of WM are rather more immature than those in MM and frequently are described as being "lymphoplasmacytoid". WM is a disease of the elderly, with a peak incidence occurring in the seventh decade of life.

Pathophysiology of WM

WM is an indolent disease which typically presents with variable combinations of weight loss, hepatosplenomegaly, lymphadenopathy and a bruising or bleeding tendency, following a long history of vague malaise, weakness and weight loss or, occasionally, of MGUS. In common with MM, most of the clinical sequelae of WM can be ascribed to malignant infiltration or the accumulation of monoclonal immunoglobulin. However, the nature of these sequelae differ markedly from those of MM. For example, osteolysis, amyloidosis and renal impairment seldom are troublesome in WM: by far the most common cause of morbidity is the hyperviscosity syndrome.

Because of the large size and chemical properties of IgM, relatively small increases in its plasma concentration can cause disproportionately large increases in viscosity. Thus, in WM, where the plasma concentration of IgM often is markedly raised, the plasma viscosity can become startlingly high. Accumulation of the monoclonal IgM can lead to a variety of clinical sequelae, including:

- **fleeting neurological symptoms** such as headache, vertigo, somnolence and, in severe cases, coma.

- **visual disturbances** secondary to retinal haemorrhage and oedema, which may cause permanent blindness

- **cardiac failure** which is exacerbated by the increased plasma viscosity which also accompanies WM

- **cryoglobulinaemia** describes the peculiar property of reversible precipitation of the monoclonal IgM in the cold, leading to peripheral vascular occlusion and Raynaud's phenomenon. This complication is present in up to 20% of cases

- **platelet dysfunction** secondary to coating of the platelets by the monoclonal IgM. The bleeding tendency is exacerbated by hyperviscosity with engorgement of the blood vessels of the nose, gastrointestinal and genitourinary tracts

- **haemostatic disturbances** secondary to inhibition of fibrin polymerisation and factor VIII activity by the monoclonal IgM

Examination of the blood reveals marked rouleaux formation and normocytic, normochromic anaemia secondary to suppression of erythropoiesis by the malignant clone, chronic bleeding and dilution by the increased plasma volume. The total white cell count may be normal or depressed but a relative lymphocytosis commonly is present. The platelet count is normal at presentation in 50% of cases. However, neutropaenia and thrombocytopaenia often become more troublesome as the disease advances.

Attempts to aspirate bone marrow frequently fail due to hypercellularity and the extremely high viscosity of the marrow blood. The malignant cells are pleomorphic: some resemble lymphocytes whereas others clearly resemble plasma cells; most, however, have an intermediate appearance and are described as being lymphoplasmacytoid. Trephine biopsy reveals three patterns of infiltration which appear to have prognostic significance: diffuse infiltration is associated with a poor prognosis, with a median survival of 17 months; nodular infiltration is associated with a much better prognosis, with a median survival of 72 months; the intermediate form of infiltration which shows features of both nodular and diffuse infiltration is associated with a median survival of 52 months.

Treatment of WM

WM behaves clinically as a low grade lymphoma and, generally treatment is palliative and conservative. Symptomatic relief from hyperviscosity syndrome is achieved most readily by repeated plasmapheresis. In many cases, little other intervention is required for many years. Progressive disease is treated with the alkylating agents chlorambucil, melphalan and cyclophosphamide.

Hodgkin's Disease

Hodgkin's disease (HD) is a malignant lymphoma and so differs from the leukaemias, myelodysplastic syndromes and non-leukaemic myeloproliferative disorders so far described in a number of important respects:

- HD arises in lymph nodes, not in bone marrow

- disease progression in HD occurs by dissemination of the malignant cells via the lymphatic circulation: involvement of blood and bone marrow occurs only as a late event in advanced disease

- the putative malignant cell in HD is known as the **Reed-Sternberg cell**. The origin of this cell and its normal equivalent remain to be established

- HD is curable in at least 70% of cases

- HD is suspected of having an infectious aetiology, at least in the younger age group

HD has an overall incidence of about 2.5/100,000/year in the UK and has a bimodal age distribution in the developed countries of the world with peaks of incidence in the third decade of life and over the age of 55 years. A different age distribution is common in developing countries, where the highest incidence of HD occurs in children and a second, smaller, peak occurs in the elderly. HD is a rare condition in young adults in developing countries. There is a slight excess incidence of HD in males.

Pathophysiology of HD

The most common presenting feature in HD is the presence of painless, asymmetrical enlargement of cervical or supraclavicular lymph nodes. Isolated axillary, inguinal or femoral lymphadenopathy also are seen occasionally. The lymphadenopathy may be accompanied by severe, generalised itching in the absence of a skin rash. In contrast to the non-Hodgkin's lymphomas, which frequently are disseminated at presentation, most cases of HD are restricted to a single anatomical site at presentation. The presence of pyrexia and drenching night sweats usually are associated with more advanced disease.

Hodgkin's disease was first described by Thomas Hodgkin of Guy's Hospital, London in 1832. His report was based on seven cases with massive lymphadenopathy and splenomegaly. Most of his colleagues thought that these were cases of tuberculosis but Hodgkin, with remarkable prescience, thought that they were clinically distinct. The name Hodgkin's disease was not coined by Hodgkin himself, he was a modest and unassuming man who would not have dreamt of such an action. The eponymous title was coined 33 years later by Samuel Wilks, also of Guy's, when he published a more detailed account of several cases of this condition.

Examination of the peripheral blood seldom affords any useful information in such cases. Most commonly, the peripheral blood is entirely normal. Occasionally, mild non-specific changes such as a mild thrombocytosis, neutrophilia or a relative eosinophilia is present. The presence of anaemia, lymphocytopaenia or leucoerythroblastosis all suggest the presence of advanced disease with bone marrow involvement, but this is uncommon at presentation.

Recognition and Classification of HD

Histological examination of an affected lymph node biopsy reveals the loss of normal follicular and sinusoidal architecture and the presence of a diffuse infiltrate of lymphocytes, histiocytes, eosinophils, plasma cells and neutrophils which are of normal appearance. Scattered among this infiltrate are variable numbers of Reed-Sternberg (RS) cells, the hallmark of HD. RS cells are not specific for HD, they also are present in some cases of infectious mononucleosis, NHL and CLL but their demonstration is mandatory for a diagnosis of HD. RS cells typically are large, with two or more large, oval nuclei, each of which contains a huge nucleolus which is separated from the thickened nuclear membrane by a clear zone.

On the basis of the pattern of lymph node infiltration, four subtypes of HD are recognised:

- **lymphocyte predominant** HD (LPHD) is characterised by a heavy infiltrate of small lymphocytes and histiocytes which have a normal morphology. The infiltrate typically is diffuse but may form loose nodules. RS cells usually are sparse. This subtype of HD is most common in young men and is associated with a rapid response to treatment and a good prognosis.

- **nodular sclerosing** HD (NSHD) involves a varying degree of sclerotic replacement of the nodal architecture, with internment of the nodular tumour infiltrate within collagenous compartments. The morphological hallmark of this form of HD is the **lacunar RS cell** in which the cell cytoplasm has contracted as an artefact of fixation, leaving an unstained zone between it and the surrounding

> The characteristic lacunae surrounding the RS cells in nodular sclerosing Hodgkin's disease are only observed in formalin-fixed tissue. Following fixation of affected lymph nodes with mercuric-based fixatives all of the other morphologic characteristics of NSHD are retained but lacunar RS cells are absent.

tissue. NSHD is the most common subtype, accounting for more than 40% of cases. It appears to be commonly associated with a thymic origin and offers a fairly good prognosis.

- **mixed cellularity** HD (MCHD) is characterised by the presence of large numbers of typical and mononuclear RS cells, scattered amidst a chaotic assortment of morphologically normal lymphocytes, histiocytes, neutrophils, eosinophils, plasma cells and fibroblasts. This subtype of HD is associated with a less favourable prognosis than either of the above subtypes.

- **lymphocyte depleted** HD (LDHD) is associated with large numbers of RS cells and atypical histiocytes, scanty lymphocytes and variable fibrosis. This subtype is the least common form of HD, and is associated with elderly subjects, who often present with advanced disease and have a poor prognosis.

The nature and origin of RS cells remains a mystery. In different subjects, RS cells have been shown to carry B lymphoid antigenic makers and to have a clonal immunoglobulin gene rearrangement or to carry T lymphoid antigenic markers and a clonal T lymphocyte receptor gene rearrangement. Consistent antigenic markers on RS cells include CD25, the IL-2 receptor, CD15 and CD30. The NSHD and MCHD are more commonly associated with T lymphoid markers while LPHD is associated with B lymphoid markers. Although it is widely agreed that RS cells are the malignant cell in HD and that there is strong evidence for a lymphoid origin, the normal counterpart of this cell remains to be identified.

Molecular analysis has revealed the presence of Epstein-Barr viral DNA in the monoclonal RS cells of about 20% of cases of HD. Coupled with the polyclonal, reactive appearance of affected lymph nodes, the differences in the pattern of incidence in developed and underdeveloped countries and the widely accepted role of EBV in Burkitt's lymphoma, this has led many to speculate about the possibility of an infectious origin for HD.

Treatment of HD

The natural history of untreated HD appears to involve the creeping advance of tumour from a single point of origin in a lymph node, first to contiguous nodes by direct contact, then to adjacent and more distant lymph nodes via the lymphatic circulatory system and, finally, to the spleen where further dissemination to the liver and bone marrow occurs via the blood circulatory system.

With this in mind, treatment selection in HD is based upon the clinical and pathological staging of the disease. Widely disseminated, advanced disease is treated more aggressively than early, unifocal disease. The most commonly used staging system, the Ann Arbor system, is summarised in Table 19.5.

SAQ 6

What is the name of the main lymphatic vessel which empties into the vena cava?

Stage	Subtype	Definition
I		Involvement of single lymph node region
	I_E	Involvement of single extralymphatic organ or site
II		Involvement of 2 or more lymph node groups on same side of the diaphragm
	II_E	Localised involvement of an extralymphatic site and one or more lymph node regions
III		Involvement of lymph node regions on both sides of the diaphragm
	III_E	As above with localised involvement of an extralymphatic site
	III_S	As above with localised involvement of the spleen
	III_{SE}	As above with localised involvement of an extralymphatic site and the spleen
IV		Diffuse or disseminated involvement of 1 or more extralymphatic organs or tissues with or without associated lymph node involvement
	A	Absence of fever, night sweats and weight loss
	B	Presence of fever, night sweats or weight loss

Table 19.5 *Ann Arbor staging system for Hodgkin's disease*

Definitive allocation of an individual case to one of the stages of the Ann Arbor system requires the histological examination of all enlarged lymph nodes, a selection of adjacent lymph nodes, the liver, the spleen and any other tissue suspected to be involved. These examinations should be performed, even if the nodes or organs are macroscopically normal, because early infiltration does not always cause gross changes. Such an exhaustive examination permits the determination of the **pathological stage (PS)** of the disease which can be expressed with precision. Staging by non-invasive techniques permits less certainty about the spread of the disease, but clearly is less traumatic. Pragmatically, invasive procedures are reserved for those cases where the identification of minimal further spread of the disease would alter treatment.

The treatment of early stage IA or IIA HD involves localised radiotherapy of the lymph nodes above the diaphragm in what is known as a **mantle field**. This includes the cervical, axillary, supraclavicular, infraclavicular, mediastinal, pulmonary hilar and upper para-aortic lymph nodes. In stage IIIA disease without splenic involvement, this is followed by irradiation of para-aortic, iliac, inguinal and femoral lymph nodes in what is known as an **inverted Y field**. The combination of mantle and inverted Y irradiation is known, erroneously, as **total nodal irradiation (TNI).** The side effects of this treatment are relatively minor and include cough, reversible myelosuppression, nausea and amenorrhoea.

The treatment of stage IB, IIB, IIIB, IIIA with splenic involvement and IV HD involves the use of combination chemotherapy with or without radiotherapy. Various combinations of drugs are used including MOPP (**M**ustine (nitrogen mustard), **O**ncovin (vincristine), **P**rocarbazine and **P**rednisone); MVPP (**M**ustine, **V**inblastine, **P**rocarbazine and **P**rednisone) and ABVD (**A**driamycin, **B**leomycin, **V**inblastine and **D**acarbazine). These combinations are associated with a range of distressing side effects such as severe nausea and vomiting, peripheral neuropathy, severe constipation, alopecia, myelosuppression and sterility. The use of alkylating agents also is associated with the development of secondary malignancy.

With modern treatment, more than 80% of cases of stage I HD and 50% of cases of stage IV HD survive for more than 10 years after presentation. Most of these can be considered to be cured.

Non-Hodgkin's Lymphomas

The term non-Hodgkin's lymphomas (NHL) encompasses a large number of quite disparate malignant clonal disorders of lymphoid tissue. Separation of NHL into smaller, more closely related groups has proved to be very difficult. As a group, NHL is the most common of the haemopoietic malignant disorders with an overall incidence of about 1 per 10,000. The incidence of NHL increases with increasing age and the median age at presentation is about 60 years. Men are affected rather more commonly than women especially, for as yet undiscovered reasons, in those under the age of 20 years.

Aetiology of NHL

The possible role of the Epstein-Barr virus and HTLV-I retrovirus in the aetiology of Burkitt's lymphoma and adult T lymphoblastic leukaemia/lymphoma is discussed in Chapter 15. Chronic suppression of the immune system such as occurs in AIDS or during long-term azathioprine therapy is associated with an increased incidence of NHL. Recent evidence has suggested that reactivation of EBV may be implicated in many of these cases. The factors involved in the aetiology of most cases of NHL are unknown. Epidemiological studies have shown a small excess of NHL among agricultural workers and rubber industry workers but the significance of this observation remains in doubt.

Cytogenetic abnormalities are present in almost all cases of NHL. The most common chromosomal rearrangement associations are t(8;14)(q24;q32) and its variants with small, non-cleaved B lymphomas, t(14;18)(q32;q21) with follicular lymphomas, +12 with small lymphocytic lymphoma and t(11;14)(q13;q32) with intermediate grade diffuse, small, cleaved cell lymphomas. These chromosomal rearrangements and the oncogenes involved are discussed in Chapter 15. Trisomy of chromosomes 2, 3, 7 or 18 is a common finding in NHL, affecting almost two thirds of cases in some studies, but there appears to be little correlation between a particular trisomy and NHL subtype.

> Although the normal function of the protein product of the *bcl-2* gene remains poorly defined, the observation that the gene shows homology with Epstein-Barr virus may be significant.

Recognition and Classification of NHL

The classification of the NHL is both confused and confusing. Several classification systems exist, each with their inherent strengths and weaknesses, but none have gained universal acceptance:

- The **Rappaport System** is based on the pattern of tumour growth within the affected lymph node and the morphology of the predominant cell. Thus, diffuse and nodular growth patterns are recognised while the accompanying morphological descriptions include poorly differentiated, well differentiated, lymphoblastic, undifferentiated and mixed types. The advantages of the Rappaport system are its simplicity and the fact that the different classes show some correlation with prognosis. However, it takes no account of immunological data which has shown that the malignant cell in most cases of "histiocytic" lymphoma has a B lymphoid origin.

• The **Lukes and Collins System** attempts to combine immunological and morphological observations. Thus, the malignant cells are classed as B lymphoid, T lymphoid or histiocytic and related on morphological grounds to the stage of differentiation of their supposed normal counterparts. Among the advantages of this system are that nodular growth is recognised to represent B lymphoid follicular growth and the use of the term histiocytic is accurate.

• The **Kiel System** also relies on a combined immunological and morphological approach and attempts to relate the malignant cell in each class of NHL to a normal counterpart. This system shows some correlation with prognosis, permitting grouping of NHL into low grade and high grade disease.

• The **Working Formulation** was drawn up in 1980 by an expert working party from North America, Europe and Japan and represents an attempt to provide a unified classification system which carries prognostic significance. In that respect, it is similar to the FAB classification of the acute leukaemias. However, it ignores immunophenotypic data and so groups together disorders which are immunologically distinct.

A summary of the different classification systems is presented in Table 19.6. The classes of NHL defined in the Working Formulation will be used in this book.

Working Formulation	Rappaport	Lukes Collins	Immunophenotype
Low Grade			
Small lymphocytic	Diffuse well-differentiated lymphocytic	Small lymphocytic	Mainly B
Follicular small cleaved	Nodular poorly-differentiated lymphocytic	Small cleaved follicular centre	B
Follicular mixed small cleaved and large cell	Nodular mixed lymphocytic & histiocytic	Small cleaved and large follicular centre cell	B
Intermediate Grade			
Follicular large	Nodular histiocytic	Large/small cleaved follicular	Mature B
Diffuse small cleaved	Diffuse poorly-differentiated lymphocytic	Small cleaved diffuse follicular centre	Mature B or T
Diffuse mixed small and large	Diffuse mixed lymphocytic & histiocytic	Small large cleaved non-cleaved follicular centre diffuse	Mature B or T
Diffuse large	Diffuse histiocytic	Large cleaved non-cleaved follicular centre diffuse	B or T
High Grade			
Large immunoblastic	Diffuse histiocytic	Immunoblastic sarcoma	B or T
Lymphoblastic	Diffuse lymphoblastic	Convoluted T cell	T
Small non-cleaved: Burkitt's	Diffuse undifferentiated	Small non-cleaved follicular centre	B
Small non-cleaved: non-Burkitt's	Diffuse undifferentiated	Small non-cleaved follicular centre	B

Pathophysiology of NHL

As already described NHL includes a large number of clinically, histologically and immunologically diverse tumours, many of which are still poorly defined. About 80% of NHL are of B lymphoid origin while almost all of the rest are of T lymphoid origin (rare examples of true histiocytic lymphomas have been described). In general, lymphomas with a follicular pattern of growth are less aggressive than those with a diffuse pattern of growth and small lymphocytic lymphomas are less aggressive than large cell lymphomas. However, in common with the acute leukaemias, some forms of high grade lymphoma are more amenable to treatment than the more indolent or chronic types. In contrast to HD, most NHL are disseminated to a greater or lesser extent at presentation.

Low Grade NHL

The typical presenting feature of low grade NHL is painless lymphadenopathy in an individual who otherwise is well. Most such NHL arise in lymph nodes and are characterised by an indolent but inexorable growth and spread.

Small lymphocytic cell lymphoma (SLL) is characterised by a diffuse infiltrate of homogeneous, small, round lymphocytes of mature appearance and an indolent growth pattern. In many respects, SLL behaves as a solid version of CLL and carries a similar immunophenotype viz weak SIgM+D, HLA DR+, CD19+, CD20+, CD21+, CD5+ and CD10-. SLL disseminates via the blood circulatory system and may be associated with heavy infiltration of the bone marrow and a leukaemic phase. In common with CLL, mild splenomegaly may be present, autoimmune haemolysis sometimes is troublesome and a small proportion of cases of SLL eventually transform to a high grade immunoblastic lymphoma.

Follicular, small, cleaved cell lymphoma (FSCL) and **follicular, mixed small, cleaved and large cell lymphoma (FML)** are more common than SLL and together account for almost one third of NHL. They share similar presenting features with SLL, and have a similarly indolent growth pattern. They differ from SLL, however, in having a greater concentration of SIgM and being CD10+, CD5-. A leukaemic phase with extensive bone marrow involvement is less common for these types of NHL but, where present, has been called **lymphosarcoma cell leukaemia**. In the early years, FSC and FML are readily treatable but up to 40% of cases eventually relapse as a high grade immunoblastic NHL which is refractory to treatment. Interestingly, clonality studies have shown identity between the original and transformed clone in most cases.

Intermediate Grade NHL

About 50% of NHL present with widespread, intermediate grade disease which commonly involves extranodal sites such as tonsils, gastrointestinal tract, bone, skin, testicles, central nervous system or salivary glands. Most cases involve cells of B lymphoid origin but, equally, most cases of T lymphoma belong to this category. In the absence of treatment, these lymphomas progress fairly rapidly and carry a median survival of a few months. With the use of aggressive chemotherapy, a durable remission can be achieved in up to 60% of cases.

High Grade NHL

About 15% of cases of NHL present with high grade disease. In contrast to the low grade lymphomas, up to 40% of high grade lymphomas present with localised disease, frequently involving an extranodal site such as the central nervous system or gastrointestinal tract. In general, these forms of lymphoma progress rapidly and, in the absence of treatment, carry a poor prognosis.

Large, immunoblastic lymphoma (LIL) is strongly associated with a history of chronic immunosuppression such as occurs in CLL, AIDS or therapeutic post-transplantation immunosuppression. As described in Chapter 17, about 5% of cases of CLL undergo immunoblastic transformation as a terminal event. More than three quarters of cases are of B lymphoid origin and the malignant cell in these cases is a plasma cell precursor. Most cases of primary lymphoma which involve the central nervous system at presentation are of this type.

Lymphoblastic lymphoma (LL) is most closely associated with teenage and young adult males and may be thought of as the solid counterpart of TALL. Typical presenting features include cervical, supraclavicular or mediastinal lymphadenopathy and, in more than 50% of cases, a mediastinal mass. This form of lymphoma disseminates rapidly to involve the bone marrow and central nervous system and carries a similar immunological phenotype to TALL.

The **small, non-cleaved cell lymphomas**, (SNCL) which include Burkitt's lymphoma, are aggressive B lymphoid malignancies of children and young adults. They are extremely fast growing and disseminate rapidly, with cell doubling times of less than 40 hours in most cases. Extranodal involvement is particularly common with this group, occurring in up to 90% of cases and most frequently involving the gastrointestinal tract, central nervous system, liver and bone marrow. The non-Burkitt's type of lymphoma is increasingly common in AIDS patients. Ironically, the high tumour growth rate makes this form of lymphoma amenable to cytotoxic chemotherapy and possible cure rates of up to 50% have been reported.

Treatment of NHL

The approach to therapy in NHL is based on a comparison of the likely outcome in the presence and absence of various forms of treatment. As described earlier in this chapter, low grade lymphomas tend to be disseminated at presentation, are associated with long survival times but, ultimately, are incurable. In contrast, high grade lymphomas often are localised at presentation, carry an appalling prognosis in the absence of treatment but are fairly amenable to treatment. Treatment selection therefore is based on a determination of the degree of dissemination of the lymphoma, using a modified form of the Ann Arbor system and on the histological classification. Using this combination, cases of NHL can be divided into three broad treatment categories:

- localised (stage I or II) disease typically is treated with localised radiotherapy, which results in significant disease regression in most cases and a durable remission in almost two thirds of cases. Where remission is incomplete, or following relapse, cytotoxic chemotherapy is required.

- disseminated (stage III or IV) disease which belongs to a good prognosis category typically is managed conservatively in the early years. Disfiguring or dangerous lymphadenopathy may be treated with localised radiotherapy but further treatment may be unnecessary for some years. When disease progression or transformation demands, the treatment choices include single-drug chemotherapy with the alkylating agent chlorambucil; COP which consists of a combination of Cyclophosphamide, **O**ncovin (vincristine) and **P**rednisolone and BACOP which is a combination of **B**leomycin, **A**driamycin, **C**yclophosphamide, **O**ncovin and **P**rednisolone. Remission rates of up to 80% are achievable using any of these approaches but the rate of relapse also is high. More than 50% of cases relapse within 2 years. Eventually, all such cases relapse, low grade lymphomas currently are considered to be incurable using radiotherapy and chemotherapy.

- Disseminated (stage III or IV) disease which belongs to a poor prognosis category typically is treated aggressively with combination cytotoxic chemotherapy. Among the protocols employed are CHOP which consists of **C**yclophosphamide, **H**ydroxydaunomycin (adriamycin), **O**ncovin and **P**rednisolone; BACOP and MACOP-B which adds methotrexate to the previous regimen. Using this aggressive approach, remission can be achieved in up to 80% of cases and cure is possible in 40% of cases.

Suggested Further Reading

Berlin, N.I. (ed.) (1975). Polycythaemia I. *Seminars in Haematology*, **12**:335-444.

Berlin, N.I. (ed.) (1976). Polycythaemia II. *Seminars in Haematology*, **13**:1-86.

Lewis, S.M. (1985). *Myelofibrosis: Pathophysiology and Clinical Management.* New York: Dekker.

Delamore, I.W. (1986). *Multiple Myeloma and other Paraproteinaemias.* Edinburgh: Churchill Livingstone.

McElwain, T.J., Lister, T.A. (eds.) (1987). The lymphomas. *Clinics in Haematology*, **16**, 1-269.

Answers to Self-Assessment Questions

1. Inhaled cigarette smoke contains large amounts of carbon monoxide which binds tightly to haemoglobin to form carboxy haemoglobin, thereby reducing the amount of haemoglobin available for oxygen delivery. The minor tissue hypoxia which results elicits an erythropoietic response. Cigarette smoking also reduces the plasma volume slightly.

2. Erythropoietin is synthesised mainly by the cortical interstitial and endothelial cells of the peritubular capillaries in the kidney. A small amount of erythropoietin is synthesised in the liver and other extrarenal tissues.

3. The dysfunctional platelets which abound in this condition pre dispose to chronic, occult blood loss which eventually leads to iron deficiency in most cases.

4. The immunoglobulin κ chain gene complex is located on chromosome 2 at 2p12 and the λ chain gene complex is located on chromosome 22 at 22q11.

5. The immunoglobulin heavy chain gene complex is located at 14q32. Translocation of proto-oncogenes into this locus results in their activation and is implicated in the aetiology of several B lymphoid malignancies.

6. The thoracic duct.

The Aplastic Anaemias

The term aplastic anaemia encompasses all forms of peripheral blood cytopaenia which are caused by a failure of haemopoiesis. Disorders such as the myelodysplastic syndromes which are characterised by bone marrow hypercellularity and ineffective haemopoiesis or hypersplenism where cytopaenia is secondary to peripheral blood cell destruction are specifically excluded by this definition. However, the term aplastic anaemia is a misnomer since a complete absence of haemopoietic activity clearly is incompatible with life. Although the terms hypoplastic or hypoproliferative anaemia are rather more accurate, they are little used. The term aplastic anaemia is firmly established and its accepted meaning is widely understood and so will be used in this book.

Aplastic anaemia is a rare condition with an overall incidence in Western Europe of about 1 per 200,000. The age-related incidence of aplastic anaemia is not uniform. It is a very rare condition in childhood, increases to a plateau of frequency between the ages of 20 and 65 years and thereafter becomes increasingly common with advancing age. The incidence of aplastic anaemia is greater in underdeveloped countries where it primarily affects children, suggesting an infectious aetiology.

SAQ 1

What is meant by the term ineffective haemopoiesis?

Classification of the Aplastic Anaemias

There is no universally agreed classification scheme for the aplastic anaemias. In this book they are classified in three steps:

- whether the aplasia affects all haemopoietic cell lines or is restricted to a single cell type

- whether they are inherited or acquired disorders

- according to their aetiology.

The classification of the aplastic anaemias is summarised in Table 20.1.

Pancytopaenia	Single Cell Line Affected
Inherited	
Fanconi's anaemia	Diamond-Blackfan syndrome
Dyskeratosis congenita	Congenital dyserythropoietic anaemia
	Congenital neutropaenias (Chapter 14)
	Congenital amegakaryocytic
	thrombocytopaenia
Acquired	
Primary (idiopathic)	Chronic acquired pure red cell aplasia
Secondary to chemical	Parvovirus infection
or physical agents	Acquired amegakaryocytic
Dose-dependent	thrombocytopaenia
Idiosyncratic	Acquired neutropaenia
Infection	
Metabolic abnormalities	
T lymphocyte-mediated	

Table 20.1 *Classification of the aplastic anaemias*

The Inherited Aplastic Anaemias

Fanconi's Anaemia

Almost one third of childhood cases of aplastic anaemia are inherited and most of these can be classified as Fanconi's anaemia. In most cases, a range of congenital abnormalities is present including patchy brown skin pigmentation, stunting of growth, microcephaly, renal and skeletal malformations and, classically, bilateral absence or underdevelopment of the thumbs. Typically, the onset of anaemia is delayed until childhood or early adolescence. Fanconi's anaemia is inherited in an autosomal recessive manner with variable penetrance. The nature of the genetic defect which leads to this disorder is unknown but is manifest as an increased number of chromosomal aberrations such as breakages and multiple complex chromatid exchanges in mitotic spreads. This feature is exploited in the antenatal diagnosis of Fanconi's anaemia. The incidence of the gene which causes Fanconi's anaemia has been estimated to be as high as 1 in 400 of the population. Some workers believe that at least some of the idiopathic aplastic anaemias described below may be more common in individuals who are heterozygous for this

Standard cytogenetic preparations of bone marrow from cases of Fanconi's anaemia typically show some increase in the number of chromosomal breakages and complex rearrangements present. However, pretreatment of the bone marrow samples with cyclophosphamide or mitomycin C increases the incidence of these abnormalities markedly. Using this technique, Fanconi's homozygotes are readily and reliably detectable. The cells of Fanconi's heterozygotes also may show an increase in the number of chromosomal aberrations but cannot be separated from normal cells with absolute certainty.

gene. However, there appears to be little directly supportive evidence for this belief.

The most common presenting features for Fanconi's anaemia are bleeding secondary to thrombocytopaenia and a request for investigation of short stature. The typical pattern for the onset of aplasia is for thrombocytopaenia to develop first as an isolated abnormality, followed some months or even years later by the development of anaemia. Neutropaenia usually is a relatively late manifestation of the disease. Bone marrow examination reveals hypocellularity with a reduction in the number of CFU-GEMM, CFU-GM and BFU-E and extensive fatty replacement of haemopoietic tissue. Dysplastic features usually are minimal and reflect the stress imposed on the dwindling haemopoietic tissue in trying to maintain circulating blood cell counts.

Fanconi's anaemia may be thought of as a premalignant condition. More than 10% of cases progress to acute leukaemia or develop a tumour of the gastrointestinal tract or skin. Allogeneic bone marrow transplantation is a successful form of treatment for aplastic anaemia but does not correct the other congenital abnormalities or the tendency to develop non-haemopoietic malignancy. Because of the increased fragility of the chromosomes in Fanconi's anaemia, the conditioning regimen needs to be markedly scaled down in these patients. In the absence of a suitable bone marrow donor, administration of high dose anabolic steroids produces a temporary recovery in peripheral blood cell counts but at the cost of development of male secondary sexual characteristics in both boys and girls, liver damage and bouts of uncontrolled hyperactivity and aggression.

SAQ 2

What is meant by the following terms, in the context of transplantation?

A. allogeneic
B. syngeneic
C. autologous

Dyskeratosis Congenita

Dyskeratosis congenita, as the name implies, is an inherited disorder which is associated with aberrant growth of skin, nails and hair. It usually is inherited as an X-linked recessive disorder although isolated reports of autosomal recessive inheritance exist. Typically, congenital abnormalities such as alopecia, abnormal sweating, telangiectasia and mental retardation are joined by the development of a progressive aplastic anaemia in early adulthood. The nature of the genetic abnormality is unknown but, in contrast to Fanconi's anaemia, dyskeratosis congenita is not associated with any apparent cytogenetic abnormality.

Diamond-Blackfan Syndrome

Diamond-Blackfan syndrome typically presents in the first two years of life as a severe anaemia and reticulocytopaenia in the presence of normal white cell and platelet counts. Bone marrow examination reveals either a complete absence of erythropoietic precursors or a maturation arrest in erythropoiesis. Frequently, this disorder is accompanied by a variety of skeletal abnormalities which may cause confusion with Fanconi's anaemia, although cytogenetic abnormalities are absent. The pattern of inheritance in most cases is consistent with an autosomal recessive condition with variable penetrance. The nature of the genetic defect is unknown.

In the absence of a suitable donor for allogeneic bone marrow transplantation, the ideal treatment, most cases of Diamond-Blackfan syndrome respond well to the administration of high dose corticosteroids or cyclosporin. Long-term corticosteroid therapy in children is associated with growth retardation, a susceptibility to infection secondary to neutrophil dysfunction and a tendency to develop diabetes. The success of corticosteroid therapy in inducing prompt and sustainable remission of the anaemia in this condition suggests an immune-mediated pathogenesis.

The Congenital Dyserythropoietic Anaemias

The congenital dyserythropoietic anaemias (CDAs) are a group of rare inherited disorders of unknown cause which are characterised by a variable degree of anaemia, reticulocytopaenia, marked ineffective erythropoiesis and erythroblast multinuclearity. Three types of CDA are recognised:

- **CDA type I** is the mildest form and is associated with a mild to moderate macrocytic anaemia, megaloblastoid bone marrow appearances and an autosomal recessive mode of inheritance. The hallmark of this form of CDA is the presence in the bone marrow of up to 3% binucleated erythroblasts with intranuclear chromatin bridges.

- **CDA type II** is the most common and most severe form and is characterised by a mild to severe normocytic anaemia, the presence of up to 50% multinucleated erythroblasts in the bone marrow, enhanced expression of Ii antigens on red cells and an autosomal recessive mode of inheritance. Mature peripheral blood red cells in this disorder classically are highly susceptible to lysis in acidified serum although, in contrast to PNH, lysis does not occur in the presence of the patient's own serum. CDA type II is also known by the descriptive title **hereditary erythroblast multinuclearity with positive acidified serum test (HEMPAS)**.

- **CDA type III** is the rarest form and is associated with a mild macrocytic anaemia, the presence of highly multinucleate erythroblasts in the bone marrow and an autosomal dominant mode of inheritance. The abnormal erythroblasts may contain up to 12 nuclei and are sometimes known as gigantoblasts.

Inherited Neutropaenias

The inherited neutropaenias are described in detail in Chapter 14 and will not be considered here.

Congenital Amegakaryocytic Thrombocytopaenia

Amegakaryocytic thrombocytopaenia is a rare condition which is inherited as an autosomal recessive disorder and is characterised by a severe thrombocytopaenia secondary to deficiency of megakaryocyte production, platelet dysfunction and, usually, bilateral absence of the bones of the lower arms. The condition is also known as the **thrombocytopaenia with absent radii (TAR) syndrome**. Haemorrhage is a major cause of mortality in the first year of life and, more especially, in the perinatal period. Interestingly, in many cases, the thrombocytopaenia gradually remits in early childhood. The nature of the underlying defect in this disorder is unknown.

In Ham's acidified serum test, patient's red cells are incubated for 1 hour at 37°C with a selection of ABO compatible acidified sera and the samples are examined for the presence of haemolysis. A "positive" result (ie haemolysis) is obtained in cases of paroxysmal nocturnal haemoglobinuria (PNH) and HEMPAS.

The Acquired Aplastic Anaemias

In about half of cases of aplastic anaemia, careful investigation reveals a likely cause for the depression in haemopoiesis such as a history of exposure to ionising radiation or to drugs or chemicals which are known to be myelotoxic. It follows that, in the remainder of cases, no clearly identifiable culprit can be found. Such cases are referred to as **idiopathic aplastic anaemias**.

Aplastic Anaemia Secondary to Chemical or Physical Agents

A wide range of chemical and physical agents has been implicated in the causation of aplastic anaemia. Broadly, these agents can be divided into two types:

- those agents which necessarily induce aplastic anaemia in all of those exposed and in whom the degree of aplasia induced typically is proportional to the degree of exposure.

- those agents which are innocuous to most of those exposed but which induce aplasia in a minority of susceptible individuals. This is the larger group, and includes a huge number of widely used drugs. In many cases, the evidence of culpability in this regard is somewhat weak.

Dose-dependent Responses to Chemical or Physical Agents

Ionising Radiation

Exposure to ionising radiation such as X-rays, γ-rays, α particles and β particles inflicts serious damage to cellular DNA, involving the introduction of strand breaks, base deletions and the promotion of inappropriate base pairing. The degree of damage inflicted typically is proportional to the dose of radiation received, although actively cycling cells are much more radiosensitive than those in G_0. Because of this, the most radiosensitive tissues are the haemopoietic stem cells, gut mucosal cells and testicular germ cells. A dose of 7 Gy or more of penetrating ionising radiation such as X-rays completely ablates the bone marrow and other rapidly dividing tissue and, in the absence of bone marrow transplantation, is uniformly fatal. With lesser doses, the effect of the radiation is dose-related. Exposure to a single, short-lived dose of ionising radiation may inflict serious damage to the bone marrow and mucosae leading to severe gastrointestinal disturbances, haemorrhage secondary to thrombocytopaenia and infectious complications secondary to neutropaenia, commonly resulting in death. However, given supportive care to maintain life, such individuals may recover following repopulation of the bone marrow by haemopoietic stem cells which were in G_0 at the time of exposure.

Chronic or repeated exposure to ionising radiation is associated with the development of profound aplastic anaemia because, as resting haemopoietic stem cells are spurred into the cell cycle to replace damaged stem cells, they too are subject to the damaging effects of the radiation. This relentlessly destructive cycle eventually leads to severe depletion of the haemopoietic stem cell pool and aplastic anaemia ensues.

Cytotoxic Chemotherapy

Long experience with the therapeutic use of cytotoxic drugs has enabled the selection of dose regimens which induce temporary bone marrow aplasia so that recovery of normal haemopoietic tissue occurs quickly after withdrawal of the drug. The rationale for this approach to cytotoxic chemotherapy is described in more detail in Chapter 15. Occasionally, prolonged use of alkylating agents such as busulphan can lead to prolonged aplasia from which recovery is slow or incomplete.

Benzene

Chronic exposure to benzene is associated with the induction of aplastic anaemia and, as described in Chapter 15, acute non-lymphoblastic leukaemia. Benzene is widely used as an organic solvent, as a cleaning agent and is added to petrol as an anti-knocking agent. It is unclear whether exposure to low levels of benzene is myelotoxic. Most recorded cases have been exposed to atmospheric concentrations of benzene in excess of 200 ppm over many years, usually at their place of work. In many cases, withdrawal of benzene exposure permits regeneration of the bone marrow without further intervention but the risk of leukaemogenesis may still be present in such cases.

A variety of chemicals have been implicated as causes of aplastic anaemia, among them carbon tetrachloride, aniline dyes and agricultural chemicals such as herbicides and insecticides.

Alcohol

Because alcohol is myelosuppressive, chronic alcoholism is associ-

---

The recent upsurge in interest about Green issues has had many effects, including the appearance of new, environmentally friendly products. One such product, lead-free petrol was made available following the publication of several studies which showed that exposure to the small quantities of lead in exhaust emissions posed a potential threat to health, particularly for those who live in the inner cities. Most motorists now use lead-free petrol in their cars, secure in the knowledge that they are helping to rid the environment of toxic pollutants such as lead. However, what is seldom publicised is that, deprived of tetraethyl lead as an anti-knocking agent, the oil companies simply increased the quantity of the known leukaemogen, benzene in their new "environmentally friendly" lead-free petrol!

ated with aplastic anaemia. Regularly drinking the equivalent of a bottle of spirits per day causes sideroblastic change with vacuolation of the erythroblasts and moderate bone marrow hypoplasia. Typically, the anaemia is complicated by the effects of hepatic cirrhosis, haematinic deficiency and other nutritional disorders. The alcohol-induced aplasia is reversible by withdrawal of alcohol.

Idiosyncratic Responses to Chemical or Physical Agents

A large number of drugs which can be used with safety in the vast majority of the population have been reported to cause unexpected aplastic anaemia in a tiny percentage of those taking them. The best known example of this type of anaemia is the antibacterial agent chloramphenicol which has been used with safety for decades. When administered in high dose, chloramphenicol therapy is associated with a very mild and transient bone marrow hypoplasia which rapidly remits on withdrawal of the drug. At the much lower doses which are in everyday use, chloramphenicol therapy is associated with no clinically significant myelotoxicity. However, certain rare individuals, estimated to be about 1 in 20,000 of the population, are exquisitely sensitive to the myelotoxic effects of this drug. In these people, chloramphenicol therapy is deadly. Even the tiny amount present in highly dilute eye drops is sufficient to cause profound and refractory aplastic anaemia, which commonly results in death. The genetic basis for this idiosyncratic response to chloramphenicol is unknown and there is no way to predict which individuals are at risk. In the last few decades, chloramphenicol has been implicated in almost one quarter of cases of acquired aplastic anaemia in the UK. Recent years have seen a marked decline in the use of chloramphenicol.

As described above, the list of drugs which have been reported to have been implicated in the causation of aplastic anaemia is extremely long. Most such reactions, however, are extremely rare and many of the reports are of dubious value. Among the drugs which are well established as potential culprits in the induction of aplastic anaemia in susceptible individuals are the analgesics indomethacin, phenylbutazone, oxyphenbutazone and diclofenac; the anticonvulsants phenytoin and trimethadione; and the anti-arthritic gold compounds. In some cases, the mechanism of myelotoxicity clearly is related to the pharmacological action of the drug and establishment of a causal relationship with aplastic anaemia is relatively straightforward. Many drugs have been implicated largely on the basis of a statistical correlation between prior drug administration and the subsequent, sometimes considerably delayed, development of aplastic anaemia. In some such cases, the putative causal relationship is underpinned by a credible biological mechanism but this is lacking in most cases and the relationship remains circumstantial.

Infection

Most infections are, to some degree, myelosuppressive. As described in Chapter 5, chronic infections may result in a refractory normocytic, normochromic anaemia known as the anaemia of chronic disorders. The aplastic crisis which is associated with chronic haemolytic states such as sickle cell disease and hereditary spherocytosis is thought to result from the myelosuppressive effects of infection on an already severely stressed bone marrow. The most common trigger of such aplastic crises is parvovirus B19 which specifically infects erythroid precursors. In the absence of chronic haemolysis, parvovirus B19 is responsible for a typical flu-like illness consisting of fever, skin rash, headache, myalgia and polyarthropathy which is variously known as **fifth disease**, **erythema infectiosum** or, more colourfully, as **slapped-cheek disease**. Similarly implicated as an occasional cause of aplastic anaemia are Epstein-Barr virus and cytomegalovirus infections.

Aplastic anaemia occasionally is associated with viral hepatitis. This rare complication is most closely associated with hepatitis C infection and can occur at any time up to 6 months after the onset of symptoms. The mechanism involved in the induction of aplasia is unknown but is thought to be immune-mediated. In the absence of a suitable bone marrow donor, this form of aplastic anaemia carries a very poor prognosis.

Metabolic Abnormalities

Aplastic anaemia is seen in association with a range of metabolic abnormalities including hypopituitarism, hyperparathyroidism and inborn errors of amino acid metabolism known as the ketotic hyperglycinaemias.

Immune Mechanisms

The evidence that immune mechanisms are involved in some cases of aplastic anaemia, although circumstantial, is considerable:

- in some identical twins, engraftment of syngeneic bone marrow transplants occurs only in the presence of pharmacologic immunosuppression

- the immunosuppressive conditioning process which is used as a preparation for bone marrow transplantation has been reported to cause disease remission in some cases

- aplastic anaemia commonly occurs in immunodeficient children following transfusion of blood which contains viable HLA-compatible lymphocytes. The mechanism here is thought to be similar to graft versus host disease.

- aplastic anaemia commonly accompanies benign thymomas

- *in vitro* culture of bone marrow from cases of aplastic anaemia is enhanced by the removal of suppressor T lymphocytes

- up to half of cases of aplastic anaemia respond favourably to the administration of antithymocyte globulin

The mechanisms of immune-mediated suppression of haemopoiesis remain obscure.

Pathophysiology and Treatment of Aplastic Anaemia

The pathogenesis of aplastic anaemia is highly diverse: some cases appear to result from a functional defect of pluripotential haemopoietic stem cells; others from a defect of the haemopoietic inductive microenvironment while, as described above, others appear to be mediated by immune mechanisms.

The presenting features of aplastic anaemia are non-specific and predictable: pallor, lassitude and exercise intolerance secondary to anaemia; frequent and recurrent bacterial and fungal infections secondary to neutropaenia and a tendency to bruise easily secondary to thrombocytopaenia. Lymphadenopathy and splenomegaly typically are absent. The diagnosis of aplastic anaemia can only be made when all other possible causes of the pancytopaenia have been excluded by careful clinical and laboratory investigation.

Examination of the peripheral blood reveals pancytopaenia, although the degree of depression of the neutrophil count typically is greater than that of the other leucocytes, and reticulocytopaenia. The concentration of foetal haemoglobin commonly is raised and may be as high as 20% of the total. Ferrokinetic studies reveal a delayed uptake and utilisation of iron from the plasma and confirm the absence of extramedullary haemopoiesis. Bone marrow aspirates are hypocellular and show replacement of haemopoietic tissue by fatty deposits. Multiple bone marrow biopsies confirm the patchy nature of reduction in haemopoiesis: some samples are extremely hypocellular whereas a few may be almost normocellular. Attempts to culture bone marrow *in vitro* reveal a deficit of haemopoietic progenitor cells such as CFU-GM, CFU-E and BFU-E, and a diminished response to haemopoietic growth factors.

In the absence of treatment, the prognosis for aplastic anaemia is poor. The two main prognostic indicators in aplastic anaemia are age and disease severity at presentation. About 25% of those cases with severe disease at presentation will die within 4 months without treatment. Of the remainder, a further 25% will die within 4-12 months, and a further 35% will succumb at some later time, usually sooner rather than later. Around 15% only will remit spontaneously, and even then the remission is more likely to be partial rather than total. Those ascribed to idiopathic causes generally do less well than those where there is a suggested cause, except where the cause is hepatitis, when the outlook is particularly bleak.

The International Aplastic Anaemia Study Group has devised a set of objective criteria which permit the recognition of cases with severe disease and a particularly poor prognosis. The criteria for severe disease are shown in Table 20.2. The median survival time in the absence of treatment for those with severe disease is 6 months: only about 20% of such cases survive much beyond a year.

Severe disease =
    Marrow cellularity < 25% of normal
or   < 50% of normal if the majority of cells are lymphoid
Plus any two of the following
    Corrected reticulocyte count < 1%
    Neutrophil count < 500/ml
    Platelet count < 20,000/ml

Table 20.2 *Definition of severe disease at presentation of aplastic anaemia*

The treatment of choice for those with severe disease is bone marrow transplantation. As discussed in Chapter 16, this form of treatment is only available to those under the age of 45 years who have an HLA-compatible donor. The age limit may be extended where an identical twin is available to act as a donor for syngeneic bone marrow transplant. Lasting restoration of haemopoiesis following bone marrow transplantation is achieved in more than 80% of cases. The success rate is somewhat lower in cases who were given blood transfusions prior to transplantation.

If a suitable donor is not available, or if the patient is too old to withstand the rigours of the transplantation process, the treatment of choice is immunosuppressive therapy. Cyclophosphamide and anti-thymocyte globulin (ATG) produce stable remission rates in more than 50% of those treated. ATG therapy is thought to act by eliminating activated suppressor T lymphocytes, thereby liberating haemopoietic stem cell growth. ATG therapy is associated with fevers, chills, skin rashes and hypotension. Long-term immunosuppressive therapy is associated with an increased susceptibility to infection and an excess of lymphoid malignancy.

An alternative treatment where bone marrow transplantation is not available is the administration of high doses of androgens such as testosterone. However, the value of this approach is questionable. Some studies have suggested that significant remissions can be obtained in almost 50% of cases whereas others have shown much poorer response rates. Androgen therapy is associated with hirsutism and virilisation in female patients.

Supportive therapy during the pancytopaenic period is extremely important. Antibiotics are required to treat established infection or, where the neutrophil count is very low, may be used prophylactically. Measures for the avoidance of infection also are important. These include avoidance of contact with infections, the use of antiseptic soaps and toiletries, the use of electric razors and soft tooth brushes, the avoidance of intramuscular injections and the avoidance of fresh fruits and vegetables. Menstrual blood losses can be prevented or minimised by the administration of oral contraceptives or anovulatory agents. Transfusion therapy should be avoided if at all possible, especially in those cases who are eligible for a bone marrow transplant.

Suggested Further Reading

Geary, C.G. (ed.). *Aplastic Anaemia*. London: Bailliere Tindall.

Nathan, D.G. and Oski, F.A. (eds.). (1994) *Hematology of Infancy and Childhood, 4th ed.* Philadelphia: WB   Saunders.

Lewis, S.M. and Verwilghen, R.L. (ed).   (1977). *Dyserythropoiesis.* London: Academic Press.

Answers to Self-Assessment Questions

1. Ineffective haemopoiesis occurs when an increased rate of haemopoiesis does not result in an increased in circulating blood cell counts due to intramedullary destruction of haemopoietic precursors. This phenomenon is seen most commonly and clearly in megaloblastic anaemia.

2. A. an allogeneic transplant utilises material from a genetically non-identical donor.
    B. a syngeneic transplant utilises material from a genetically identical donor ie an identical twin.
    C. an autologous transplant utilises material from the recipient eg bone marrow harvested during remission of leukaemia may be transplanted following relapse.

Chapter 21

Haemostasis: an Overview

Haemostasis may be defined as that process which maintains the flowing blood in a fluid state and confined to the circulatory system. The haemostatic mechanism is not a single biological pathway, but the product of the complex interactions of a number of distinct systems:

- the vascular system

- blood platelets

- the blood coagulation system

- the fibrinolytic system

- the Complement system

- the kinin system

- inhibitors of the above systems

This chapter presents an overview of the processes involved in maintaining optimal haemostasis. Knowledge of this chapter is assumed in the following chapters.

The Vascular System

The blood circulatory system can be divided into three subsystems:

- the **systemic circulation** which is responsible for the delivery of oxygenated arterial blood from the **left ventricle** of the heart to the body tissues and the return of deoxygenated venous blood to the **right atrium** of the heart.

- the **pulmonary circulation** which is responsible for the delivery of deoxygenated blood from the **right**

ventricle of the heart to the lungs and the return of oxygenated blood to the **left atrium** of the heart.

- the **portal systems** which act as venous conduits, transporting important substances such as nutrients and hormones between various sites within the body. The largest portal system of the body is the **hepatic portal system** which connects capillaries in the intestine and spleen, via the **portal vein**, to the **hepatic sinusoids** of the liver. This arrangement facilitates the utilisation of newly absorbed nutrients by the liver and the removal of particulate debris by the phagocytic Küpffer cells of the liver. The hepatic sinusoids drain into the **hepatic veins** and, from there, into the **vena cava** which carries the blood directly into the right atrium of the heart.

> **SAQ 1**
>
> From which blood cell type are Küpffer cells derived?

The systemic and pulmonary circulatory systems are depicted schematically in Figure 21.1.

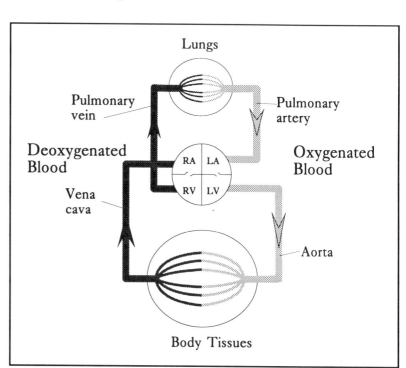

Figure 21.1 *The systemic and pulmonary circulatory systems*

Blood Vessel Structure

Blood vessel walls are composed of three distinct, concentric layers as shown in Figure 21.2:

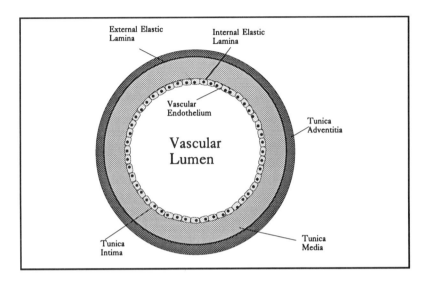

Figure 21.2 *The structure of a muscular artery. Other types of blood vessel structure differ as described in the text*

- the **intima** forms the inner layer and consists of a thin monolayer of flat vascular endothelial cells. Vascular endothelial cells are non-thrombogenic and contain microtubules called **Weibel-Palade bodies**. The vascular endothelium is mounted upon an internal elastic membrane, which is largely composed of collagen fibres.

- the **media** forms the central layer and is the most variable component of the blood vessel wall. In elastic arteries, such as the aorta, the media is mainly composed of elastic fibres arranged in concentric, circumferential layers. This arrangement helps to absorb the huge changes in pressure between systole and diastole. In muscular arteries, which are further from the heart, the media is composed of a layer of smooth muscle cells which are under autonomic nervous control, permitting rhythmic contraction and relaxation of the artery which helps to maintain blood pressure. In arterioles and veins, the media is thin and of much less functional importance.

- the **adventitia** forms the exterior coat and largely is composed of collagen with a scattering of smooth muscle cells. The border between the media and the adventitia may be marked by a collection of elastic fibres which form the **external elastic lamina**.

Contribution of Vascular System to Haemostasis

Constriction of the injured blood vessel to limit early blood loss is a primary means of securing haemostasis; a process which is under local neural and hormonal control. The latter probably is the most important and may be mediated by various compounds, including adrenaline, ADP, kinins and thromboxanes. Many of these vasoactive substances are derived from blood platelets.

The metabolic activities of vascular endothelial cells play an important role in haemostasis. These cells are the major source of **von Willebrand factor (vWF), thrombomodulin** and **tissue factor pathway inhibitor (TFPI)**. The contribution of these substances to haemostasis is discussed later in this chapter. vWF also is synthesised by megakaryocytes. Endothelial cell prostaglandin metabolism produces **prostacyclin (PGI$_2$)** which is a very potent inhibitor of platelet aggregation and also acts as a vasodilator.

When the integrity of the vascular endothelial layer is breached, the subendothelial layers provide a surface for platelet activation and aggregation as well as activation of the intrinsic coagulation system via coagulation factors XII and XI. More importantly, the adventitial cells are constitutive expressors of **tissue factor**, which is now thought to be the primary activator of blood coagulation.

Blood Platelets

Platelet Structure

SAQ 2

What unique form of cell division do megakaryocytes undergo?

Platelets are formed from the cytoplasm of bone marrow megakaryocytes and are the smallest of the blood cells. The normal platelet count lies between 150 and 400 x 10^9/l. They are disc-shaped, anucleate cells with a relatively complex internal structure reflecting the specific haemostatic functions of the platelet. The ultrastructure of the blood platelet is shown in Figure 21.3.

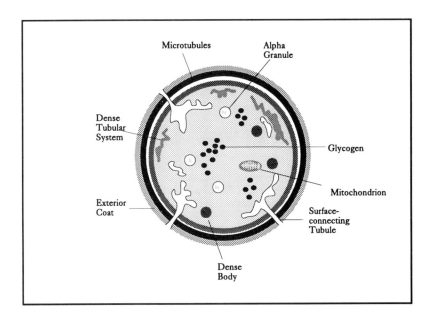

Figure 21.3 *Normal platelet ultra-structure*

Of particular importance are the two major types of intracellular granule, the α **granules** and the **dense granules**. The α granules contain the platelet glycoprotein **thrombospondin** as well as **fibrinogen, fibronectin, platelet factor 4 (PF4), vWF, β-thromboglobulin (β-TG), platelet-derived growth factor (PDGF)** and coagulation factors V and VIII. The dense granules, so called because of their appearance on electron microscopy, contain ADP, ATP and **serotonin (5-hydroxytryptamine, 5-HT)**. The contents of both the α and dense granules may be released, via a system of surface-connecting tubules, during platelet function. These granular contents have a variety of important biological activities as shown in Table 21.1.

Location	Compound	Function
α granule	Platelet factor 4	neutralises heparin effect
	β thromboglobulin	promotes fibroblast chemotaxis
	Platelet derived growth factor (PDGF)	mitogenic for fibroblasts, chemotactic for neutrophils, fibroblasts and smooth muscle cells
	vWF	adhesion, carrier for VIII
	PAI-1	fibrinolytic inhibitor
	Fibronectin	adhesion of platelets and fibroblasts
	Thrombospondin	promotes platelet-platelet interaction
Dense bodies	ADP	aggregation of platelets
	ATP	source of ADP
	Serotonin	vasoconstriction

Table 21.1 *Platelet granule constituents and their most important biological functions*

Both the blood platelets and the vessel wall contain biochemical pathways for the metabolism of **arachidonic acid** (Figure 21.4). This polyunsaturated fatty acid is mainly present bound to membrane phospholipids, but can be released by the enzyme phospholipase A_2 in activated platelets. The newly liberated arachidonic acid is converted to **thromboxane A_2 (TXA$_2$)** by the actions of the enzymes **cyclo-oxygenase** and **thromboxane synthetase**. TXA$_2$ is a powerful inducer of platelet aggregation, but has a very short half-life (around 30 secs), being rapidly converted to the stable derivative TXB$_2$. Arachidonic acid metabolism within vascular endothelium results in the generation of PGI$_2$ via the intermediates PGG$_2$ and PGH$_2$. PGI$_2$ is a potent inhibitor of platelet aggregation.

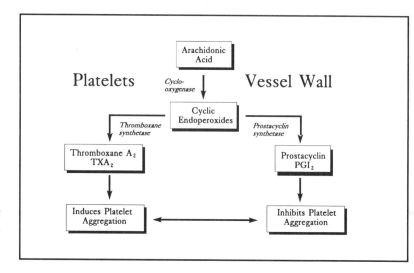

Figure 21.4 *Arachidonic acid metabolism in vascular endothelium and platelets*

Platelet Function

During primary haemostasis, platelets generally display four distinct properties as illustrated schematically in Figure 21.5.

- adhesion to a surface

- shape change

- release of granule contents

- aggregation

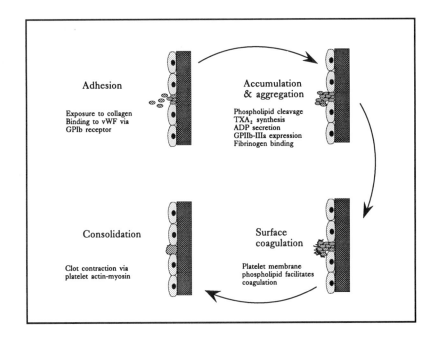

Figure 21.5 *Primary haemostatic plug formation*

Adhesion

Blood platelets may be activated by contact with a range of physiological and non-physiological substances, including subendothelial tissue, foreign or charged surfaces, ADP, thrombin, TXA_2 and bacterial endotoxin. *In vivo* damage to the vessel wall causes exposure of subendothelial fibres and results in the rapid adherence of circulating platelets to the surface of the wound. Normally, sufficient platelets would be present to cover completely the damaged area. The importance of platelet adhesion *in vivo* is illustrated by the relatively easy bruising and enhanced capillary fragility seen in patients with thrombocytopaenia.

Platelet adhesion largely is dependent on the interactions of specific platelet membrane receptors, structural components of the subendothelium and the von Willebrand factor (vWF). The process of vWF-mediated platelet adhesion is essential for platelet interactions with an injured vessel wall, especially at the high shear rates which prevail in stenosed arteries and the microcirculation. There are two binding sites for vWF on the platelet membrane, viz **glycoprotein Ib (GPIb)** and **glycoprotein IIb/IIIa (GPIIb/IIIa)**. Platelet GPIb binds to high molecular weight vWF in the presence of calcium ions. The subendothelial receptor remains to be unequivocally identified. However, collagen is particularly potent in inducing platelet adhesion and types I, II and III have all been shown to be active in this respect. Occupation of the GPIb receptor causes the exposure of the hitherto cryptic GPIIb/IIIa receptor which acts as a secondary vWF binding site.

Shape Change

Platelet adhesion usually is accompanied by a transformation in platelet shape from the normal discoid form to one of irregular outline with numerous cytoplasmic projections, the echinocytic configuration. In the early stages of platelet activation the shape changes are reversible, but with increased and continued stimulation the change becomes irreversible and is associated with centralisation of the cytoplasmic granules and ultimately with degranulation and release of granule contents.

Spiculated blood cells are called echinocytes because of their supposed resemblance to the spiny sea urchin *Echinus esculenta*.

Release of Granule Contents

Platelet degranulation (release reaction) occurs largely as a result of the fusion of the cytoplasmic granules with the surface-connected tubular system. The contents of the α and dense granules are thus made available at the platelet surface where they facilitate further local platelet adhesion and aggregation, thrombin generation and wound healing. Degranulation is accompanied by enhanced phosphatidyl inositol and arachidonic acid metabolism, both of which promote platelet aggregation.

Aggregation

The platelet release reaction usually is followed by aggregation of the platelets. The initial attachment of platelets to each other largely is mediated by plasma fibrinogen which acts as a bridge between adjacent stimulated platelets. The fibrinogen molecules bind, via their γ chains, to the platelet membrane glycoprotein IIb/IIIa receptor. Each half of the fibrinogen molecule contains two domains which can interact with platelet receptor sites, and fibrinogen is therefore clearly capable of acting as a divalent platelet-platelet bridge.

A variety of compounds are capable of inducing platelet aggregation. For example, ADP is a powerful aggregator, but at physiological calcium concentrations, causes aggregation without inducing degranulation. Collagen and thrombin on the other hand, are potent inducers of platelet release and aggregation. Collagen causes aggregation by inducing the release of ADP and generation of TXA_2. The latter is a particularly potent platelet activator and can rapidly induce shape change, degranulation and aggregation. Arachidonic acid and cyclic endoperoxides cause platelet aggregation via TXA_2 production. Most platelet functions seem to depend on the mobilisation of intracellular calcium ions, and platelet aggregating agents act by modifying the free calcium ion concentration.

The key modulator of intraplatelet function is **cyclic AMP (cAMP)**. This compound combines with a cAMP-dependent protein to generate kinase activity, leading to the phosphorylation of a receptor protein which then binds calcium ions. The resulting reduction in free calcium ion concentration renders the platelet less susceptible to aggregation and adhesion. Adrenaline, thrombin, collagen and serotonin all inhibit the enzyme adenylate cyclase which converts ATP to cAMP. The reduction in intraplatelet cAMP concentration which results from binding of these agonists to the platelet surface leads to an increased free calcium ion concentration and platelet hyperaggregability. Calcium ions activate the platelet contractile system and may be required to bind an aggregation agonist such as ADP to its receptor. Thus, calcium channel blocking drugs may interfere with intracellular calcium movement and thereby interfere with platelet function. Aspirin and other non-steroidal anti-inflammatory drugs (NSAIDs) interfere with arachidonic acid metabolism and impair ADP release from platelets.

> The most commonly prescribed antiplatelet drug is aspirin (acetylsalicylate) which acts by acetylating the enzyme cyclooxygenase, thereby inhibiting TXA_2 production. Low-dose aspirin therapy can be used as an effective prophylactic measure in cases of established thromboembolic disease.

The ADP released from activated platelets and damaged red cells at sites of injury stimulates the activation of adjacent platelets, which undergo the release reaction and subsequently join the growing aggregate. This self-propagating activation rapidly results in the formation of a **primary haemostatic plug** which physically blocks the breach in the vessel wall, thereby staunching blood loss.

Consolidation of the Platelet Aggregate

The plug formed at the site of vessel wall damage is relatively fragile. If it is not reinforced quickly, the plug breaks down and bleeding recommences. The consolidation of the primary haemostatic plug is brought about by the enzymatic conversion of fibrinogen to fibrin and the subsequent stabilisation of the resultant fibrin molecules by blood coagulation factor XIII. The activation and regulation of the blood coagulation system is discussed in greater detail below, although it should be remembered that the platelets themselves are capable of providing many of the components of this system at the local level.

The Blood Coagulation System

The blood coagulation system is composed of a series of functionally specific plasma proteins (coagulation factors). These proteins interact in a highly ordered and predetermined sequence with the sole object of converting the soluble protein fibrinogen to an insoluble network of fibrin which consolidates and stabilises the primary haemostatic plug. The coagulation factors are, by convention, referred to by an internationally agreed system of Roman numerals. These numbers are related to the order of discovery of the individual coagulation factors; they bear little relationship to the order in which they take part in the coagulation process. Each coagulation factor also has one or more synonyms which may be used, particularly in the earlier literature. The Roman numeral system for coagulation factor identification and the corresponding synonyms are listed in Table 21.2.

Factor	Most Commonly Used Synonym
I (not normally used)	Fibrinogen
II	Prothrombin
III (not used)	Tissue factor (thromboplastin)
IV (not used)	Calcium ions
V	Labile factor
VII	Stable factor
VIII	Anti-haemophiliac factor
IX	Christmas factor
X	Stuart-Prower factor
XI	Plasma thromboplastin antecedent
XII	Hageman factor
XIII	Fibrin stabilising factor
None assigned	Prekallikrein
None assigned	High molecular weight kininogen

Table 21.2 *Nomenclature of the coagulation factors*

The coagulation factors are synthesised primarily in the liver, although von Willebrand factor is produced by endothelial cells and megakaryocytes. Platelets also contain some coagulation factors, viz von Willebrand factor, fibrinogen and factors V and XIII. Some factors are present in both plasma and serum, but others (eg factors V and VIII) are completely consumed during coagulation.

There are two main types of coagulation factor:

- **zymogens** which are inactive plasma proteins (proenzymes), and which, after cleavage by a specific enzyme, are themselves transformed into active enzymes. Coagulation factors which fall into this category include factors II, X, XI, XII and XIII. Most of the coagulation enzymes are **serine proteases** ie the active site of the proteolytic enzyme contains a serine residue. The single exception to this rule is activated factor XIII which, as detailed below, acts as a transglutaminase.

- accelerators which are not converted to an active enzyme during the coagulation process but act as accelerators or catalysts for other enzymatic reactions. Factors V and VIII fall into this category.

Two coagulation factors, fibrinogen and factor VII, cannot strictly be classified as either zymogens or accelerators. Fibrinogen is converted to fibrin which has no enzymatic properties, and factor VII normally circulates as an active enzyme, although as described below its activity is considerably potentiated by tissue factor. By convention, activated coagulation factors are denoted by the suffix a eg XII_a is the activated form of factor XII.

Components of the Blood Coagulation System

Fibrinogen consists of three pairs of polypeptide chains termed Aα, Bβ and γ, and has a molecular weight of 338,000. The chains are held together by inter- and intra-chain disulphide bonds as shown in Figure 21.6. The conversion of fibrinogen to fibrin is achieved by thrombin which cleaves specific arginine-glycine bonds in the N-terminal ends of the Aα and Bβ chains. During this process, small peptides, known as **fibrinopeptides A and B**, are released from the ends of the Aα and Bβ chains respectively. The presence of these

---

Key dates

1686 First separation of blood clot fibres from cells and serum

1731 Observation that clots stem blood loss

1803 Recognition of sex-linking in haemophilia

1819 First observation of the procoagulant effect of tissues (tissue factor)

1845 Recognition that fibrin formed from plasma fibrinogen

1905 Morawitz theory of blood coagulation

1926 Description of von Willebrand's disease

1935 Development of one stage prothrombin time by Quick

1935 Description of the anti-haemorrhagic properties of vitamin K

1944 Recognition that Xmas disease is distinct from haemophilia

1947 Description of serum inhibitor to tissue thromboplastin

1964 Waterfall hypothesis of coagulation proposed

1971 Use of ristocetin to diagnose vWD

1977 Purification of tissue factor

1982- **Present** Development of monoclonal antibody and molecular techniques lead to improved understanding of haemostasis

1987 Pathways of blood coagulation revised to take account of central roles of tissue factor and TFPI

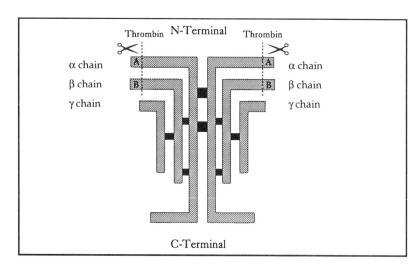

Figure 21.6 *Structure of the fibrinogen molecule*

fibrinopeptides in plasma therefore is indicative of the action of thrombin on fibrinogen. The resultant **fibrin monomers** spontaneously polymerise to form a visible fibrin polymer which subsequently is stabilised and rendered insoluble by the action of factor XIII.

Prothrombin is a single-chain zymogen which requires vitamin K for its synthesis. Prothrombin is activated by factor Xa to yield thrombin, the most potent of all the coagulation enzymes, in a reaction accelerated by factor V. Thrombin, a two-chain serine protease, is the natural coagulant of fibrinogen, but has several other important functions in haemostasis, including:

- the potentiation of the activity of factors V and VIII at low thrombin concentration

- the inhibition of the activity of factors V and VIII at high thrombin concentration

- the activation of factors XI, XIII and protein C

- the stimulation of platelet aggregation

Calcium ions are essential for most steps in the blood coagulation process, with the possible exceptions of the initiation of coagulation by a foreign surface and the initial conversion of fibrinogen to fibrin. Calcium is particularly important in the activation of factor X, prothrombin and factor XIII.

Factor V is a single-chain glycoprotein which also is found in platelets. Its main function is to accelerate the activation of prothrombin by factor X_a, in a reaction markedly accelerated by calcium ions, phospholipid and trace amounts of thrombin.

Factor VII is a member of the vitamin K-dependent group of coagulation factors. As mentioned above, factor VII circulates as an active enzyme, albeit of relatively low potency, which probably accounts for its very short plasma half-life (around 4 hours). The ability of factor VII to activate factor X is greatly increased by the presence of tissue factor.

Factor VIII, historically, is one of the most important coagulation factors. Hereditary deficiency of factor VIII, or haemophilia A, was first documented over 1700 years ago. Although the presence of factor VIII in plasma was first demonstrated in 1911, its detailed biochemical and structural characteristics have only recently been elucidated. Factor VIII circulates in plasma complexed to von Willebrand factor. Before this fact was clearly recognised, there was considerable confusion over nomenclature and understanding of the separate roles in haemostasis of these factors. These problems have now been resolved as shown in Table 21.3.

Factor	Correct Designation
Factor VIII protein	FVIII
Factor VIII procoagulant activity	FVIII Act
Factor VIII antigen	FVIIIAg
von Willebrand factor	vWF
von Willebrand factor antigen	vWFAg

Table 21.3 *Nomenclature of the components of the factor VIII complex*

The term **ristocetin cofactor** also is used to describe the attribute of vWF required for platelet aggregation by the antibiotic ristocetin. However, the use of specific terminology to indicate functional activities of vWF is not recommended. The major role of the factor VIII procoagulant is to act as an accelerator of factor X activation by factor IXa in a reaction potentiated by calcium ions, phospholipid and trace amounts of thrombin. Newly generated factor IXa forms a complex with factor VIIIa in the presence of calcium ions and phospholipid. This complex activates factor X by cleaving the same bonds that are hydrolysed by the tissue factor-factor VIIa complex (see later). The mechanism by which factor VIII functions in this process is poorly understood. It has no enzymatic activity of its own but accelerates the reaction some 200,000-fold. Factor VIII is proteolytically activated by factor Xa and thrombin to yield factor VIII_a. By analogy with factor V, it is likely that factor VIII_a accelerates the proteolysis of factor X by factor IX_a on a phospholipid surface to facilitate a conformational change that favours catalysis.

von Willebrand factor is a multimeric glycoprotein which has a dual role in haemostasis:

- vWF acts as a carrier protein for factor VIII. In this capacity, vWF protects factor VIII from degradation by proteolytic enzymes and from inactivation by activated protein C.

- vWF acts as a mediator of platelet adhesion to the subendothelium. vWF is the most important adhesive protein at high shear, mediating both platelet adhesion and thrombus formation. Its direct interaction with subendothelium results in binding to platelet GpIb followed by binding to platelet GpIIb/IIIa. Thus, vWF acts as a bridge between platelets and subendothelium (via GpIb) and between adjacent platelets (via GpIIb/IIIa).

vWF is synthesised in vascular endothelial cells and megakaryocytes as a large precursor molecule containing a signal peptide and the vWF subunit. These molecules associate to form dimers and the signal peptide is cleaved off. Further self-association produces a series of multimeric forms of vWF which have molecular weights ranging from 5×10^5 to more than 1.5×10^7. vWF is stored in the Weibel-Palade bodies of endothelial cells and the α granules of platelets. The efficient role of vWF in haemostasis is a function of its multiple localisation in platelet α granules, plasma, endothelial cells and subendothelium.

Factor IX is a vitamin K-dependent coagulation factor which is converted to its active form by factor XI_a. It may also be activated by plasma kallikrein and factor VII, and factor IX_a may also act in a feedback mechanism to activate further factor IX.

Factor X occupies an important central role in the blood coagulation cascade, being capable of activation by both intrinsic and extrinsic pathways. Whichever activation pathway is employed, the main role of factor X_a is to activate prothrombin. The mechanics of this process are described in greater detail below.

Factor XI is converted to its active form following limited cleavage by factor XII_a during contact activation of the coagulation pathway. Factor XI_a then activates factor IX, but is also capable of amplifying the enzymatic reactions by feedback activation of factor XII.

Factor XII is a single chain zymogen which is capable of being adsorbed on to a variety of negatively charged surfaces. This results in a conformational change in the molecule, increased susceptibility to cleavage by plasma kallikrein and exposure of an active site. Activated factor XII activates factor XI and also, by reciprocal proteolysis, activates further factor XII.

Factor XIII is a relatively large molecule which shows a strong affinity for fibrinogen. It is a tetrameric molecule, composed of two pairs of dissociable subunits (a_2b_2) and is activated by thrombin in the presence of calcium ions. Factor XIII functions as a transglutaminase, stabilising the fibrin clot by catalysing the formation of covalent crosslinks between the ε-amino groups of lysine and the γ-amino groups of glutamine on adjacent fibrin molecules. The crosslinking reaction requires the presence of calcium ions and occurs rapidly at the C-terminal ends of the γ chains, and somewhat more slowly between α chains leading to the formation of large, multimeric chain-like structures. The overall solubility of the fibrin is mainly dependent on the degree of α chain crosslinking.

Factor XIII is found in platelets and other tissues, for example placenta, and may also be present in blood monocytes. It may also be involved in wound healing, fibroblast proliferation and the maintenance of normal gestation.

Prekallikrein (PK) is a serine protease zymogen which is activated by factor XII_a. The active product, kallikrein, acts as a major link between the various haemostatic processes in its ability to activate the kinin, complement and fibrinolytic pathways. It is also a potent activator of surface-bound factor XII.

High molecular weight kininogen (HMWK) is a member of a family of large proteins which give rise to the production of potent vasoactive peptides called kinins. HMWK may be converted to bradykinin by kallikrein. HMWK functions in the contact activation

In 1955 a railway worker named John Hageman required surgery for a peptic ulcer but laboratory tests showed that his blood clotting time was prolonged. Further investigation revealed that he was deficient in a hitherto unknown plasma protein which was involved in contact activation of coagulation. This protein was named Hageman factor. Ten years later, several members of a family called Fletcher were shown to have similarly prolonged clotting times and to be deficient in another plasma protein involved in contact activation. This factor subsequently was called Fletcher factor. A further 10 years passed before Fitzgerald factor was discovered when a Mr Fitzgerald, being treated for gunshot wounds, was shown to have a defect of contact activation and to be deficient in the eponymous plasma protein.

All three cases, separated by 20 years, have one important facet in common: gross prolongation of laboratory clotting times but an absence of any bleeding tendency. This apparent anomaly cannot be explained by classical blood coagulation theory.

Hageman factor is now known as factor XII, Fletcher factor as prekallikrein and Fitzgerald factor as high molecular weight kininogen.

process by reversibly associating with prekallikrein and factor XI and acting as an accelerator of the activation of factor XI by surface-bound factor XIIa.

Tissue factor (TF) is the protein that accelerates blood coagulation following the addition of various tissue extracts to plasma. Under these conditions, the so-called intrinsic pathway may be bypassed. The existence of this protein has been recognised since the 1800s but has only been purified and characterised in the last 15 years. TF is a large lipoprotein complex found in a wide variety of tissues, although it is particularly concentrated in brain, lung and placenta. Functionally, the tissue distribution of TF is illuminating. It is not normally found in cells in contact with circulating blood, although blood monocytes and endothelial cells, given appropriate stimulation can synthesise TF. It is, however, selectively expressed in different tissues including epidermis, mucosal epithelium, myocardium, vascular adventitia and organ capsules. Based on its distribution, it appears that TF acts as a "haemostatic envelope" ready to rapidly activate blood coagulation in the event of blood vessel damage. Haemostasis in sensitive organs such as brain, lung and placenta is particularly vital, explaining the relatively high levels found in these tissue. As discussed in a later section TF is now held to be the major physiological initiator of coagulation. No case of congenital TF deficiency has been described and it is likely that such a condition would be incompatible with life.

Tissue factor is a single chain polypeptide which is synthesised as a cell membrane integral protein. The amino acid sequence of this protein has been determined and consists of a short (21 residues) C-terminal domain separated from a much larger amino-terminal domain by a stretch of hydrophobic residues. These areas represent the cytoplasmic, extracellular and transmembrane portions of the molecule respectively. The cytoplasmic domain has no coagulation function and is thought to be involved in cell signalling. There are no other structurally similar proteins known but it appears that TF may be a member of the cytokine receptor family, the prime function of which is to act as a receptor for plasma factor VII/VII$_a$ via sites in the extracellular domain. The regulation of TF expression on cells is complex and not fully understood. There are little or no intracellular stores of TF but rapid synthesis can be induced by a variety of cytokines including interleukins and tumour necrosis factor. The phospholipid configuration of the membrane is vital for procoagulant activity and changes in membrane state may well represent a basic mechanism for the cellular regulation of TF activity.

SAQ 3

How would severe factor XIII deficiency be likely to be manifest?

Plasma contains a specific inhibitor to TF-induced coagulation activation and the role of this protein is discussed in a later section.

The Role of Vitamin K in Blood Coagulation

The importance of vitamin K in the maintenance of normal blood coagulation has long been recognised. It is now well established that coagulation factors II, VII, IX and X as well as proteins C and S are dependent on vitamin K for their normal function. In essence, these factors are synthesised in an inactive form which cannot bind calcium ions. This ability is conferred by a post-translational modification which involves γ-carboxylation of glutamic acid residues. Vitamin K is an essential cofactor for the carboxylase enzyme responsible for the γ-carboxylation of these factors.

At the molecular level, vitamin K-dependent carboxylation involves the cyclic interconversion of reduced vitamin K and its epoxide. Thus, the carboxylation of precursors of the vitamin K-dependent coagulation factors is coupled to the epoxidation of vitamin K; the epoxide cycle being essentially a salvage pathway for this vitamin. For prothrombin, this step involves the γ-carboxylation of 10 glutamic acid residues within the preformed molecule. In the absence of vitamin K, the acarboxy forms of these factors are released into the circulation. Although they are immunologically identical to the normal proteins, these **P**roteins **I**nduced by **V**itamin **K** **A**bsence or **A**ntagonism (PIVKA) cannot bind calcium ions, and thus lose their ability to bind to phospholipid surfaces. Because of this, they are activated much more slowly than their normal counterparts and this gives rise to the anticoagulant effect, seen for example, following oral anticoagulant therapy. PIVKA also are not adsorbed on to aluminium hydroxide and barium salts; properties characteristic of the normal vitamin K-dependent coagulation factors. They can, however, be activated *in vitro* with the venom of certain snakes such as *Echis carinatus* and this property can form the basis for their laboratory measurement.

During the winter of 1921-22 herds of Canadian cattle suffered an epidemic of haemorrhagic disease which was related by Schofield, a vegetarian veterinary surgeon, to the ingestion of spoiled sweet clover. The coagulation defect was identified as prothrombin deficiency. A subsequent outbreak in the USA led a suffering farmer to persuade a Wisconsin chemist, Karl Paul Link, to investigate the problem. This led to the extraction of the agent responsible, bis-hydroxy-coumarin (dicoumarol) and its eventual use as a rat poison and oral anticoagulant for the treatment of thromboembolic disease, under the name of warfarin.

Warfarin acts by inhibiting the vitamin K-dependent carboxylation of factors II, VII, IX and X and proteins C and S, without which they are inactive.

Mechanisms of Blood Coagulation

The Classical Blood Coagulation Cascade

Classical blood coagulation theory has divided the coagulation process into the **intrinsic pathway** and the **extrinsic pathway** as shown in Figure 21.7. It remains convenient to discuss the process in these

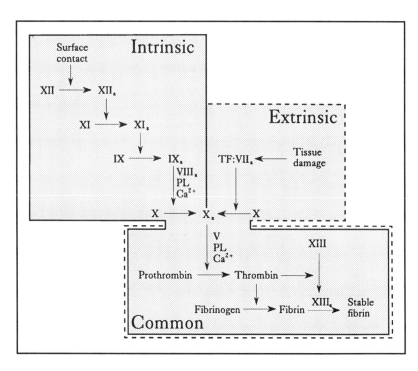

Figure 21.7 *The classical coagulation cascade illustrating the division into intrinsic, extrinsic and common pathways of coagulation. This theory ascribes the major physiological role to surface contact activation via the intrinsic pathway. PL - phospholipid surface*

terms, although it will become clear that the current concept of the coagulation cascade is rather more complex, and that these pathways are not completely independent.

The Intrinsic Pathway

Intrinsic blood coagulation is initiated by contact of the flowing blood with a foreign surface. A variety of foreign surfaces, both physiological (eg collagen, basement membranes and lipopolysaccharides) and non-physiological (eg glass, kaolin and celite) are capable of activating blood coagulation via this pathway. Surface activation plays a key role in initiating many of the component pathways of the haemostatic system (Figure 21.8), although recent evidence, discussed below, has suggested that coagulation activation via this route may be of lesser physiological importance.

Exposure of a negatively charged surface to blood causes adsorption of factor XII which then undergoes a conformational change and activates a limited amount of prekallikrein. The kallikrein so formed converts further surface-bound factor XII to its activated form (reciprocal proteolytic activation). The resultant factor XII_a then converts factor XI to XI_a. The factor XI zymogen for this reac-

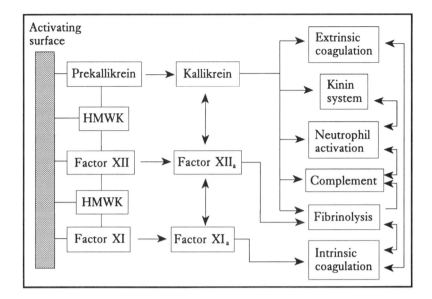

Figure 21.8 *The role of contact activation in the activation of coagulation and other pathways related to haemostasis. HMWK - high molecular weight kininogen*

tion is also bound to the activating surface, together with prekallikrein, by HMWK. This enables the major contact activation product, factor XI_a, to remain localised at the activation site, although kallikrein molecules freely dissociate into the surrounding plasma. Prekallikrein and HMWK circulate as a complex with a 1:1 molar stoichiometry. The complex binds to an activating surface, and when factor XIIa and kallikrein are generated, HMWK is digested to release the vasoactive peptide bradykinin. Surface-dependent activation of factor XII can occur in the absence of prekallikrein, albeit more slowly. In contrast, factor XII-deficient plasma does not activate on surface contact, suggesting that factor XII plays the central role and prekallikrein acts as an accelerator of this process. An important feature of the contact system is the ability of factor XII to auto-activate, ie the ability of factor XII_a to activate more factor XII zymogen. These interactions are detailed in Figure 21.9.

Factor XIa activates factor IX in a process requiring two proteolytic cleavages. Factor IX_a then forms a complex with factors VIII and X, calcium ions and phospholipid derived largely from platelet membranes, which results in the activation of factor X. This complex sometimes is referred to as the **tenase complex**. The resultant factor X_a forms a complex with factor V, prothrombin, calcium ions and phospholipid in a manner analogous to the formation of the factor X-activating complex. This complex sometimes is referred to as the

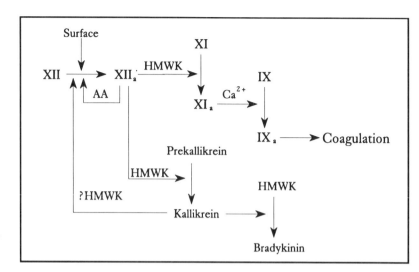

Figure 21.9 *Mechanisms of contact activation. HMWK - high molecular weight kininogen. AA - autoactivation*

prothrombinase complex. In these reactions, factors V and VIII act as accelerators, the activity of which is greatly increased by trace amounts of thrombin. However, at higher thrombin concentrations, factors V and VIII are degraded, thereby reducing the rate of reaction and slowing down the natural amplification of the process.

The prothrombinase complex converts the phospholipid-bound prothrombin to the active enzyme, **thrombin.** The primary function of thrombin is the conversion of fibrinogen to fibrin. The removal of fibrinopeptides A and B from the fibrinogen molecule reduces the overall negative charge of the molecule and allows the spontaneous polymerisation of the fibrin monomers. At this stage, however, the fibrin clot is held together by hydrophobic and electrostatic bonds alone and is therefore relatively unstable. The final stage of blood coagulation is the stabilisation of the fibrin clot by thrombin-activated factor XIII. This enzyme acts as a transglutaminase by catalysing the formation of $\varepsilon(\gamma$-glutamyl)lysine bonds between adjacent fibrin molecules.

The Extrinsic Pathway

In the presence of calcium ions, tissue factor binds both zymogen factor VII and factor VII_a with equal affinity, markedly altering the coagulant activity of these factors:

- TF-bound factor VII is rapidly converted to factor VII_a by trace amounts of factor X_a, although cleavage can also be mediated by factor IX_a, XII_a and thrombin. The activation of factor VII by factor XII_a explains the shortened activated partial thrombo-plastin times sometimes seen in plasmas exposed to cold.

•   The enzymatic activity of factor VII_a is greatly increased by complexing with TF. The resultant complex is capable of activating both factor IX and factor X. The exact sequence of events is still controversial but it is clear that TF promotes the conversion of factor VII to VII_a and then serves as a cofactor for factor VII_a in the activation of factors IX and X.

Following factor X activation, coagulation proceeds as described above. The extrinsic pathway of coagulation activation is regulated by the specific inhibitor **tissue factor pathway inhibitor** whose role is discussed in a later section.

The classical concept of blood coagulation remains convenient, particularly in the interpretation of laboratory screening tests of coagulation. However, it has become increasingly evident that such a division does not exist *in vivo* and that tissue factor is the major physiological activator of blood coagulation. In particular, the observation that subjects deficient in factor XII, high molecular weight kininogen or kallikrein do not have the expected severe bleeding disorder is difficult to explain by these means. The modern concept of the coagulation cascade is described later in this chapter.

Inhibitors of Blood Coagulation

As described above, the blood coagulation system is a multifactorial biological pathway consisting of zymogens and accelerators. Because of the natural amplification of the enzyme products of the coagulation cascade there is always a danger that the process may get out of hand and develop systemic proportions. Therefore, in order to contain the fibrin clot to the site of vessel damage the haemostatic system provides a variety of inhibitory mechanisms. The major inhibitors of the blood coagulation pathway are **antithrombin III**, **heparin cofactor II**, activated **protein C** and **tissue factor pathway inhibitor**.

Antithrombin III

Antithrombin III is a single chain glycoprotein of molecular weight 61,000. It is synthesised in the liver and endothelium. The term antithrombin is rather a misnomer; ATIII is not only the main physiological inhibitor of thrombin, but also of all the other activated serine protease coagulation enzymes (IX_a, X_a, XI_a and XII_a). The importance of ATIII in the inhibition of blood coagulation is clearly demonstrated by the high incidence of venous thrombosis in patients with congenital ATIII deficiency. ATIII reacts irreversibly with thrombin and other serine proteases to form a complex in which both components are inactivated. This reaction is greatly accelerated (about 2000-fold) by the presence of heparin and this represents the molecular basis for the anticoagulant activity of heparin. Heparin promotes the formation of a ternary complex with antithrombin and thrombin in which the active site of the protease is brought into close contact with the reactive site of antithrombin. The process of binding produces a conformational change in the ATIII molecule which further enhances heparin binding.

The reaction of heparin with ATIII is clearly of clinical significance in anticoagulant treatment. Heparin usually is absent from the vasculature and the major physiological role of ATIII must therefore be seen as regulating the generation of coagulation enzymes. However, a similar mechanism may operate *in vivo* through heparan sulphate proteoglycans present on the surfaces of endothelial cells. Because of the relationship between the presence of heparin and ATIII, the latter is sometimes known as **heparin cofactor I**.

Heparin Cofactor II

Heparin cofactor II is a single chain glycoprotein of molecular weight 65,000, which is synthesised in the liver. It complexes with thrombin in a 1:1 stoichiometric ratio, thereby inactivating the protease. In contrast to ATIII, heparin cofactor II is specific for thrombin, having no inhibitory activity against the other serine proteases. The activity of heparin cofactor II is amplified 1000-fold by the presence of heparin.

The Protein C Inhibitor Pathway

Four components are involved in the protein C inhibitor pathway;

- protein C

- thrombomodulin

- protein S

- C4b binding protein

There is also at least one specific inhibitor of this pathway.

Protein C

Protein C is one of the more recently discovered of the vitamin K-dependent haemostatic proteins. It is a two chain molecule of molecular weight 62,000. The light chain has a molecular weight of 22,000 and carries the γ-carboxylated glutamyl residues while the heavy chain has a molecular weight of 40,000 and carries the active serine site. Protein C plays a dual role in haemostasis by inhibiting blood coagulation on the one hand and stimulating fibrinolysis on the other. Activation of protein C occurs when the heavy chain is cleaved by thrombin, in the presence of calcium ions, exposing the active site. In the absence of thrombomodulin, protein C is activated only slowly.

Thrombomodulin

Thrombomodulin has a molecular weight of 68,000 and is present in tight association with vascular endothelium. As its name suggests, thrombomodulin complexes with thrombin in a 1:1 stoichiometric ratio and modulates its activity in two ways:

- when complexed with thrombomodulin, thrombin is capable of activating protein C several thousand times faster than in the uncomplexed state

- complexed thrombin does not clot fibrinogen, activate factors V and VIII or aggregate platelets

Thrombomodulin-bound thrombin can, however, still be inhibited by antithrombin III. Activation of protein C involves the formation

Factor	Activator	Cofactor
Factor X	Factor IX_a	Factor VIII
Factor X	Factor VII_a	Tissue Factor
Prothrombin	Factor X_a	Factor V
Protein C	Thrombin	Thrombomodulin

Table 21.4 *Activation of the vitamin K-dependent coagulation factors*

of a complex with thrombomodulin, thrombin and calcium ions in a process analogous to the activation of the other vitamin K-dependent coagulation factors (Table 21.4).

Protein S

Protein S is a single chain glycoprotein of molecular weight 69,000 which is synthesised in the liver and by endothelial cells. It is a vitamin K-dependent protein but, unlike protein C, is not a serine protease. Activated protein C, in the presence of calcium ions, forms a complex with protein S, which is present on endothelium, platelets and possibly other cells. Activated protein C inhibits the coagulation cascade by inactivating factor VIII_a and factor V_a. This process is greatly amplified by complex formation with protein S. As factors V_a and VIII_a act as accelerators earlier in the coagulation process, their inactivation has the effect of reducing the rate of thrombin generation.

C4b Binding Protein

Normally, about 60% of the circulating protein S is bound to C4b-binding protein and is therefore unavailable for complexing with protein C.

The protein C inhibitor pathway may be altered by disease states in several ways. Levels of protein C and S are dependent on vitamin K for their synthesis. They therefore tend to decrease together with factors II, VII, IX and X in conditions of vitamin K absence or antagonism, thus maintaining the balance between procoagulant and anticoagulant effects. However, in major inflammatory events especially, agents such as interleukins, tumour necrosis factor and endotoxin may suppress the expression of thrombomodulin on the endothelial cell surface and the plasma concentration of C4b binding protein rises leading to a reduction in free protein S concentra-

Protein C derives its name from the chromatographic separation of the vitamin K-dependent factors from plasma. Using this method, 4 peaks are obtained, and these are labelled A, B, C and D. Protein C is the major constituent of the third peak.

Protein S is named after the city of its discovery, Seattle.

SAQ 4

How would a deficiency of protein S be manifest?

tion. Coupled with the production of tissue factor stimulated by the same agents, this may give rise to a marked procoagulant state.

Tissue Factor Pathway Inhibitor

The existence of an inhibitor of tissue factor was suggested by the early observation that the procoagulant activity of tissue extracts could be inhibited by serum. It is now known that plasma contains an inhibitor which binds and inhibits factor X_a directly. This inhibitor is now known as tissue factor pathway inhibitor (TFPI) although in older literature it is also referred to as extrinsic pathway inhibitor (EPI) and lipoprotein-associated coagulation inhibitor (LACI).

In plasma, TFPI circulates bound to lipoproteins, mainly the low density type. Platelets contain about 10% of the blood pool of TFPI and this can be released by thrombin stimulation. Plasma TFPI levels increase 2-4-fold during heparin infusion. This additional TFPI appears to be bound to heparan sulphate and similar molecules on the surface of endothelial cells, the site of synthesis of this inhibitor. The liver does not appear to contribute significantly to the synthesis of TFPI.

TFPI binds to factor X_a and inhibits its activity. The TFPI-factor X_a complex then binds to the tissue factor-factor VII_a complex thereby inhibiting its proteolytic activity as shown in Figure 21.10. Artificially induced TFPI deficiency has been shown to greatly increase susceptibility to TF-induced coagulopathy. The central importance of this coagulation inhibitor is suggested by the fact that no cases of congenital deficiency of TFPI have been described.

Current Concept of the Coagulation Cascade

The relatively recent discovery of tissue factor pathway inhibitor coupled with the need to explain the lack of a bleeding tendency in factor XII deficient subjects and the severe bleeding tendency in haemophiliacs has given rise to the revised scheme of blood coagulation shown in Figure 21.10.

In this scheme, coagulation is initiated when factor VII or VII_a in flowing blood comes into contact with tissue factor constitutively expressed by subendothelial cells exposed at sites of vascular dam-

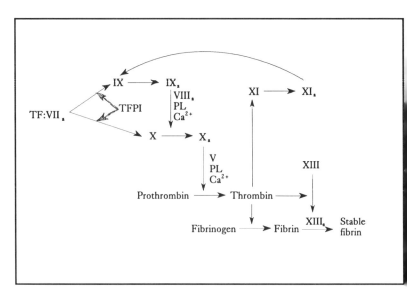

Figure 21.10 *A simplified overview of the modern concept of coagulation. The inhibitory action of TFPI is shown in grey*

age. Factor VII binds to TF where it is rapidly activated to factor VII_a. The resultant TF-VII_a complex activates some factor X to X_a and some factor IX to IX_a. The generation of factor X_a results in the intervention of TFPI which binds factor X_a and then forms a quaternary complex with factor VII_a and TF, effectively blocking further factor X_a generation through this route. Subsequently, additional factor X_a can only be generated through the action of factor IX_a on factor X. This process is still thought to occur via complex formation as described above. Once the initial factor IX_a generated by the action of TF-VII_a has been exhausted, supplemental factor IX_a is supplied by the action of factor XI_a. Factor XI, now placed at the terminal end of the coagulation cascade is activated by thrombin. Contact activation via factor XII, prekallikrein and HMW kininogen plays no role in this model of the coagulation cascade. It is likely that the importance of these factors lies in orchestrating other inflammatory responses such as Complement, kinin and fibrinolytic activation.

In this way, TFPI-mediated feedback inhibition of the TF-factor VII_a complex explains the clinical importance of both "intrinsic" and "extrinsic" coagulation factors. Further, it appears that the tissue factor-factor VII pathway is responsible for the rapid generation of thrombin sufficient to cause localised platelet aggregation and activation of the critical cofactors factor V and factor VIII. Continuing haemostasis, however, certainly requires ongoing generation of factor X_a through the actions of factors VIII and IX, thereby explaining the clinical importance of these coagulation factors.

The Fibrinolytic System

The major function of the fibrinolytic system is the degradation and dissolution of formed fibrin within the circulation. The enzyme responsible for this activity, **plasmin**, has been recognised for over 40 years, but the normal, physiological role of the fibrinolytic pathway remains to be accurately defined. It has been widely assumed that fibrinolysis is required to degrade small quantities of fibrin which are continually being deposited within the circulation, and is therefore the body's first line of defence against thrombosis. Although the evidence for this hypothesis remains equivocal, it is widely held that there is a balance between the coagulation and fibrinolytic pathways *in vivo*.

As shown in Figure 21.11, the fibrinolytic system has four main components:

- plasminogen activators

- plasminogen

- plasmin

- fibrinolytic inhibitors

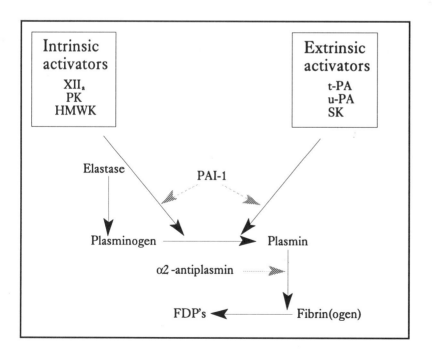

Figure 21.11 *The fibrinolytic system. Inhibitory pathways are shown in grey*

Plasminogen activation may occur via an intrinsic pathway, possibly mediated by components of contact activation or via an extrinsic mechanism involving activators released from the blood vessel wall. Plasminogen activators are present in many different human and animal tissues and secretions. The plasminogen activator found in blood appears to represent vascular activator which has been released from the vessel wall. This form is known as **tissue-type plasminogen activator (t-PA)**. The other major type of activator is found predominantly in urine and is known as **urokinase-type plasminogen activator (u-PA)**.

Plasminogen Activators

Tissue Plasminogen Activator

Tissue plasminogen activator has a molecular weight of 70,000 and its N-terminal region is composed of several domains which have structural similarities with other proteins, eg fibronectin, human epidermal growth factor precursor and plasminogen. It functions as a serine protease whose main physiological function is to cleave a specific arginine-valine bond in the plasminogen molecule. However, the important property which distinguishes t-PA from u-PA is the former's strong affinity for fibrin. In the absence of fibrin, t-PA activates plasminogen relatively slowly. For example, at physiological plasminogen concentrations, one molecule of t-PA takes approximately 30 minutes to activate one molecule of plasminogen. In the presence of fibrin, however, this process may take less than five seconds. Fibrin accelerates plasminogen activation by increasing the affinity of plasminogen for fibrin-bound t-PA rather than by enhancing the enzymatic activity of the activator.

This property ensures that fibrinolysis is mainly localised to the fibrin clot where the specific binding of t-PA results in a complex which has high affinity for circulating plasminogen. Locally-generated plasmin is then free to digest the fibrin with relatively little interference from circulating fibrinolytic inhibitors which ensures rapid and specific fibrinolysis with minimal degradation of circulating fibrinogen or other coagulation factors.

t-PA is synthesised and stored by vascular endothelial cells, ready for release into the bloodstream when required. Various stimuli can elicit release of t-PA including prolonged strenuous exercise, venous occlusion, thrombin and the vasoactive peptide DDAVP.

Urokinase-type Plasminogen Activator

Urokinase (u-PA) is a trypsin-like protease which is synthesised in the kidney and hence is found mainly in urine. It occurs in both single-chain (scu-PA, prourokinase) and two-chain (tcu-PA) forms, although scu-PA is a much weaker activator of plasminogen. Urokinase converts plasminogen directly to plasmin in a reaction which does not require the presence of fibrin. u-PA and t-PA may be distinguished immunologically and on the basis of functional assays with and without added fibrin.

Plasminogen and Plasmin

Plasminogen is a single-chain glycoprotein with a molecular weight of about 92,000. The molecule contains five homologous triple loop structures known as **kringles**. These loops contain lysine binding sites, which mediate interaction with fibrin and fibrinogen via lysine residues in the substrate molecule. Fibrinolytic inhibitors also bind to plasminogen via these lysine binding sites. Prior to activation, the N-terminal amino acid of the plasminogen molecule is a glutamic acid. This form is known as **glu-plasminogen**.

Physiological activators of glu-plasminogen act by cleaving a specific arginine-valine bond, forming a two chain molecule of **glu-plasmin**. This form of plasmin is inert because the lysine binding sites, which reside on the heavy chain, remain hidden and unable to bind to fibrin. The serine centre of plasmin resides on the light chain. Glu-plasmin subsequently undergoes a further cleavage at a specific lysine-lysine bond which results in the loss of 76 amino acids (the pre-activation peptide) from the N-terminal end of the heavy chain. The resulting molecule has a lysine residue at its N-terminal end and is known as **lys-plasmin**. This form of plasmin has a strong affinity for fibrin and therefore is the physiologically active form.

Both forms of plasmin attack glu-plasminogen and remove the pre-activation peptide, resulting in the formation of **lys-plasminogen**. The strong affinity for fibrin of the lys- forms of plasminogen and plasmin also helps to localise fibrinolysis to the site of clot formation.

Inhibitors of Fibrinolysis

As with the coagulation system, uninhibited proteolytic activity is potentially dangerous, and the fibrinolytic pathway is similarly

In addition to the physiological activators of fibrinolysis, a number of exogenous activators exist. For example, streptokinase is derived from β haemolytic streptococci and has been used as a therapeutic agent for the treatment of established thrombi for many years. However, streptokinase therapy is difficult to control and complicated by the antigenicity of bacterial products. It is likely to be superseded by genetically engineered tissue plasminogen activator, although currently this is extremely expensive.

equipped with inhibitory mechanisms. The major physiological inhibitor of plasmin is α2-antiplasmin; enzyme activity which exceeds the capacity of this inhibitor is neutralised by the high molecular weight plasma protein α2-macroglobulin or **histidine-rich glycoprotein**. Inhibition of fibrinolysis is also mediated by inhibition of plasminogen activators via **plasminogen activator inhibitor 1 (PAI-1)** and **plasminogen activator inhibitor 2 (PAI-2)**.

α2-antiplasmin is a single-chain glycoprotein of molecular weight 70,000 which is synthesised in the liver. This inhibitor circulates in an inactive form until attacked by plasmin, whereupon lysine binding sites are exposed. Activated α2-antiplasmin inhibits fibrinolysis in two ways:

- by forming a 1:1 stoichiometric complex with plasmin, thereby destroying its proteolytic activity

- by binding to plasminogen and fibrin, via its lysine binding sites, thereby inhibiting binding of plasminogen to those same sites

α2-macroglobulin is an inhibitor that reacts more slowly with plasmin, but over a longer period can inactivate a greater amount of enzyme. It acts by forming a 1:1 stoichiometric complex with plasmin which retains minimal proteolytic activity but is removed rapidly by the liver.

Histidine-rich glycoprotein has a molecular weight of 75,000 and inhibits fibrinolysis by occupying the lysine binding sites of plasminogen.

Multiple mechanisms are involved in the inhibition of t-PA in plasma. Plasminogen activator inhibitor-1 (PAI-1) is a specific, rapid-acting inhibitor, and is the primary inhibitor of t-PA and u-PA in plasma. It has a molecular weight of 52,000 and is synthesised by endothelial cells and megakaryocytes. PAI-1 reacts with both single and two-chain t-PA and with tcu-PA, but not with scu-PA or the exogenous plasminogen activator streptokinase. PAI-1 is released from platelet α-granules during platelet activation resulting in a 10-fold increase in plasma levels. PAI-2 inhibits tcu-PA, although less efficiently than PAI-1 but, similarly, does not affect scu-PA.

Mechanisms of Fibrinolysis

Fibrinolysis may be activated by several mechanisms which are closely linked to the activation of the coagulation pathway. Tissue plasminogen activator, released from the vessel wall, binds to newly formed fibrin along with the fibrinolytic zymogen, plasminogen. Thus, the fibrin clot is produced already equipped with the mechanisms for its own dissolution. Plasminogen may also be activated by kallikrein and factor XIa, providing further links with the intrinsic coagulation system. Plasminogen activation may be accelerated by leucocytes; a mechanism which may have particular relevance *in vivo*.

Irrespective of the pathway involved, plasminogen activation results in the generation of plasmin. The main physiological target of this highly potent serine protease is fibrin but, if its action remains unchecked, plasmin will also cleave intact fibrinogen and other coagulation proteins.

The degradation of a fibrin clot begins with the cleavage of a number of peptides from the C-terminal end of the α chains and one from the N-terminal end of the Bβ chain. This removes approximately 20% of the original molecule, leaving a fragment known as **fragment X** as shown in Figure 21.12. Further proteolysis of this fragment may yield a variety of intermediate-sized fragments of molecular weight 100-200,000, but under physiological conditions, degradation of fragment X leaves the smaller **fragment Y**, while the remaining portion is termed **fragment D**. Further plasmin cleavage of fragment Y results in the generation of **fragment E** and a second fragment D. These fragments, known as **fibrin degradation products (FDP)** are easily measured in plasma or urine and are indicative of the activation of the coagulation and fibrinolytic pathways. The exact structure of FDP vary according to whether the substrate for plasmin action is fibrinogen, non-crosslinked fibrin or factor XIII-stabilised fibrin. In particular, plasmin degradation of cross-linked fibrin yields a unique fragment known as **D-dimer** comprising a pair of D-fragments from adjacent fibrin molecules. The development of specific monoclonal antibodies has made it possible to distinguish accurately between fibrin- and fibrinogen-derived degradation products.

SAQ 5

How would a deficiency of $\alpha 2$ antiplasmin be likely to be manifest?

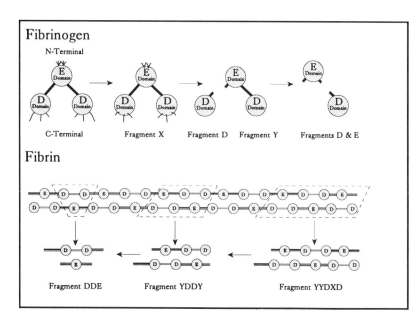

Figure 21.12 *Formation of fibrin (ogen) degradation products caused by the stepwise degradation of fibrin or fibrinogen by plasmin*

Role of Blood Cells in Haemostasis

The major contribution of the cellular components of blood is that of the platelets as described above. However, the plasma haemostatic factors come into contact with a variety of other cell types and it would be surprising if some of these did not also play a role in the haemostatic process.

Blood monocytes and tissue macrophages are capable of expressing tissue factor and thereby creating or enhancing a prothrombotic state. TF expression by monocytes requires *de novo* synthesis of the protein and it appears that cooperation by other cells, mainly platelets and T-helper lymphocytes, are required in this process. Increased monocyte expression of TF may be observed in, for example, cancer and sepsis, and appears to contribute to the coagulation activation in such conditions. Endothelial cells may also express TF although these two cell types respond differently to stimuli suggesting that different cellular regulatory mechanisms exist.

Neutrophils contain a variety of hydrolytic enzymes and are closely involved with the inflammatory response to injury. Among the many enzymes produced by the neutrophil, **elastase** has been the best studied with regard to its interactions with haemostatic pathways and has been shown to exert several effects:

- cleavage of many of the coagulation proteins, especially fibrinogen, reducing their ability to participate in normal coagulation

- cleavage of glycoproteins Ib and IIb/IIIa from the platelet membrane, thereby inhibiting platelet function

- modification of the plasminogen molecule to make it more readily activated by plasminogen activators

- inactivation of plasminogen/plasmin inhibitors

Interestingly, a significant proportion of neutrophil elastase release is mediated by kallikrein, providing a link between this and other aspects of the contact-mediated inflammatory response as shown in Figure 21.8. Other neutrophil enzymes such as the **cathepsins** may have additional effects and all these pathways may be important in regulating haemostasis at the local (wound) level.

Haemostasis is a complex process, in which several distinct but closely related biological systems act together to limit blood loss and aid tissue repair following injury. Although this review has been limited to a brief overview of the procoagulant, anticoagulant and fibrinolytic systems, it should be remembered that these pathways are closely linked to the inflammatory response and must therefore be regarded as relative to events at the tissue, vascular, platelet and leucocyte level.

Suggested Further Reading

Bloom, A.L. and Thomas D.P. (eds) (1987). *Haemostasis and Thrombosis.* (2nd ed).Edinburgh: Churchill Livingstone.

Broze, G.J. Jr. (1992). The role of tissue factor pathway inhibitor in a revised hypothesis coagulation cascade, *Seminars in Haematology,* **2:** 72-77.

Francis, J.L. (ed.) (1988). *Fibrinogen, Fibrin Stabilisation and Fibrinolysis.* Chichester: Ellis Horwood.

Answers to Self Assessment Questions

1. Küpffer cells are derived from blood monocytes.

2. Megakaryocytes undergo asynchronous endomitotic replication. Mature (platelet producing) megakaryocytes may have up to 64n chromosomal complement.

3. Factor XIII is responsible for stabilising pre-formed fibrin clots. Thus, factor XIII deficient subjects stop bleeding normally but, because the clots formed are friable, have a tendency to bleed recurrently from a single wound.

4. Protein S is an important inhibitor of coagulation. Thus deficiency of protein S is manifest as a tendency to thrombosis, often at a very young age.

5. $\alpha 2$ antiplasmin acts as an inhibitor of fibrinolysis. In its absence, therefore, fibrinolysis is unrestrained and a bleeding tendency develops.

Hereditary Disorders of Haemostasis

As described in the previous chapter, optimal haemostasis requires the interaction of numerous components of the blood vessel wall, platelets, coagulation system and the fibrinolytic system. Defects affecting any of these mechanisms can predispose to a haemorrhagic or thrombotic diathesis. This chapter deals exclusively with hereditary defects which predispose to haemorrhage or thrombosis. The acquired disorders of haemostasis are discussed in the next chapter.

Inherited Haemorrhagic Disorders

The haemostatic mechanism can be thought of as a dynamic equilibrium between clot-promoting or coagulant activities and clot-preventing or anticoagulant activities. A haemorrhagic diathesis results from any alteration in the haemostatic balance which either impairs clot promoting activities or potentiates clot prevention. A variety of such defects exist including:

- structural defects of the vascular system, resulting in easy disruption

- quantitative (thrombocytopaenia) or qualitative (thrombopathy) defects of platelets, resulting in impaired platelet plug formation

- deficiency or dysfunction of coagulation factors (coagulopathy), resulting in impaired clot formation

- deficiency or dysfunction of fibrinolytic inhibitors, resulting in hyperfibrinolysis

The fact that coagulation of the blood is an important prerequisite to the cessation of bleeding has been recognised for centuries. However, the nature of the processes involved in the stimulation remained a complete mystery until relatively recently. The ancient Greek philosopher Plato suggested that blood contained solid fibres which were dormant at body temperature but which triggered rapid coagulation when cooled. The innovative microscopist Malpighi apparently confirmed the presence of these fibres when, in 1666, he examined the fibrin meshwork of newly-formed clots. Other theories which have enjoyed some prominence include the suggestions that coagulation is triggered by exposure to air, rough surfaces, stasis and acidity. Even with the benefit of modern methods of investigation, many of the mysteries surrounding haemostasis remain.

Inherited Structural Defects of the Vascular System

Hereditary Haemorrhagic Telangiectasia

Hereditary haemorrhagic telangiectasia (HHT), also known as **Osler-Rendu-Weber syndrome**, is inherited as an autosomal dominant condition and is characterised by a defect of angiogenesis which results in the widespread formation of malformed, thin-walled capillaries which are highly susceptible to rupture. These tiny malformations, known as **telangiectases**, are most obvious as bright red lesions around the borders of the tongue, on the lips and on the nose but they occur throughout the body. HHT typically presents few problems until adolescence or early adulthood by which time the progressive enlargement of the telangiectases which occurs with increasing age may lead to recurrent epistaxis or occult gastrointestinal blood loss with concurrent iron deficiency. In some cases, enlargement and coalescence of telangiectases leads to the formation of pulmonary or cerebral arteriovenous fistulae which may be life-threatening. No treatment is available for HHT other than correction of the recurrent anaemia and cautery of troublesome bleeding points.

Ehlers-Danlos Syndrome

Ehlers-Danlos syndrome embodies a heterogeneous group of collagen disorders which are characterised by extreme elasticity of the skin, which often can be drawn out from the body for several inches, skin fragility, hypermobility of the joints and a bruising or bleeding tendency. In the most serious variant of this disorder, type III collagen, the form which predominates in blood vessels, is deficient. This leads to a liability to acute and severe internal bleeding or sudden death secondary to arterial rupture. Other sequelae include recurrent joint problems and scarring of the face and weight-bearing joints such as elbows and knees.

Kasabach-Merritt Syndrome

A **haemangioma** is a benign tumour of vascular tissue which may grow rapidly to giant proportions and threaten the function of neighbouring tissues. Because of their highly vascular nature, mechanical injury to haemangiomas may result in severe bleeding.

Further, abnormalities of the vascular endothelium within these massive tumours may trigger a localised DIC with thrombocytopaenia and consumption coagulopathy, thereby worsening the bleeding tendency. Strictly, the term Kasabach-Merritt syndrome relates to the presence of localised DIC in a giant, cavernous haemangioma. Treatment of haemangiomas involves surgical removal, if possible, or localised radiotherapy to induce tumour regression coupled with injection of fibrinolytic inhibitors to promote occlusive thromboses within the tumour.

Inherited Defects of Platelets

A deficiency of the contribution of platelets to the prevention of haemorrhage may be caused by severe thrombocytopaenia or defective platelet function. The inherited aplastic anaemias and thrombocytopaenias are described in Chapter 20 and will not be discussed further here.

Inherited Thrombopathies

The clinical manifestations of congenital platelet disorders all follow a similar pattern. Most commonly, these consist of easy bruising, petechial rash, mucous membrane bleeding (epistaxis, gastro-intestinal bleeding, menorrhagia) or excessive bleeding following minor trauma. The severity of these symptoms varies from a severe, life-long haemorrhagic diathesis to a much milder condition, depending upon the nature of the defect. The standard panel of laboratory investigations shown in Table 22.1 can differentiate between most of the congenital platelet abnormalities.

Bernard-Soulier Disease

Bernard-Soulier disease (BSD) is a rare, autosomal recessive trait which is characterised by the presence of giant platelets, variable thrombocytopaenia, impairment of vWF-mediated platelet adhesion, prolonged bleeding time and a bleeding tendency of variable severity. The first case of Bernard-Soulier disease was reported in 1948 by two French physicians, Jean Bernard and Jean-Pierre Soulier, in a 5 month old child with recurrent haemorrhagic problems.

Bernard-Soulier platelets are deficient in platelet membrane glycoproteins Ib, IX and V (GPIb, GPIX and GPV). GPIb is a two-chain

Petechiae are pin-point haemorrhages which represent blood which has leaked from intact capillaries because of increased vascular permeability or failure of platelet function. Petechiae typically occur in clusters.

Purpura describes the appearance of confluent patches of petechiae.

Ecchymoses, are commonly known as bruises and represent larger amounts of extravasated blood under the skin.

A **haematoma** is a large ecchymosis which involves subcutaneous tissue or muscle, producing localised swelling and deformity.

Haemarthrosis describes haemorrhage into a joint.

Disorder	Platelet Morphology	Bleeding Time	ADP	Epinephrine	Aggregation with Collagen	Ristocetin	Arachidonate	Platelet Nucleotides
Glanzmann's thrombasthenia	Normal	Prolonged	Absent 1° and 2° aggregation	Absent or markedly reduced	Absent	Normal	Reduced	Normal
Bernard-Soulier syndrome	Large platelets present	Prolonged	Normal	Normal	Normal	Reduced	Normal	Normal
δ-storage pool disease	Normal size dense granules deficient	Usually Prolonged	Deficient 2° aggregation	Reduced	Reduced	Normal	Normal	Normal
α-storage pool disease	Large platelets α granules deficient	Usually normal	Normal/ reduced	Normal/ reduced	Normal/ reduced	Normal	Normal	Normal
von Willebrand's disease	Normal	Usually Prolonged	Normal	Normal	Normal	Reduced	Normal	Normal
Aspirin defect	Normal	Usually prolonged	Deficient 2° aggregation	Reduced	Reduced	Normal	Absent or markedly reduced	Reduced ADP:ATP ratio

Table 22.1 *Investigation of the inherited thrombopathies*

molecule composed of a heavy chain of molecular weight 145,000, designated Ibα, and a light chain of molecular weight 22,000, designated Ibβ, which probably are encoded by separate autosomal genes. GPIb acts as a binding site for vWF and thrombin. GPIX, which has a molecular weight of 18,000, exists on the platelet membrane in non-covalent association with GPIb. GPV has a molecular weight of 82,000 and is thought to mediate the interaction between platelets and thrombin, although it does not function as a thrombin receptor. GPV appears to be loosely associated with the GPIb:GPIX complex. It is thought that the assembly of a stable GPIb:GPIX:GPV complex requires the presence of all of the component parts and that deficiency of any component leads to a secondary deficiency of the complete complex as occurs in Bernard-Soulier disease. A number of secondary defects exist in the platelets of Bernard-Soulier disease including a shortened platelet lifespan, impaired adhesion to vascular endothelium, hypertrophy of the surface-connected canalicular and dense tubular systems and an increase in the number of dense granules.

Recognition of BSD requires the demonstration of the characteristic platelet aggregation pattern of an impaired response to ristocetin with a normal response to other agonists, a pattern which also is typical of von Willebrand's disease. BSD can be differentiated from von Willebrand's disease by measuring the platelet aggregation response to ristocetin following the addition of a small amount of normal, platelet-poor plasma. A normal aggregation response suggests the presence of a plasma defect which is typical of von Willebrand's disease, whereas the persistence of the defective response suggests the presence of a platelet defect which is typical of BSD.

There is no specific curative treatment for BSD. Supportive therapy includes red cell transfusions to combat anaemia, hormonal control of ovulation to minimise menorrhagia and platelet transfusions when required by acute bleeding. Generally, platelet transfusions are kept to an absolute minimum because of the danger of alloantibody stimulation to the deficient platelet glycoproteins.

Pseudo von Willebrand's Disease

Pseudo von Willebrand's disease (pseudo vWD) is inherited as an autosomal dominant condition and is characterised by mild thrombocytopaenia, moderately reduced vWF concentration due to a selective deficiency of higher multimers, increased sensitivity to ristocetin and a prolonged bleeding time. Platelet-derived vWF has a normal structure. Pseudo vWD is thought to be caused by an abnormality of the platelet GPIb:GPIX:GPV complex which results in an increased avidity for higher multimers of vWF. Subsequent removal of these abnormal platelets from the circulation also selectively removes the higher multimers of vWF. The exact structural abnormality of the platelet GPIb:GPIX:GPV complex has not been identified.

Glanzmann's Thrombasthenia

Glanzmann's thrombasthenia is inherited as an autosomal recessive trait and is characterised by a normal platelet count and morphology, impairment or absence of clot retraction, absence of aggregation responses to virtually all agonists except ristocetin and a profound deficiency or defect of the platelet membrane glycoprotein GPIIb:GPIIIa complex. GPIIb exists as a 2-chain molecule composed of a heavy chain, designated IIbα, of molecular weight 120,000 and a light chain, designated IIbβ of molecular weight 23,000. GPIIIa is a single-chain molecule of molecular weight 110,000. The GPIIb:GPIIIa complex exists as a calcium-dependent dissociable complex which, following platelet activation, mediates aggregation responses by functioning as a surface receptor for fibrinogen, fibronectin, vWF and vitronectin. The GPIIb:GPIIIa complex in Glanzmann's thrombasthenia is incapable of binding fibrinogen and vWF, resulting in the near absence of aggregation responses. Although Glanzmann's thrombasthenia is a very uncommon disorder it is one of the most frequently encountered inherited qualitative platelet defects.

δ-Storage Pool Disease

δ-storage pool disease (δ-SPD) is inherited in an autosomal dominant fashion and typically is associated with relatively mild clinical features. Characteristic findings include an absence of secondary wave platelet aggregation following exposure to ADP or epinephrine, a reduced or absent aggregation response to collagen and a normal aggregation response to arachidonic acid. δ-SPD is caused by a deficiency of platelet dense granules with a consequent decrease in platelet ADP and serotonin concentration. As well as being a primary finding, δ-SPD has been described in association with a variety of other disorders such as **Hermansky-Pudlak syndrome, Chediak-Steinbrink-Higashi syndrome, Wiskott-Aldrich syndrome** and **thrombocytopaenia with absent radii syndrome.**

Adhesion between cells and various substrates is mediated by adhesion molecules such as the ICAMs (intercellular adhesion molecules eg fibrinogen) and SAMs (substrate adhesion molecules eg vWF). These and virtually all adhesive molecules contain the amino acid sequence arginine-glycine-aspartic acid which is known as the **RGD triptych** and functions as the recognition site for a large family of receptors known as the **integrins**. The platelet GPIIb:GPIIIa complex is a member of the integrin receptor family.

Grey Platelet Syndrome (α-SPD)

The grey platelet syndrome, or α-SPD, is a rare autosomal dominant disorder which is characterised by clinically mild disease and a profound deficiency of platelet α granules. The term grey platelet syndrome arises from the appearance of the platelets when stained with Romanowsky dyes and viewed by light microscopy: the absence of granulation results in a uniform grey appearance. Deficiency of α granules obviously causes a deficiency of α granule constituents such as platelet factor 4, β thromboglobulin and thrombospondin and a secondary increase in their plasma concentrations secondary to failure of incorporation.

Some SPD cases exhibit a combined deficiency of both α granules and dense bodies. Interestingly, the bleeding tendency in these αδ-SPD cases is no more severe than in δ-SPD or α-SPD alone.

Cyclo-oxygenase and Thromboxane Synthetase Deficiencies

Although very rare, deficiencies of both cyclo-oxygenase and thromboxane synthetase have been described. Differentiation between these two disorders can be made by measuring the platelet aggregation responses to the prostaglandin endoperoxides PGG_2 and PGH_2. As shown in Figure 22.1, the presence of these endoperoxides can bypass a cyclo-oxygenase deficiency, resulting in platelet aggregation but cannot prompt such a response if thromboxane synthetase is deficient. Distinguishing between true cyclo-oxygenase deficiency and that which is secondary to aspirin ingestion represents a major diagnostic challenge. Both cyclo-oxygenase and thromboxane synthetase deficiencies appear to be associated with a relatively mild bleeding tendency.

Defective Arachidonic Acid Mobilisation

A few cases have been described of defective release of arachidonic acid from membrane-bound phospholipids. Thromboxane A_2 production in these individuals in response to ADP or thrombin is reduced but normal in response to arachidonic acid, suggesting that the defect lies in the liberation of arachidonic acid and not in its subsequent catabolism.

Miscellaneous Congenital Platelet Disorders

Many reproducible but poorly defined congenital platelet defects have been reported. A heterogeneous group of patients appear to have a defective response to weak agonists such as adrenaline, ADP and platelet activating factor (PAF) but normal responses to the stronger agonists thrombin and collagen. Other defects reported include a reduced response to the calcium ionophore A23187 and thromboxane A_2. Another poorly defined group of deficiencies are associated with abnormal interaction of platelets with the coagulation system. Formation of the prothrombinase complex involves the interaction of the platelet surface with the clotting factors X, V and prothrombin. The platelet factor 3 availability test is probably still the only method of screening for this type of abnormality. Better characterisation of these defects must await the development of more sensitive diagnostic tools.

Inherited Coagulopathies

The inherited coagulopathies are rare, with an overall incidence of about 2 in 10,000 of the population. Despite their comparative rarity, disorders such as haemophilia are both scientifically and clinically important. Much of our current knowledge of the physiology of coagulation has been derived by studying the pathophysiology of cases of isolated coagulation factor deficiency. Haemophilia, in the absence of early recognition and treatment, is a highly disabling condition.

von Willebrand's Disease

As described in the previous chapter, von Willebrand factor (vWF) and coagulation factor VIII normally circulate in plasma as a non-covalently bound complex. Formation of this complex is essential for the survival of factor VIII in plasma. There are two inherited disorders associated with an abnormality or deficiency in a component of this complex, von Willebrand's disease (vWD) which is caused by a deficiency or defect of vWF and haemophilia A which is caused by a deficiency or defect or factor VIII.

Von Willebrand's disease probably is the most common inherited haemorrhagic disorder with a worldwide distribution and a particularly high incidence in the Scandinavian countries. It was first described in a five year old Finnish girl by Eric von Willebrand in 1926 and, at that time, was thought to be either a platelet or a vascular defect. However, in 1953, a deficiency of factor VIII was demon-

> Von Willebrand's disease was first described in 1926 as an apparently inherited haemorrhagic condition in several members of a Finnish family from the Aland Islands in the Gulf of Bothnia. This new condition was readily distinguished from haemophilia by the presence of a prolonged bleeding time test. Von Willebrand suspected that the condition which he named pseudohaemophilia but later came to bear his name was a disorder of platelet function. The true nature of von Willebrand's disease is only now becoming clear.

strated in vWD and four years later it was shown that the addition of normal plasma could correct the haemostatic defect. Later, in 1971, Zimmerman *et al* discovered that an antigen related to the factor VIII complex, and hence termed **factor VIII related antigen, VIIIRag,** was deficient in vWD. In the same year, detection of vWD was further facilitated by the observation by Howard and Firkin that **ristocetin,** an antibiotic isolated from *Nocardia lurida* triggered platelet aggregation in the presence of vWF but not in its absence.

The prevalence of vWD in the general population has been estimated as between 8 and 10 cases per 1,000 in the population, but it is possible that this is an underestimate since very mild cases may never be detected.

Classification of vWD

Early attempts to classify vWD were complicated by the extreme variability of the clinical severity and the results of laboratory investigations observed in affected individuals. However, the discovery that vWF normally exists in plasma in a series of multimeric forms, and the development of sensitive techniques for multimeric analysis, provided the first steps in the ongoing process of unravelling the heterogeneity of vWD. Briefly, in normal human plasma vWF consists of an aggregate of 250kDa subunits which are held together by disulphide bonds to form a series of multimers which vary in size from a dimer to oligomers containing up to 50 subunits. Acrylamide/agarose gel electrophoresis permits the separation of the various multimers according to molecular weight. Using this technique, each multimer appears as a triplet band structure composed of an intensely-staining central band with two satellite bands. Assessment of alterations in multimeric structure, when combined with other standard laboratory investigations, has enabled the division of vWD into three major types and more than 20 different subtypes, as shown in Table 22.2.

Type	FVIII Act	vWFAg	vWFRCo	Multimeric pattern
I	Reduced	Reduced	Reduced	All multimers present
II	Normal/ reduced	Normal/ reduced	Reduced	Largest multimers absent
III	Very low	Absent	Absent	Absent

Table 22.2 *Classification of von Willebrand's disease*

Broadly, types I and III represent a quantitative deficiency of a functionally normal vWF while type II variants represent the presence of a qualitatively abnormal vWF. Type I is the most common form of vWD, accounting for more than 70% of cases. The molecular basis of the type I deficiencies is unknown, most of the current molecular research associated with vWD is directed at the type II variants.

The most common type II (dysfunctional) variant is type IIA which accounts for about 15% of cases. Type IIB is the second most common qualitative defect and is characterised by a selective deficiency of higher multimers in the plasma, mild thrombocytopaenia and an increased aggregation response to ristocetin. The deficiency of higher multimers in type IIB vWD is secondary to their increased affinity for the platelet membrane GPIb:GPIX:GPV complex and the subsequent removal by the spleen of the vWD-coated platelets which result.

Subtle multimeric changes have been used to form the current complex classification of type II variants, many of which are very rare. The more "common" variants are described in Table 22.3.

Table 22.3 *Classification of von Willebrand's disease*
FVIII Act = procoagulant factor VIII, vWFAg = von Willebrand factor antigen, vWFRCo = von Willebrand factor ristocetin cofactor activity

Subtype	Mode of Inheritance	FVIII Act	vWFAg	vWFRCo	Multimeric Pattern
IA	Dominant	Reduced	Reduced	Reduced	Normal
IB	Dominant	Reduced	Reduced	Reduced	All present/larger multimers reduced relative to other forms
IC	Dominant	Normal/ Reduced	Normal/ Reduced	Reduced	No flanking bands
IIA	Dominant	Normal/ Reduced	Normal/ Reduced	Reduced	Absent large and intermediate forms
IIB	Dominant	Normal/ Reduced	Normal/ Reduced	Normal/ Reduced	Larger multimers absent in plasma, normal in platelets
IIC	Recessive	Normal/ Reduced	Normal/ Reduced	Reduced	Larger multimers absent, smaller multimers increased. Flanking bands abnormal. Same abnormality in platelets
III	Recessive	Markedly reduced	Absent	Absent	Absent
Pseudo	Dominant	Normal	Normal	Reduced	Larger multimers absent

Type III vWD represents a severe, life-long haemorrhagic disorder which is clinically similar to severe haemophilia apart from the added complication of platelet dysfunction secondary to deficiency of vWF. This form of vWD, in common with type IIC, is inherited as an autosomal recessive trait, whereas all other types are inherited in an incompletely dominant fashion.

Pseudo vWD is a rare disorder which, in common with type IIB vWD, is characterised by thrombocytopaenia and a selective absence of higher molecular weight vWF multimers. However, in pseudo vWD the defect lies within the platelet GPIb:IX:V complex, which has an increased affinity for the higher molecular weight vWF multimers. Pseudo vWD can be distinguished from the type IIB variant by mixing experiments using plasma and platelets.

Pathophysiology of vWD

The vWF gene is located on the short arm of chromosome 12 while a partial vWF pseudogene, which consists of a duplication of the central portion of the functional vWF gene, is located on chromosome 22. The characterisation of the specific molecular defects associated with vWD has been the focus of much research in recent years, but progress has been hampered by the enormous size and complexity of the vWF gene which is 178 kb in length and is split into 52 exons. The greatest progress has been made in the identification of the specific mutations associated with type II vWD, particularly subtypes IIA and IIB. In type IIA vWD, many of the point mutations identified so far tend to cluster within the A2 homologous region of exon 28. Two distinct subgroups of type IIA vWD have been identified in which the absence of high molecular weight multimers of vWF can be traced to a defect of intracellular transport of vWF or to selective proteolysis in plasma following secretion by endothelial cells and megakaryocytes. The two subgroups can be distinguished by the presence of a normal vWF multimeric pattern within platelets in the latter subgroup.

Four different point mutations have been implicated in more than 90% of cases of type IIB vWD. All are located in exon 28 between codons 449 and 728, an area of the gene which encodes the GPIb binding region. It is hoped that the accumulation of knowledge of the molecular bases of the various subtypes of vWD will simplify the classification of this disease.

A variety of gene mutations have been demonstrated in type III vWD, including deletions, the creation of premature stop codons and the loss of vWF mRNA expression.

Because vWF is involved in both primary and secondary haemostasis, the bleeding problems associated with vWD are highly heterogeneous. Severe type III vWD is associated with spontaneous bleeding into joints, or **haemarthrosis**, and into muscles, or **haematoma**, and with severe and prolonged bleeding following trauma. In other words, severe vWD is clinically very similar to defects of secondary haemostasis such as haemophilia. Most cases of vWD, however, are relatively mild and significant bleeding problems may be absent. Where present, bleeding usually is manifest as mucous membrane bleeding including recurrent epistaxis, menorrhagia and easy bruising. Bleeding from coincident pathology such as duodenal ulcers may be unusually heavy and prolonged. Mild vWD is clinically similar to platelet disorders such as Bernard-Soulier disease.

Until recently, antenatal diagnosis of vWD required specific assays of vWF to be performed on foetal blood samples obtained by foetoscopy. However, because of the generally mild nature of the disease, and the significant inherent risks of foetal blood sampling, antenatal diagnosis was seldom performed. Increasing knowledge of the molecular defects associated with vWD and the use of polymerase chain reaction (PCR) technology has extended the applicability of antenatal diagnosis of vWD.

Treatment of vWD

With the exception of the type III variants, vWD is a relatively mild haemorrhagic disorder and treatment is only required for post-traumatic bleeds and to cover elective surgery. The most common form of treatment involves the use of the vasopressin analogue **DDAVP (1-desamino-8-D-argininylvasopressin)** which triggers the release of vWF from the Weibel-Palade bodies of vascular endothelium. However, DDAVP treatment is not universally applicable: types I and IIA vWD usually respond well to this substance but type III variants typically do not respond at all. DDAVP therapy is contra-indicated in type IIB vWD because the sudden release of high molecular weight vWD which it triggers can induce acute and severe thrombocytopaenia. DDAVP therapy is suitable as a short-term measure only, the endothelial stores of vWF are exhaustible, following which further treatment is ineffective. Types IIB and III vWD can be treated by replacement therapy using cryoprecipitate which is rich in vWF.

Haemophilia A

Haemophilia A is the second most common inherited haemorrhagic disorder, occurring in all ethnic groups. The incidence of this X-linked recessive disorder in the UK is approximately 5 per 100,000. Haemophilia A is characterised by a decreased plasma concentration of functionally active factor VIII.

Classification of Haemophilia A

Haemophilia A is classified according to the plasma concentration of factor VIII which correlates inversely with the clinical severity of the condition as shown in Table 22.4.

FVIIIAct	Classification	Incidence	Manifestations
<0.01	Severe	40	Spontaneous haem-arthroses & haematomas
0.01-0.05	Moderate	35	Bleeding after relatively minor trauma
>0.05	Mild	25	Bleeding after major trauma eg surgery

Table 22.4 *Classification of haemophilia A*

The clinical severity of haemophilia A is highly variable but, in contrast to vWD, typically is constant within a given family. The normal plasma concentration of factor VIII Act ranges from 0.5-2.0 units/ml. Haemophiliacs can be classified as being severe (<0.01 units/ml factor VIII Act), moderate (0.01-0.05 units/ml factor VIII Act) or mild (>0.05 units/ml factor VIII Act). Recognition of haemophilia A typically is straightforward, provided that the possibility of severe vWD is excluded. A comparison of the distinguishing features of these two disorders is given in Table 22.5.

Disorder	FVIIIAct	vWFAg	vWFRCo	Platelet Count
Haemophilia	Low	Normal	Normal	Normal
von Willebrand's	Low	Low	Low	Normal
Bernard-Soulier	Normal	Normal	Low	Low

Table 22.5 *Differential diagnosis of von Willebrand's disease, haemophilia A and Bernard-Soulier disease*

Haemophilia probably has been recognised as a distinct disease since antiquity. The earliest written evidence of its recognition comes in the Babylonian Talmud which records a decision that the fourth-born son of a particular woman should be exempt circumcision because her first three sons had all bled to death following this ritual. It seems likely that this case describes a haemorrhagic disorder which is transmitted vertically to males by symptom-free carrier females.

Genetics of Haemophilia A

The gene which encodes factor VIII is located on the tip of the long arm of the X chromosome at Xq28-Xqter. Haemophilia A is caused by mutations of this gene and so is inherited as an X-linked recessive disorder. This mode of inheritance is associated with several clearly defined features:

- hemizygous males express the disease

- heterozygous females typically are symptomless carriers

- homozygous females express the disease

- the sons of a hemizygous male are normal

- the daughters of a hemizygous male are **obligate carriers**

- the sons and daughters of a carrier female have a 50% chance of inheriting the mutant gene

Molecular characterisation of the factor VIII gene and its mutations also has been hampered by its large size and considerable complexity. The gene has been shown to span 186 kb, to comprise 26 exons which range in size from 69 to 3,106 bp and are separated by 25 introns, and to occupy almost 0.1% of the X chromosome. The largest exon encodes the central B domain of factor VIII which is excised during thrombin activation of the molecule. The factor VIII gene appears to be highly susceptible to mutation, more than 100 different mutations of the factor VIII gene have been characterised, most unique to an individual family and up to 30% of cases result from novel spontaneous mutations. Precise characterisation of genetic defects enables a greatly increased level of accuracy in the detection of female carriers and in antenatal diagnosis of haemophilia A.

Carrier Detection in Haemophilia A

One of the most common tasks of the haemostasis laboratory is to offer an assessment of the likelihood that an individual female is a carrier of haemophilia. Typically, such an investigation progresses through up to four phases:

- formal **counselling** of the possible carrier prior to any laboratory investigation. Among the issues which must be explored are the possible implications of the results which might be obtained; the type of tests available for carrier detection and the possibility that the results might be inconclusive and the potential impact of any results on other family members.

- **family study**. The construction of as complete a family pedigree chart as possible may identify the subject as an obligate carrier, in which case no further assessment is required. Obligate carriers include daughters of confirmed haemophiliacs, mothers of at least two haemophiliac sons, born at separate deliveries, and mothers of one haemophiliac son where definite evidence of haemophilia in other members of the family exists. Possible carriers need further investigation. Using the pedigree chart, a probability of carrier status can be derived by examining the relationship of the subject to the closest affected family member and applying a factor of 0.5 for each vertical or horizontal step. For example, in the pedigree chart shown in Figure 22.2, the probability that the subject (III2) is a carrier is 0.5 x 0.5 ie 0.25.

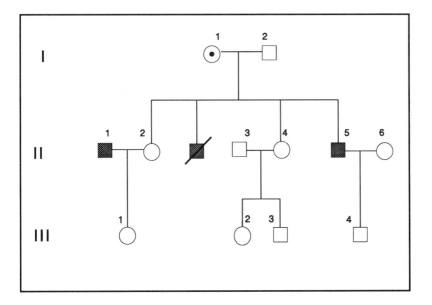

Figure 22.2 *Family study in haemophilia A*

I1 is an obligate carrier because she has two haemophiliac sons (one of whom is dead)
II1 is an unrelated haemophiliac
II2 and II4 have a 50% chance of being carriers
III2 is the subject of the study
III4 is normal (son of haemophiliac)

- **phenotypic assessment**. In theory, a female carrier of haemophilia should have approximately 50% of the normal plasma concentration of factor VIII. In practice, however, the range of values obtained is wide and overlaps with the normal range. However, measurement of the plasma concentrations of FVIII Act and vWFAg on a number of occasions permits the calculation of the probability of carrier status using the method of bivariate linear discriminant analysis. The probabilities obtained from the family study and the phenotypic assessment can be combined to produce a more refined assessment of the likely carrier status.

Restriction endonucleases are named according to their bacterial source. Thus, EcoR1 is derived from *E. coli* and Hpa II is derived from *H. parainfluenzae*.

- **genotypic assessment**. In the absence of specific knowledge regarding the factor VIII gene mutation, **restriction fragment length polymorphism (RFLP) linkage analysis** can be used to track the mutation through the family. Briefly, electrophoretic analysis of the results of restriction enzyme digestion and polymerase chain amplification may permit the identification of the haemophilia-associated allele within the family under investigation. Commonly used restriction enzymes include Bcl I, Xba I and Bgl II. The CA repeat sequences within introns 13 and 22 have proven to be of particular value. Using these markers, more than 95% of Caucasian females are informative, although there is considerable ethnic variation. Application of the methods outlined here for the determination of carrier status are illustrated in Figures 22.2 and 22.3.

However, RFLP linkage analysis suffers from a number of important shortcomings. It can only be used to track the defective gene within a given family, it does not identify the mutation nor does it provide information which can be applied to other families. There is an absolute requirement for a sample of DNA from at least one affected male. This is difficult to obtain in many cases because of the high incidence of HIV-related death in affected males and the high incidence of spontaneous mutation. For these reasons, the identification of the specific mutation within a family is still required to provide carrier risk assessment in non-informative families. Recent refinements in molecular genetic techniques such as PCR coupled with chemical cleavage mismatch detection and single

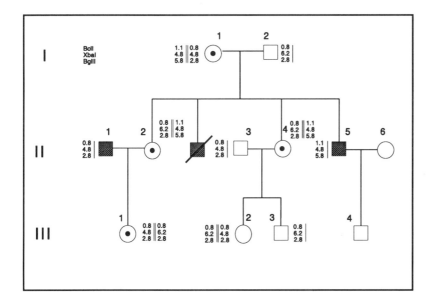

Figure 22.5 *Genotypic analysis in haemophilia A*

From examination of II5 and I1, the mutant allele is 1.1,4.8,5.8, therefore II2 and II4 are both carriers.
III2 has not inherited the mutant allele from her carrier mother and so is normal.
III1 has not inherited the mutant allele from her mother but has inherited that from her father. She therefore is a carrier

stranded conformational polymorphism analysis have greatly improved the accuracy of carrier detection.

Antenatal Diagnosis in Haemophilia A

Antenatal diagnosis should only be undertaken in centres with full genetic, haematological and obstetric expertise in such matters. The steps involved in the antenatal diagnosis of haemophilia A are similar to those required for carrier detection. Careful pre-investigation counselling of both parents regarding the implications and limitations of possible results is extremely important. Similarly, examination of a family pedigree chart may obviate the need for investigation.

Phenotypic assessment can be performed during the second trimester of pregnancy using direct assay of FVIII Act and FVIII Ag in foetal blood obtained by cordocentesis. Assays of factor V are also performed to check for sample integrity.

Genotypic assessment can be performed in the first trimester of pregnancy using foetal DNA obtained by placental biopsy (chorion villus sampling, CVS) or, later, by amniocentesis. Using PCR, the results of genotypic investigations typically are available within 2 days. For those families who are not informative for any available DNA probe or who present during the second trimester of preg-

Prospective parents who are at risk of conceiving a haemophiliac son but who are unwilling to undergo antenatal diagnosis may be able to take advantage of recent developments in *in vitro* fertilisation. It has recently become possible to sex pre-implantation conceptuses and to select only females for implantation. Using this approach, half of the children will be entirely unaffected and half will be symptom-free carriers. It is currently impossible to screen conceptuses for haemophilia.

nancy, foetal blood sampling is still the method of choice. Some parents prefer to wait until the second trimester of pregnancy when ultrasound foetal scanning at 16-20 weeks can sex the foetus and so avoid invasive testing of females. Possible future developments for antenatal genetic diagnosis of haemophilia A include screening of pre-implantation embryos as part of the *in vitro* fertilisation programme and the use of foetal cells derived from the maternal circulation.

Pathophysiology of Haemophilia A

Primary haemostasis is normal, even in severe haemophiliacs. Accordingly, bleeding from minor cuts and abrasions seldom is troublesome. More substantial tissue damage, which elicits activation of secondary haemostasis, results in the formation of weak clots which are highly susceptible to mechanical or fibrinolytic breakdown. This explains the classical pattern of bleeding into joints and deep tissues which is delayed for some hours after trauma. Most apparently spontaneous bleeds probably result from some ill-remembered minor trauma in the preceding hours.

The most common sites of haemorrhage in haemophilia A are the weight-bearing joints such as knees, elbows, ankles, shoulders, wrists and hips. In addition to bearing much of the strain of everyday movement, these joints are particularly susceptible to the knocks and bumps of everyday life. Recurrent bleeding into joint spaces, or **haemarthroses,** is extremely painful and results in irreversible tissue damage such as thickening and roughening of the synovium, erosion of joint cartilage and bone resorption and eventually leads to a chronic arthropathy which is characterised by an inability to straighten fully the affected joint and progressive wasting of attached muscle. Haemophilic arthropathy is a major cause of morbidity in haemophiliacs and frequently necessitates joint replacement.

In addition to recurrent haemarthroses, severe haemophiliacs are plagued by frequent, painful bleeding episodes which most commonly involve the large, weight-bearing muscles of the thigh and calf, the iliacus and psoas muscles which connect the trunk and femur and are responsible for flexing the hip, posterior abdominal wall and the gluteal muscles which connect the pelvis and femur. Haematomata may take several months to resolve and the affected muscle frequently is permanently damaged with collagen fibrotic replacement of muscle fibres, and progressive contraction and loss of power. Rarely, failure of resolution may result in the formation of a **pseudotumour** within the muscle which, as it grows, may become infected and cause severe erosion of surrounding tissue, eventually requiring amputation of the affected limb. Two types of deep tissue bleed are worthy of special mention:

- a right-sided iliopsoas bleed causes severe abdominal pain and tenderness which can mimic acute appendicitis but is differentiated by sensory loss in the knee and weakness in the quadriceps muscle which is absent in appendicitis.

- a sublingual haematoma can cause upward displacement of the tongue and may track into the neck, leading to respiratory obstruction. Urgent medical attention is required in such cases to prevent death.

Other common bleeding manifestations in haemophiliacs include both macroscopic and microscopic haematuria, cerebral bleeds which commonly are fatal, recurrent epistaxis and gastrointestinal haemorrhage.

The pattern of bleeding in haemophilia differs according to age. Provided that delivery is not traumatic, bleeds in the first few months of life are uncommon. However, as the child becomes mobile and increasingly adventurous, the falls and bumps which characterise this period of life frequently are accompanied by extensive traumatic bruising and haematoma formation and may result in unjust accusations of non-accidental injury. Bleeding in haemophiliacs is not faster than normal but typically continues for longer and may recur several times after cessation. For example, dental extractions may bleed intermittently for several weeks. With experience, however, the haemophiliac learns to avoid hazardous situations and to seek medical attention early, thereby limiting the damaging effects of haemorrhage. However, this variation is caused by alteration in behaviour, not by changes in the nature of the disease, which remains constant throughout life.

Treatment of Haemophilia A

Treatment of haemophilia A currently involves the infusion of freeze-dried and heat-treated factor VIII concentrate to limit established bleeding. Prompt and early treatment is essential if sec-

Recently, the human factor VIII gene has been cloned and expressed in mammalian cells in culture. This raises the prospect of a limitless supply of pure factor VIII concentrate for therapeutic use which is free of the possibility of viral contamination. Recombinant factor VIII concentrate is currently undergoing clinical trials.

The successful insertion and subsequent expression of the human factor factor VIII gene also raises hopes that gene therapy for haemophilia may one day be possible.

ondary tissue damage is to be avoided following a bleed, so most severe haemophiliacs are taught how to administer factor VIII concentrate to themselves at home. Infusion of sufficient concentrate to achieve haemostasis is required twice daily until symptoms subside. Surgical cover may necessitate treatment for as long as 21 days post-operatively. During this period regular FVIII Act assays are mandatory. Ancillary methods of treatment include the use of fibrinolytic inhibitors such as tranexamic acid and the injection of DDAVP to bring about a transient increase in the circulating concentration of factor VIII by stimulating the release of vWF from the vascular endothelium.

Additionally, regular examinations are required to monitor general health and, in particular, liver function and HIV status because of the risks of viral transmission associated with the use of blood products. The human factor VIII gene has been cloned and expressed in mammalian cells, raising the prospect of unlimited availability of recombinant human factor VIII concentrate which is guaranteed to be free of the risks of viral contamination. Further, because a comparatively small rise in the plasma level of factor VIII can significantly alter the clinical severity of haemophilia A, this disorder is a likely candidate for the early exploitation of gene therapy. Genetic, social and psychological services also form an important part of the overall care of the haemophiliac and his family.

Haemophilia B

Haemophilia B, also known as **Christmas disease**, results from a deficiency or defect of factor IX, occurs with a frequency of about 15-20 per 1,000,000 and is clinically indistinguishable from haemophilia A.

Classification of Haemophilia B

The initial classification of haemophilia B mirrors that of haemophilia A: severe cases have less than 0.01 units/ml of factor IX Act; moderate cases have up to 0.05 units/ml of factor IX Act and mild cases have more than 0.05 units/ml of factor IX Act. The majority of cases of haemophilia B fall into the severe category. A further subclassification of the severe form is dependent upon the immunological detection of factor IX (FIXAg) in plasma. Those individuals with a normal level of FIXAg are designated as cross-reacting material positive (CRM$^+$ or haemophilia B$^+$) while those

The possibility that haemophilia might consist of more than one defect of coagulation was first raised in 1944 when Argentinian investigators showed that the plasma of two haemophiliacs was mutually corrective. Several similar studies followed until, in 1952, Biggs *et al.* published a report of several patients with the variant form of haemophilia. Since one of the patients was called Christmas and the report appeared in the Christmas issue of the *British Medical Journal*, the name adopted for this condition almost chose itself!

with no detectable FIXAg are designated CRM⁻ or haemophilia B⁻ and those with an intermediate level of FIXAg are designated CRM^R. Inhibitors to factor IX tend to occur within the CRM⁻ group. A further subtype, designated haemophilia B$_M$ is characterised by the prolongation of the prothrombin time test when bovine thromboplastin is used but a normal time when thromboplastin of human origin is used.

Genetics of Haemophilia B

The factor IX gene spans approximately 33.5 kb of the X chromosome at the terminus of the long arm in the Xq27 region, close to the fragile X locus and the factor VIII gene. More than 50 different mutations of the factor IX gene have been characterised, including both point mutations and gross deletions. Most CRM⁻ cases result from gross deletions whereas the CRM⁺ variants result from any of a large number of different point mutations. Many of these point mutations have been fully characterised and have helped to advance knowledge regarding structure-function relationships in coagulation factors. For example, factor XI$_a$ is known to activate factor IX by cleaving the molecule at the arginine residues at positions 145 and 180. The substitution of a histidine residue for an arginine residue at position 145 renders the factor IX molecule impervious to the proteolytic action of factor XI$_a$ at that point and results in a failure of activation. This CRM⁺ variant is known as factor IX$_{Chapel Hill}$.

Carrier Detection and Antenatal Diagnosis in Haemophilia B

The basic approach and underlying principles of carrier detection in haemophilia B are identical to those already described for haemophilia A. The only significant difference is that the routine use of immunological assays of FIXAg is of no proven benefit and so univariate linear discriminant analysis using factor FIX Act assays are used.

In those cases where the molecular defect is known precisely, carrier detection and antenatal diagnosis are greatly simplified. However, in most cases RFLP analysis is still the mainstay of such investigations. In haemophilia B, the use of the restriction enzymes TaqI, XmnI, DdeI, HhaI and MnlI will be informative in approximately 80% of Caucasian females.

Treatment of Haemophilia B

The mainstay of treatment for haemorrhage in haemophilia B is replacement therapy using heat-treated factor IX concentrate. This product also contains traces of activated factors II, IX and X and its use carries a risk of thrombotic complications. This danger can be minimised by the apparently paradoxical subcutaneous administration of the anticoagulant heparin.

Inhibitor formation is a much less common event following treatment for haemophilia B than it is in haemophilia A. There is a strong correlation between the presence of gross gene deletions and inhibitor formation in haemophilia B. This relationship is not present in haemophilia A.

Fibrinogen

In the early decades of the 19th century, debate raged about the site of synthesis of fibrinogen within the body. Theories abounded with many workers suggesting that they could show that fibrinogen was synthesised by red cells, white cells, within the plasma or even that it formed the basis of muscle! The fact that fibrinogen is synthesised within the liver was not recognised until the turn of that century.

The fibrinogen molecule is composed of three non-identical polypeptide subunits, designated Aα, Bβ and γ, which are encoded by three separate genes which are closely linked on chromosome 4 at the 4q31 location in the order 5' γ, α, β, 3'. The γ chain gene comprises 10 exons and spans 10 kb, the β chain gene comprises eight exons and spans 8 kb and the α chain gene comprises five exons and spans 8 kb of DNA.

The overall incidence of inherited defects of fibrinogen is unknown. Until recently, this group of autosomal recessive disorders was believed to be very rare but, with improvements in technology and in knowledge about the structure and behaviour of the fibrinogen molecule, it now appears that both quantitative and qualitative defects of fibrinogen are relatively common. Significant clinical sequelae typically are absent until the functional plasma fibrinogen concentration falls to less than 0.6 g/l. For this reason, heterozygotes typically are asymptomatic, only compound heterozygotes and homozygotes have clinically significant haemorrhagic or thrombotic problems.

Quantitative Defects of Fibrinogen

The quantitative defects of fibrinogen can be divided into the **afibrinogenaemias** where circulating fibrinogen is absent and the **hypofibrinogenaemias** where the plasma concentration of fibrinogen persistently is less than 1 g/l. As in the haemophilias the clinical severity of the disorder within a single family is proportional to the depression in the plasma fibrinogen concentration.

The overall incidence of the gene mutations which cause quantitative defects of fibrinogen in the general population probably is relatively low: more than half of symptomatic cases are associated with consanguinity. Severe hypofibrinogenaemia results in a life-long haemorrhagic tendency but spontaneous haemorrhage is rare. Common haemorrhagic manifestations include recurrent bleeding from the umbilical stump in neonates, intracranial haemorrhage following minor trauma which frequently is fatal, gastrointestinal bleeding, epistaxis and, less commonly, menorrhagia. This pattern of bleeding reflects the impairment of coagulation and the secondary platelet dysfunction which results from a fibrinogen deficiency. Quantitative defects of fibrinogen are not associated with thromboembolic disease. The molecular basis of fibrinogen deficiency is obscure but there remains the possibility that, in some cases at least, the underlying defect is impaired hepatic secretion rather than a mutation of the Aα, Bβ or γ chain genes.

Qualitative Defects of Fibrinogen

The qualitative defects of fibrinogen are known collectively as the **dysfibrinogenaemias**. Many dysfibrinogenaemias are clinically silent and are only discovered by chance during a routine screening procedure. This group of abnormalities is highly heterogeneous and may be manifest in several ways:

- as a bleeding disorder eg **fibrinogen Rouen**

- as a thrombotic tendency eg **fibrinogen Naples**

- as impaired wound healing eg **fibrinogen Paris I**

- as a clinically silent mutation eg **fibrinogen Milano I**

Much of our current understanding of the structure and functional domains of the fibrinogen molecule has been derived by investigation of the dysfunctional mutants. A wide variety of aberrant behaviour has been described in the dysfibrinogenaemias and many have been traced to alteration in the amino acid sequences of specific functional domains within the fibrinogen molecule:

> Of the quantitative defects of fibrinogen, congenital afibrinogenaemia was discovered first in 1920 by Rabe and Solomon. The earliest description of congenital hypofibrinogenaemia was made 15 years later by Risak. Qualitative defects of fibrinogen were not accurately defined until 1958 when Imperato and Dettori published their description of a confirmed case.

- absent or delayed release of fibrinopeptides eg **fibrinogen Baltimore I**

- delayed polymerisation eg **fibrinogen Milano**

- enhanced polymerisation eg **fibrinogen Oslo I**

- defective thrombin binding eg **fibrinogen New York I**

- defective plasminogen binding eg **fibrinogen Chapel Hill III**

- defective aggregation eg **fibrinogen Haifa**

- defective cross-linking eg **fibrinogen Paris I**

- defective tPA binding eg **fibrinogen Dusart**

- defective secretion from hepatocytes

Most cases of dysfibrinogenaemia and all but the most severe cases of hypofibrinogenaemia are free of symptoms for much of the time. Replacement therapy therefore is unnecessary until such time as a haemorrhagic or thrombotic event occurs. When required, infusion of cryoprecipitate or fresh frozen plasma to achieve a circulating fibrinogen level of greater than 1 g/l usually is sufficient to restore haemostatic balance.

Prothrombin

Prothrombin deficiency is one of the rarer hereditary coagulation defects. This disorder is transmitted as an autosomal recessive trait; heterozygotes express a subnormal plasma concentration of prothrombin but are clinically silent. Homozygotes and compound heterozygotes can have a life-threatening haemorrhagic condition. Haemarthrosis has been reported but is unusual. Detection of heterozygotes within a known pedigree is relatively straightforward, involving the demonstration of subnormal levels of prothrombin activity.

Defects of prothrombin synthesis fall into two broad types; decreased synthesis of a normal protein, known as **hypoprothrom-**

binaemia and production of a structurally abnormal, dysfunctional molecule, known as **dysprothrombinaemia**. Numerous defects of the prothrombin molecule have been reported including defective binding of calcium ions, factor V_a or factor X_a. Although the structure of the prothrombin gene is known, few abnormal kindred have been investigated at the genetic level.

Factor V

Factor V deficiency is also known as **parahaemophilia** and was first described in 1947 by Owren. It is a rare, autosomal recessive disorder with about 150 cases reported. Consanguinity commonly is present in affected families. The bleeding manifestations exhibited by homozygotes and compound heterozygotes are highly variable, but often are relatively mild and include easy bruising, epistaxis, menorrhagia and post-traumatic bleeding. Haemarthrosis, although reported, is rare.

Occasional kindred with thromboembolic disease associated with factor V deficiency have been reported. Factor V deficiency has also been reported in combination with factor VIII deficiency, with and without von Willebrand factor involvement. As both the factor V and factor VIII genes share a high degree of sequence homology a common gene defect may be implicated. It has been proposed that this combined deficiency is a secondary finding, with the primary defect being a deficiency of protein C inhibitor. This may indeed be true for some cases but there are documented instances of combined V and VIII deficiency with normal or near normal protein C inhibitor levels. The haemorrhagic manifestations associated with combined factor V and VIII deficiency generally are mild but other congenital abnormalities such as mental retardation and dwarfism are common.

> Factor V deficiency was described independently by the American Armand Quick and the Norwegian Paul Owren, two giants of haemostasis. During World War II, Owren used his medical skills to aid the Norwegian resistance movement. In these less than ideal circumstances, he was called upon to investigate a woman with a lifelong haemorrhagic diathesis. Owren successfully showed that her prothrombin time was prolonged but was corrected by prothrombin-deficient plasma. He therefore concluded that his patient was lacking a hitherto unknown coagulation factor, the fifth to be discovered. This factor has had many names over the years but is best known nowadays as factor V.

Factor VII

Factor VII deficiency is a rare haemorrhagic disorder which is inherited as an autosomal recessive trait with high penetrance and variable expression. The pathophysiology of factor VII deficiency and overproduction is complex and incompletely understood. The clinical manifestations, which include epistaxis, easy bruising and menorrhagia, are highly variable in severity and correlate poorly with the circulating factor VII concentration. Some families with factor VII deficiency experience thromboembolic complications instead of the expected haemorrhagic problems. An increased plasma concentration of factor VII is associated with an increased risk of arterial thrombosis.

Further characterisation of factor VII gene lesions and correlation with structural and functional abnormalities in the protein product is expected to improve understanding of the phenotypic heterogeneity of factor VII deficiency. The factor VII gene, which has been mapped to chromosome 13q34-qter, close to the factor X gene, consists of nine exons and eight introns. The degree of sequence homology and intron-exon organisational similarity between the factor VII gene and those of factor IX, factor X and protein C suggests that they share a common ancestral gene which has undergone duplication. Carrier detection in known kindred can be achieved using functional and antigenic measures of factor VII. Both type I deficiency, where reduced synthesis of normal protein results in low plasma levels, and type II deficiency where a functionally abnormal protein is produced have been reported, with approximately 20% falling into the latter category. Some variants such as **factor VII Padua** show variable clotting activity dependent upon the species source of thromboplastin used in the functional assay. The deficiency in this case is most pronounced with rabbit brain thromboplastins and normal when ox brain thromboplastins are used. In view of this, a range of thromboplastin reagents should be used to assess factor VII deficiency.

Treatment of factor VII deficiency requires replacement therapy using specific factor VII concentrate. However, the short *in vivo* half-life of factor VII (6 hours) requires that infusions of factor VII concentrate need to be given frequently to maintain haemostasis.

Factor X

Factor X deficiency is a rare haemorrhagic disorder which is inherited as an autosomal recessive trait. The clinical manifestations are typical of congenital procoagulant defects and include epistaxis, easy bruising and menorrhagia with haemarthrosis reported in severely affected individuals. A number of different molecular variants of factor X have been described, indeed the two index cases (the Stuart and Prower families) appear to be different variants. There are many different approaches to the assay of factor X and many variants show a unique pattern of results, reflecting the

In common with so many of the other haemostatic proteins, factor X was unknown until cases of inherited deficiency were discovered. Two cases of factor X deficiency were described independently and almost simultaneously by Hougie *et al.* and Telfer *et al.* in 1956. The two index cases were a lay preacher called Stuart and a young woman called Prower. Each team of investigators called their "new" coagulation factor after their patients. When it later became clear that Stuart factor and Prower factor were really one and the same, the name Stuart-Prower factor was proposed. This synonym for factor X is little used these days.

heterogeneity of this condition. It is important to distinguish an inherited deficiency of factor X from the much more common acquired deficiency states which are associated with vitamin K deficiency or amyloidosis.

Contact Factors

Deficiencies of each of the four contact factors have been reported, but prekallikrein, or Fletcher factor, deficiency and high molecular weight kininogen, or Fitzgerald factor, deficiency are very rare. The pathophysiology of factor XI deficiency and factor XII deficiency appears to be very different. Factor XI deficiency, first described in 1953 by Rosenthal *et al.*, is inherited as an autosomal incompletely recessive trait and is associated with a mild bleeding tendency. The reported incidence of consanguinity is relatively low, suggesting that the gene exhibits a high rate of spontaneous mutation. Interestingly, haemorrhagic manifestations are seen in both homozygotes and heterozygotes and the severity of the symptoms correlates poorly with the plasma factor XI concentration. Factor XI deficiency is seen most commonly in Ashkenazi Jews; only isolated cases have been reported in other ethnic groups.

Factor XII deficiency, first described in 1955 by Ratnoff and Calopy in a patient called Hageman, appears to be associated with thromboembolic rather than haemorrhagic problems, presumably reflecting the importance of this factor in the initiation of fibrinolysis. In some reports, the incidence of factor XII deficiency within selected thrombotic populations is as high as 14%. Factor XII deficiency is inherited as an autosomal incompletely recessive trait. It appears that factor XII deficiency in isolation is insufficient to trigger thrombosis but that it acts in concert with other risk factors to produce thrombophilia. The majority of cases of factor XII deficiency are type I deficiencies, few variant molecules have been reported.

Factor XIII

Factor XIII deficiency was first described by Duckert et al in 1961. Since then over 150 cases have been reported. The protein is composed of two subunits, designated a and b, and it is likely that at least two genes are involved in the synthesis and activation of factor XIII. It appears that three categories of factor XIII deficiency exist as shown in Table 22.6.

	Incidence	FXIIIAct	Factor XIII antigens	
			Subunit b	Subunit a
Type I	Rare	Low	Absent/ very low	Absent/ very low
Type II	Frequent	Low	Normal/ near normal	Absent/ very low
Type III	Rare	Low	Absent	Low

Deficiency of factor XIII or fibrin-stabilising factor was first reported as a distinct disease entity in 1961 by Duckert *et al.* This deficiency is not detectable by routine tests of coagulation which use fibrin formation as their end-point. Instead, factor XIII deficiency is screened for by placing pre-formed clots in 1% monochloroacetic acid and watching for dissolution of the clot. Homozygous factor XIII deficiency results in clots which dissolve within minutes, whereas normally stabilised clots do not dissolve, even after 24 hours incubation.

Subunit b is essential for the survival of subunit a in plasma thus explaining the fact that the combination of a deficiency of subunit b with a normal concentration of subunit a is not seen. The clinical manifestations of factor XIII deficiency characteristically reflect delayed and recurrent bleeding and poor healing of wounds. Common complications include recurrent bleeding from the umbilical stump in neonates, easy bruising, haematomata, delayed bleeding after surgery or dental extraction and spontaneous abortion.

Replacement therapy using specific factor XIII concentrate is relatively straightforward because the plasma half-life of factor XIII is 4 days.

Inherited Hyperfibrinolysis

Hyperfibrinolysis is almost always a secondary phenomenon, although a congenital deficiency of the inhibitor α2-antiplasmin has been linked to a haemorrhagic disorder.

α2-Antiplasmin

α2-antiplasmin is the main physiological inhibitor of plasmin. Although rare, inherited deficiency of α2-antiplasmin has been reported and is associated with a haemorrhagic tendency of variable severity. Typically, homozygotes exhibit severe haemorrhagic problems with spontaneous haemarthroses and prolonged post-traumatic bleeding, almost certainly secondary to premature lysis of fibrin. About 40% of heterozygotes experience a mild haemorrhagic tendency but the remainder are clinically silent. The majority of inherited α2-antiplasmin deficiencies described are the result of a quantitative deficiency but a few reports exist of qualitative defects which result in a serious haemorrhagic condition. One such defect, **α2-antiplasmin Enschede**, has been characterised at the molecular level and identified as an insertion within the reactive site of the protein.

Tissue Plasminogen Activator

An increase in the plasma concentration of tissue plasminogen activator (tPA) has been reported in association with a mild haemorrhagic tendency in at least two families. Extensive investigations have failed to reveal any alternative explanation for the haemostatic failure in those affected. The pathogenesis of this abnormality remains obscure.

Inherited Thrombotic Disorders

An inherited thrombotic tendency results from any alteration in the haemostatic balance which impairs the capacity of the body to combat clot formation. As described in the previous chapter, the two main mechanisms which oppose clot formation are the naturally occurring anticoagulants such as antithrombin III and proteins C and S and the fibrinolytic mechanism. Overall, the inherited thrombophilias are estimated to be about three times more common than the inherited bleeding disorders. The pathogenesis of arterial and venous thrombosis is described in the next chapter.

Inherited Defect of the Naturally Occurring Anticoagulants

The naturally occurring anticoagulants include antithrombin III, proteins C and S, heparin cofactor II, tissue factor pathway inhibitor and the recently discovered and as yet poorly characterised protein C cofactor. The normal function of each of these is discussed in the previous chapter.

Antithrombin III

Antithrombin III (ATIII) is an important member of the class of natural anticoagulants which act as **serine** protease coagulation factor inhibitors, or **serpins**. Its main anticoagulant action is directed against thrombin and factor X_a but it is also capable of inactivating

The earliest description of antithrombin III deficiency as a cause of a thrombotic tendency was published by Egeberg in 1965. His report described a Norwegian family with an increased incidence of venous thrombosis which appeared to be associated with trauma, inflammation or pregnancy. Investigation showed that the affected individuals all had an antithrombin III level which was 50% of normal as measured by immunological and functional assays.

factors IX_a, XI_a and XII_a. ATIII acts by forming an irreversible 1:1 stoichiometric complex via an arginine residue on the ATIII molecule and the active serine centre of the relevant serine protease. This action is greatly accelerated by the presence of the therapeutic anticoagulant heparin or *in vivo* heparin-like substances such as endothelial heparan sulphate.

ATIII deficiency is a relatively common autosomal dominant disorder with an estimated incidence of about 1 in 2000. The disorder is manifest as a susceptibility to recurrent deep venous thrombosis or pulmonary embolism, which is exacerbated by pregnancy, surgery or oral contraceptive use. In the normal population, thromboembolic problems most commonly are associated with middle and old age whereas in ATIII deficient individuals, thrombotic complications typically start in the second or third decade of life. Thromboses in infancy or early childhood are uncommon sequelae of ATIII deficiency.

The human ATIII gene is located at 1q21.1-q24 and has been fully characterised. A variety of mutations have been identified and some have been fully characterised. **Type I ATIII deficiency** results from mutations such as short deletions and insertions which interfere with the rate of synthesis of ATIII. This form of deficiency is characterised by a relative lack of ATIII as measured by both functional and immunological assays. Typically, a thrombotic tendency results when the circulating ATIII concentration falls to less than 50-60% of normal. Up to 80% of cases of inherited ATIII deficiency are of this type. **Type II ATIII deficiency** results from point mutations within the ATIII gene which encode the synthesis of a structurally abnormal and functionally impaired molecule. This form of deficiency is characterised by a lack of ATIII as measured by functional assays but a normal concentration as measured by immunological assays. Some of the type I defects are associated with the retarded synthesis of a structurally abnormal protein and are designated type Ib defects. This situation is analogous to the haemoglobinopathies described in Chapters 7 and 8 where thalassaemia represents retarded synthesis of structurally normal globin (cf type I ATIII defects), the structural haemoglobinopathies represent the synthesis of variant molecules (cf type II ATIII defects) and the thalassaemic haemoglobinopathies represent deficient synthesis of a structurally abnormal product (cf type Ib ATIII defects). Type II defects can be further subdivided according to the behaviour of the aberrant ATIII molecule. Type IIa ATIII defects are characterised by impairment of their molecular interaction with both heparin and thrombin whereas in type IIb only thrombin reactivity and in type IIc only heparin reactivity is affected.

Once the presence of inherited ATIII deficiency is established, treatment typically takes one of three forms:

- counselling about avoidable factors which are known to predispose to venous thrombosis such as obesity, venous stasis and the use of oral contraceptives which are known to lower the circulating ATIII concentration further. In the absence of thrombosis, counselling may be the only action required.

- acute thrombotic events may be managed with a combination of heparin and the androgenic steroid danazol which induces a transient rise in circulating ATIII concentration. Prophylactic coumarin therapy usually is instigated as quickly as possible and may be required as a long-term measure.

- unavoidable elective surgery can be covered by replacement therapy using specific ATIII concentrates.

Heparin Cofactor II

In contrast to ATIII, heparin cofactor II (HCII) has a very narrow substrate specificity, with thrombin being the only substrate so far identified. Following the discovery that dermatan sulphate elicits activation of HCII but has no effect on antithrombin III, it was possible to develop functional assays for HCII. The first description of HCII deficiency in association with a thrombotic tendency appeared in 1985 and several others have followed. However, a number of families with inherited HCII deficiency have been described which exhibit no evidence of thrombophilia, leading some to doubt the importance of HCII as a natural anticoagulant. HCII deficiency is much less common than ATIII, protein C or protein S deficiency.

Protein C

Protein C is a vitamin K-dependent serine protease which plays the dual roles in haemostasis of inactivating coagulation factors V_a and

VIII$_a$ and stimulating fibrinolysis. The anticoagulant properties of protein C are markedly enhanced by the presence of thrombomodulin and protein S.

Protein C deficiency was first described as an autosomal dominant disorder in 1981. Since then, the human protein C gene has been fully characterised. Considerable sequence/structural homology exists between protein C and the other vitamin K-dependent coagulation factors. The incidence of protein C deficiency is the subject of great controversy with estimates ranging between 1 in 16,000 and 1 in 200. Greater reliance can be placed on the observation that up to 8% of individuals with recurrent venous thrombosis have been shown to be protein C deficient, a slightly higher incidence than that for ATIII. Protein C deficiency represents an array of genetic defects of the protein C gene which, in common with ATIII, are classified as type I (quantitative) and type II (qualitative) defects. Heterozygous protein C deficiency typically is associated with a reduction in the plasma concentration of this protein to between 30 and 60% of normal and is accompanied by recurrent venous thrombosis. However, an individual with homozygous protein C deficiency has recently been described who exhibited no evidence of thrombophilia, suggesting that the nature of the molecular defect and other risk factors are important determinants of disease severity.

In addition to the expected venous thrombotic tendency, which typically is manifest from the second decade of life, protein C deficiency is associated with two other manifestations:

In 1960, Mammen, Thomas and Seegers reported the presence of an inhibitor of coagulation which they named autoprothrombin IIa because they thought that it was a degradation product of thrombin. Sixteen years later, Stenflo isolated a novel vitamin K-dependent factor from bovine prothrombin complex, and named it protein C because it eluted in the third peak of a DEAE chromatographic separation. Protein C was subsequently shown to be identical to the previously described autoprothrombin IIa. The determination of the anticoagulant and fibrinolytic-promoting properties of protein C followed and the first description of an inherited deficiency as the cause of a thrombotic tendency was published by Griffin *et al.* in 1981.

- the occurrence of thrombohaemorrhagic skin necrosis at the start of coumarin anticoagulant therapy. The *in vivo* half-life of protein C is of the order of 7 hours and therefore the plasma concentration of this protein falls rapidly during the early stages of coumarin therapy. Because the *in vivo* half-life of the vitamin K-dependent coagulation factors II, IX and X is much longer, this produces a marked shift in the haemostatic equilibrium and prompts the formation of thrombotic skin lesions. As the therapeutic anticoagulant effect of the coumarin takes hold in the ensuing days, the skin lesions become haemorrhagic. The tissue damage which results from this process may be severe enough to require amputation. Induction of coumarin anticoagulant therapy in protein C deficient individuals needs to be covered by heparin therapy if this ruinous complication is to be avoided.

- homozygous protein C deficiency is associated with a severe thrombohaemorrhagic state known as **neonatal purpura fulminans** which is manifest in the first days of life as severe and extensive skin necrosis and cerebral thrombosis and commonly is fatal. The immediate treatment of this condition requires extensive replacement therapy. The only prospect of long-term relief lies with hepatic transplantation.

Treatment of protein C deficiency mirrors that of ATIII deficiency. In the absence of thrombosis, counselling about the disorder and its associated problems may be all that is required. Prophylactic anticoagulant therapy usually is withheld until the first thromboembolic event, because some heterozygotes may never have a thrombosis. Surgical cover can be managed using fresh frozen plasma or specific protein C concentrate.

Protein C Cofactor

Recent work from Dahlback and Griffin has shown that factor V, in addition to its procoagulant effect, also acts as a cofactor of protein C. The coagulant effect is mediated by the activated form of factor V whereas activated protein C (APC) appears to require native factor V for optimal activity. A defect in the anticoagulant response to APC has been demonstrated in up to 64% of cases of recurrent venous thrombosis in whom no other abnormality could be detected. This appears to be caused by the presence of an abnormal factor V molecule which is capable of functioning in its procoagulant but not its anticoagulant role.

Protein S

Protein S is a vitamin K-dependent protein which circulates in the plasma in two forms. About 40% circulates as a free and haemostatically active protein while the remainder is bound to C4b-binding protein, a regulatory protein of the Complement system, and has no recognised haemostatic activity. The role of protein S as a cofactor is associated with its ability to bind protein C at phospholipid surfaces, although at present, the site of interaction between protein S and protein C is unknown. The overall incidence of protein S deficiency in the general population is unknown but, in a selected thrombotic population, the incidence has been reported as between 1 and 8%.

Protein S deficiency is clinically indistinguishable from protein C deficiency with recurrent venous thrombosis in heterozygotes and neonatal purpura fulminans in a recently described homozygote. The protein S gene has been partially characterised and comprises 15 exons which encode a similar domain structure to the other vitamin K-dependent haemostatic proteins. However, the presence of a pseudogene with homology to exons II to VIII and a 3' untranslated region has made molecular analysis of this gene difficult. As a result, few protein S mutations have been characterised at the molecular level. About 70% of cases of protein S deficiency exhibit type I deficiency.

Tissue Factor Pathway Inhibitor

Assays have recently been described for the measurement of tissue factor pathway inhibitor (TFPI) which mediates the inhibition of the factor VII_a:tissue factor complex. A number of TFPI deficient individuals have been described but any increased thrombotic tendency has yet to be proven.

Inherited Deficiency or Defect of Fibrinolysis

Hypofibrinolysis may be the result of impaired activation of plasminogen activation secondary to a variety of causes:

- deficiency of tissue plasminogen activator synthesis or release

- an increased concentration of plasminogen activator inhibitor (PAI-1)

- deficiency of plasminogen

- fibrinogen abnormalities which are resistant to fibrinolysis

- defects within the factor XII-dependent pathway of fibrinolytic activation

- an increased plasma concentration of histidine-rich glycoprotein.

Tissue Plasminogen Activator and Plasminogen Activator Inhibitor

The rate of synthesis and release of tissue plasminogen activator (tPA) into the plasma from the vascular endothelium can be assessed following prolonged venous occlusion or DDAVP infusion. Impaired tPA release commonly is present in association with thrombophilia, but familial links are difficult to prove and follow-up investigations often prove negative. The clinical importance of a transient impairment of tPA release is difficult to assess and whether the finding is a primary or a secondary event is uncertain. Similarly, a raised plasma concentration of plasminogen activator inhibitor (PAI-1) is common in post-thrombotic individuals but a positive correlation remains unproven.

Plasminogen

Plasminogen is a single-chain glycoprotein which is attacked by tPA to form the proteolytic mediator of fibrinolysis, plasmin. Plasminogen deficiency is inherited as an autosomal dominant characteristic and affects up to 3% of individuals with recurrent venous thrombosis. Both type I (quantitative) and type II (qualitative) defects of plasminogen have been described. Type II plasminogen defects appear to be more common than type I defects. For example, **plasminogen Tochigi I** is associated with an Ala^{600} to Thr mutation within the plasminogen reactive site and has been identified in 3.6% of a Japanese population. This polymorphism, although linked to thromboembolic disease in three Japanese families appears to be benign in the other individuals, suggesting that plasminogen deficiency represents a thrombotic risk factor but that other risk factors are important in determining the overall thrombotic risk. Several other dysplasminogenaemias have been characterised including **plasminogen Chicago I** which is associated with impairment of activator binding.

Histidine-rich Glycoprotein

Histidine-rich glycoprotein (HRG) inhibits fibrinolysis by occupying the lysine binding sites of plasminogen, thereby impairing the binding of fibrinogen. An increased plasma concentration of HRG is a theoretical risk factor for venous thrombosis. This is supported by the observation that up to 9% of a selected thrombotic population have an increased plasma concentration of HRG and by the discovery of a number of families in whom raised HRG concentration is accompanied by a thrombotic tendency. However, in both cases, the correlation between HRG concentration and apparent thrombotic risk is poor.

Suggested Further Reading

Bloom, A.L. and Thomas, D.P. (eds). *Haemostasis and Thrombosis.* Edinburgh: Churchill Livingstone.

Nathan, D.G. and Oski, F.A. (eds). *Hematology of Infancy and Childhood.* (4th ed). London: W.B. Saunders.

Belluci, S. and Caen, J.P. (1988) Congenital platelet disorders. *Blood Reviews.* **2**:16.

Thomas, D.P. (1985) Venous thrombogenesis. *Annual Review of Medicine* **36**:39.

Acquired Disorders of Haemostasis

Acquired disorders of haemostasis are far more common than the inherited conditions described in the previous chapter. In contrast to the inherited haemostatic disorders, the acquired disorders of haemostasis typically are multifactorial and are associated with varying assortments of thrombocytopaenia, platelet dysfunction, coagulation abnormalities and vascular involvement. Because of this, no attempt will be made in this chapter to classify these disorders as related to one particular component of haemostasis. Instead, the interrelatedness of the haemostatic process is emphasised. The acquired disorders of haemostasis will be considered under the following headings:

- disseminated intravascular coagulation

- haemostatic disorders associated with malignant conditions

- haemostatic disorders associated with liver disease

- haemostatic disorders associated with renal disease

- treatment-associated haemostatic disorders

- haemostatic disorders of pregnancy and the neonatal period

- acquired purpuras

- acquired inhibitors

- acquired thrombophilia

Disseminated Intravascular Coagulation

Disseminated intravascular coagulation (DIC) is a common complication of a wide range of disorders and is characterised by the

Pioneering experiments designed to investigate the role of tissue damage in haemostasis were conducted during the 19th century and revealed two apparently paradoxical findings: rapid injection of tissue extract into animals was immediately fatal, apparently secondary to widespread thrombosis while slow infusion of tissue extract rendered the blood of the experimental animal incoagulable, and prompted death due to uncontrolled haemorrhage. These we now recognise as two facets of disseminated intravascular coagulation (DIC). It was not until the 1950's that the first reports of DIC associated with human clinical conditions appeared.

widespread activation of the haemostatic mechanisms including procoagulants, anticoagulants, fibrinolysis, platelets and the vascular system. Paradoxically, although the early result of DIC is thrombosis, the most obvious feature in most cases is haemorrhage secondary to the consumption of coagulation factors and platelets. Thrombosis is manifest as the formation of occlusive microthrombi throughout the microcirculation, but especially in the kidneys, leading to widespread ischaemic damage. Bleeding manifestations typically involve the gastrointestinal tract and the sites of venepunctures, surgical wounds or indwelling catheters. Subcutaneous and deep tissue haematomas also are common. DIC may present as an acute, life-threatening thrombohaemorrhagic condition or may follow a chronic, less malevolent, course.

Pathophysiology of DIC

As shown in Table 23.1, DIC is seen in association with a wide range of conditions. The most common triggers of DIC are infection, malignancy and obstetric complications.

Despite the myriad associated disorders, the triggering of DIC occurs in response to varying combinations of three mechanisms:

- **Release of procoagulant material into the circulation**. The release of tissue factor or similar procoagulant material into the circulation stimulates the activation of the coagulation cascade as described in Chapter 21. This is the predominant triggering mechanism of DIC associated with obstetric complications, surgery, trauma, malignancy, chemotherapy, transfusion reaction, liver disease, *P falciparum* malaria, tissue rejection and some snake bites. Some tissue extracts contain additional, uncharacterised activators of coagulation.

- **Damage to vascular endothelium**. Exposure of the subendothelium results in contact activation of platelets, coagulation, fibrinolysis, Complement and the kinin system and, in severe cases, can trigger DIC. Endothelial damage of sufficient severity is associated with vasculitis, extensive burns, Gram negative septicaemia, acute viral infections, tissue necrosis and prolonged hypoxia.

Obstetric Complications

    Amniotic fluid embolism
    Placental abruption
    Retained dead foetus
    Eclampsia
    Septic abortion

Malignancy

    Disseminated carcinoma
    Acute leukaemia (especially APL)

Infections

    Septicaemia (especially meningococci and other Gram neg)
    Viral (CMV, HIV, hepatitis, yellow fever)
    Protozoa (especially *P falciparum* malaria)

Trauma

    Surgical (especially thoracic)
    Crush injuries (especially penetrating brain injuries)
    Burns

Liver Disease

    Acute hepatocellular failure
    Chronic liver disease
    Obstructive jaundice

Miscellaneous

    Tissue necrosis (eg necrotising enterocolitis)
    Anaphylactic shock
    Acute anoxia
    Graft rejection
    Extracorporeal circulation eg cardiopulmonary bypass
    Acute intravascular haemolysis
    Incompatible blood transfusion (especially ABO)
    Vasculitis
    Snake bite (eg *Crotalus adamanteus*)
    Heat stroke

The most common cause of DIC world-wide is snake bite. The venoms of a variety of poisonous snakes act by inducing disseminated activation of coagulation. Ironically, many of these venoms have proven to be useful in the investigation of defects of coagulation.

X activation
    Vipera russeli

Prothrombin activation
    Oxyuranus scutellatus
    Echis carinatus
    Notechis scutatus

Fibrinogen activation
    Bothrops atrox
    Agkistrodon rhodostoma
    Crotalus adamanteus
    Agkistrodon contrortix

Fibrinogenolysin
    Crotalus atrox

Platelet activator
    Bothrops jararaca

Table 23.1 *Acquired conditions associated with DIC*

-     **Direct activation of platelets** with concomitant triggering of DIC can occur in some forms of septicaemia or acute viral infections, in the presence of immune complexes and during cardiopulmonary bypass. Obviously, secondary platelet activation occurs in response to all forms of DIC.

Whatever the triggering event, the pathophysiology of DIC remains the same. The generation of thrombin results in the cleavage of fibrinopeptides A and B from fibrinogen, forming fibrin monomers which polymerise to form long strands of fibrin. At this stage, the fibrin clot is held together by hydrophobic and electrostatic bonds alone and is therefore relatively unstable. Stabilisation of the fibrin clot is mediated by factor XIII_a, a transaminase which catalyses the formation of $\varepsilon(\gamma$-glutamyl)lysine bonds between adjacent fibrin molecules. Simultaneous activation of platelets results in the formation of platelet aggregates. Normally, these processes are localised to the area of tissue damage but in DIC they assume systemic proportions. The deposition of microthrombi of fibrin and platelet aggregates throughout the body leads to widespread occlusion of the microcirculation and results in ischaemic tissue damage. This is exacerbated in the renal circulation by glomerular filtration. Occlusion of the microcirculation of the brain and lungs by microthrombi may be life-threatening. Thus, the primary events in the pathogenesis of DIC are thrombotic.

Widespread activation of platelets and generation of fibrin rapidly and progressively lead to thrombocytopaenia and a drop in the circulating levels of coagulation factors. The widespread generation of thrombin also leads to the progressive depletion of circulating antithrombin III, secondary to the clearance of thrombin-antithrombin complexes by the reticuloendothelial system. Fibrin deposition and local endothelial injury trigger secondary fibrinolysis (fibrinolysis may already have been initiated directly by the primary disorder), resulting in the generation of plasmin. This proteolytic enzyme acts by cleaving arginine-lysine bonds and is not specific for fibrin. In the normal, controlled haemostatic process plasmin generation is restricted to the site of thrombus formation by the inhibitor $\alpha 2$-antiplasmin but in DIC systemic plasmin release results in the degradation of fibrinogen, the coagulation cofactors V and VIII, and a range of other plasma proteins. Fibrin(ogen) degradation products released by the action of plasmin interfere with fibrin polymerisation and platelet function. To cap it all, widespread activation of the Complement and kinin systems leads to an increase in vascular permeability, hypotension and shock. These secondary events in the pathogenesis of DIC explain the apparently paradoxical thrombohaemorrhagic state which typifies this condition. The pathogenesis of DIC is depicted schematically in Figure 23.1.

As described above, once triggered, DIC can rapidly spiral out of control and result in death. The emphasis, then, must be on speed of recognition, assessment of severity and the prompt institution of

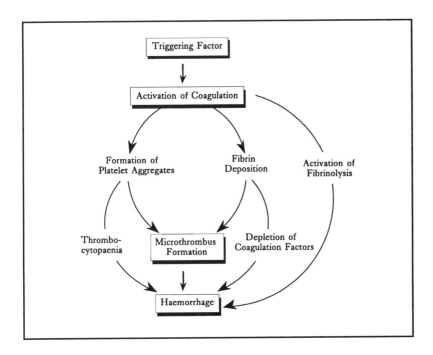

Figure 23.1 *The pathogenesis of DIC*

effective therapy. The minimum laboratory assessment for a suspected case of DIC should include:

- estimation of haemoglobin concentration to assess the transfusion requirement

- estimation of the platelet count to assess the degree of thrombocytopaenia

- measurement of the prothrombin time which is most sensitive to the depletion of factors V, II and I

- measurement of the activated partial thromboplastin time which is most sensitive to the depletion of factors VIII, V, II, I

- measurement of the thrombin time which is sensitive to the depletion of fibrinogen and the elevation of fibrin(ogen) degradation products

- an assay of fibrinogen to assess the replacement requirement

- estimation of fibrin degradation products to assess the severity of the DIC

- examination of a blood film to check for signs of microangiopathic haemolytic anaemia

As shown in Table 23.2, a large number of other tests are available which can aid in the recognition of DIC but these are time-consuming and seldom form part of the emergency diagnostic strategy. Conditions which may be confused with DIC include severe liver disease which presents as a generalised haemostatic defect with impairment of clearance of activated coagulation factors and enzyme-inhibitor complexes and primary fibrinolysis.

As well as the acute and calamitous events described above, many conditions are associated with a chronic, compensated DIC. This state results from a weak, but sustained, stimulus, where the increased consumption of coagulation factors and platelets is compensated by an increase in their production. The pathophysiology of the chronic condition is identical to that of acute DIC. Conditions associated with chronic DIC include intrauterine death, leukaemia, disseminated carcinoma, graft rejection and vasculitis.

Treatment and Management of DIC

Many aspects of the treatment of DIC are highly controversial, partly because the complexity and heterogeneity of the pathophysiology of this disorder make rational treatment selection and objective assessment of efficacy very difficult. There is universal agreement that the primary aims of treatment are to eliminate the triggering mechanism for the DIC as quickly and as completely as possible and to maintain life in the meantime by replacement therapy and, in some cases, anticoagulant therapy.

Replacement therapy typically involves the administration of large quantities of fresh frozen plasma which is a valuable source of coagulant factors and natural anticoagulants, cryoprecipitate which is rich in factor VIII, von Willebrand factor, fibrinogen, factor XIII and fibronectin, platelet concentrates, red cell concentrates and volume expanders such as human albumin solution. The efficacy of replacement therapy should continuously be assessed using the simple laboratory tests described above.

Variable	Alteration	Comment
Coagulation factors		
I	Low	Consumption or degradation
II	Low	Conversion to thrombin
V	Low	Activation and degradation
VIII	Low	Activation and degradation
XIII	Low	Activation and consumption in fibrin cross-linkage
Natural anticoagulants		
ATIII	Low	Clearance of thrombin-ATIII complexes
Protein C	Low	Activation and consumption
Protein S	Low	Activation and consumption
Fibrinolysis		
Plasminogen	Low	Conversion to plasmin
Plasminogen activator	Variable	Increased release from endothelium and consumption as activator/inhibitor complex
α2-antiplasmin	Low	Clearance of plasmin-antiplasmin complexes
Platelets		
Plt count	Low	Consumption in aggregation
Plt function	Abn	High levels of FDP and action of plasmin
β-TG, PF4	Raised	Increased platelet turnover
Thrombospondin	Raised	Increased platelet turnover
Activation products		
Thrombin-AT complex	Raised	
Fragment F1.2	Raised	
Plasmin-AP complex	Raised	
Fibrinogen fragment E	Raised	
Fibrinopeptide A	Raised	
FDP, XDP	Raised	
Fragment Bβ15-42	Raised	

Table 23.2 *Laboratory features of DIC*

The administration of a powerful anticoagulant such as heparin to a bleeding patient whose blood apparently is incoagulable may seem to be paradoxical. The rationale for this manoeuvre is that interruption of coagulation should also slow consumption of platelets and secondary fibrinolysis and permit restoration of haemostatic function. This approach clearly is effective in cases of chronic DIC. Its efficacy is much less certain in acute DIC, however, particularly where septicaemia is involved. In certain cases of severe DIC where standard replacement therapy has proved ineffective, the use of antithrombin III concentrates may be successful.

Haemostatic Disorders Associated with Malignancy

Disturbances of haemostatic function secondary to malignant conditions which predispose to thrombosis or haemorrhage have been recognised for more than a century. Numerous abnormalities have been described, including:

- prostatic tumours have been shown to promote local fibrinolytic activity

- increased expression of thrombomodulin which correlates with disease severity has been described in association with both pancreatic and colorectal tumours. The relevance of this finding to the high incidence of DIC seen in association with these tumours remains to be established

- pancreatic tumours can secrete a trypsin-like enzyme which activates haemostasis through non-specific proteolytic digestion

- circulating heparin-like substances have been described in association with some leukaemias and solid tumours

- dissemination of a malignancy often results in an elevation of acute phase reactants such as the factor VIII:vWF complex and fibrinogen

- elevated fibrinogen levels also are associated with squamous cell carcinomas, Hodgkin's disease and testicular tumours

- soluble immune complexes from tumour antigens can stimulate monocyte and macrophage procoagulant activity

- some solid tumours activate platelets via thrombin generation or as a result of ADP or prostaglandin release

DIC in Malignant Conditions

The most common haemostatic disturbance in malignant conditions is DIC. A chronic, compensated DIC commonly accompanies a variety of malignant conditions such as gastrointestinal, lung and breast tumours and frequently is associated with a thrombotic tendency. In such cases, the only abnormal laboratory variable may be an elevation in the level of circulating fibrin(ogen) degradation products. Acute DIC may be precipitated in these cases by circumstances which promote haemostatic stress such as surgery or infections.

Acute promyelocytic leukaemia also is associated with chronic DIC at presentation but cytotoxic chemotherapy typically triggers acute DIC secondary to the release of procoagulant material from the lysosomal granules causing extrinsic activation of coagulation. A urokinase-type plasminogen activator also is released and may stimulate primary fibrinolysis. In the absence of prophylactic anticoagulant therapy before and during cytotoxic chemotherapy up to 25% of cases of APL experience potentially life-threatening haemorrhage secondary to DIC.

Procoagulant Expression by Malignant Tumours

Expression of procoagulant activity in the form of tissue factor is associated with renal, gastric and colonic tumours and commonly causes a thrombotic tendency. Tissue factor expression by tumour cells is thought to act as a protective mechanism by shielding them from immune recognition and attack. A more direct activation of coagulation in association with tumour cell expression of a cysteine protease which acts upon factor X has been described

Malignant Paraproteinaemias

As described in Chapter 19, conditions such as multiple myeloma and Waldenström's macroglobulinaemia are characterised by the autonomous production of monoclonal immunoglobulin. This paraprotein can interfere with haemostasis in several ways:

- by interfering with fibrin polymerisation

- by coating platelet surfaces, thereby obscuring surface receptors and preventing normal function. This is seen more commonly in association with IgM paraproteinaemia

- by binding to circulating coagulation factors, thereby increasing their rate of clearance. Acquired vWF deficiency has been described by this mechanism

- amyloid deposits, which occur in about 10% of cases of multiple myeloma and Waldenström's macroglobulinaemia, adsorb factor X from the plasma and can produce a deficiency state

- accelerated clot lysis with depletion of $\alpha2$– antiplasmin and an increase in circulating plasmin-antiplasmin complexes has been described in association with paraproteinaemia

- the increased blood viscosity, coupled with the restricted mobility of the elderly population which these conditions affect, also contributes to an increased thrombotic risk

Hepatic Tumours

The haemostatic abnormalities associated with hepatic tumours are similar to those found in chronic liver disease which is discussed later in this chapter, with the exception that fibrinogen levels almost always are elevated. Rare disorders such as Dubin-Johnson syndrome or Gilbert and Rotor syndrome have been described with isolated factor VII deficiencies.

Platelet Dysfunction

As described previously in this book, many haematological malignancies are associated with defective platelet function, usually as a result of defective thrombopoiesis. The most common defects are an acquired storage pool disease or an abnormality of glycoprotein-associated surface receptors.

Haemostatic Disorders Associated with Liver Disease

The liver is the site of synthesis of virtually all of the coagulation factors and natural anticoagulants, although factor VIII appears to be synthesised independently of the others. It is hardly surprising, therefore, that liver disease is associated with many severe and diverse abnormalities of haemostasis, including:

- decreased synthesis of normal haemostatic proteins

- synthesis of functionally abnormal haemostatic proteins

- DIC and primary fibrinolysis

- thrombocytopaenia

- failure to clear activated clotting factors

- failure to clear enzyme-inhibitor complexes

Acute Hepatocellular Failure

Acute hepatocellular failure is associated with a failure of synthesis of coagulation factors and with an increased incidence of DIC and primary fibrinolysis. In the absence of DIC, the levels of circulating coagulation factors, particularly factor V, correlate well with the severity of the hepatocellular damage. The vitamin K-dependent proteins II, VII, IX, X, protein C and protein S are all reduced in concentration due to a combination of decreased synthesis and impaired γ-carboxylation. Synthesis of abnormal and dysfunctional coagulation factors may be present. In particular, dysfibrinogenaemia with impaired fibrin polymerisation and increased catabolism commonly is present. In contrast, the level of circulating factor VIII:vWF complex frequently is raised, especially during acute exacerbations. There is some conflicting evidence that suggests that the factor VIII:vWF complex also may be dysfunctional.

Because the clearance of activated coagulation factors and plasminogen activators is seriously impaired in acute hepatocellular failure, DIC and primary fibrinolysis are relatively common complications. However, recognition of the presence of these complications and the assessment of their severity is hampered by the fact

Liver transplantation is fraught with difficulties, many associated with gross derangement of haemostasis. In essence, the procedure involves subjecting an already haemostatically compromised individual to major surgery which involves the removal of the organ responsible for the production of most of the coagulation proteins. Severe coagulopathy occurs during the anhepatic and reperfusion phases of the operation due to both dilutional and consumptive processes. During the anhepatic phase there is rapid consumption of clotting factors and normal clearance of activated products ceases. Reperfusion of the ischaemic donor liver results in a further DIC stimulus secondary to contact with the damaged endothelium. The clinical management of these patients before, during and after surgery requires continual monitoring of haemostatic function and represents a major challenge to the haemostasis laboratory.

that the haemostatic disturbances which characterise them mirror those of the underlying hepatocellular failure. For example, hypofibrinogenaemia in the presence of a raised circulating FDP level could be explained equally well by impaired synthesis secondary to hepatocellular failure, dysfibrinogenaemia with increased catabolism, DIC, primary fibrinolysis or a combination of any or all of these. One pointer to the existence of DIC would be a circulating factor V level below that of factor VII.

Thrombocytopaenia is a common finding in liver disease and may be associated with DIC or hypersplenism. Defects of platelet function also are relatively common.

Chronic Liver Disease

Chronic liver disease is associated with thrombocytopaenia, platelet dysfunction, failure of synthesis of coagulation factors, dysfibrinogenaemia and increased fibrinolytic activity. In general, the severity of the haemostatic disturbance reflects the severity of the liver disease. For example, in early disease the circulating fibrinogen level may be normal or increased. As the disease progresses, fibrinogen levels typically fall and the presence of dysfunctional fibrinogen becomes ever more apparent. As in acute hepatocellular failure, the circulating level of factor VIII and vWF typically are raised. The vWF multimeric pattern often is abnormal as a result of proteolytic degradation.

Obstructive Jaundice

Obstructive jaundice causes impairment of the vitamin K-dependent carboxylation of γ-glutamic acid residues on coagulation factors II, VII, IX, X, protein C and protein S and results in a reduction in the circulating levels of the functional counterparts of these proteins. All other haemostatic proteins typically are normal or elevated. The presence of acarboxy vitamin K-dependent haemostatic proteins (PIVKA) in the plasma represents one of the earliest and most sensitive markers of hepatic failure.

Haemostatic Disorders Associated with Renal Disease

Both chronic and acute renal disease are associated with thrombocytopaenia, platelet dysfunction and various changes to coagulation and fibrinolytic factors, all of which commonly cause a bleeding tendency.

Platelet dysfunction is caused by the accumulation of metabolites which normally are excreted via the kidneys such as urea, guanidinosuccinic acid and hydroxyphenolic acids. The presence of these substances in high concentration leads to impairment of platelet adhesion and aggregation responses, abnormal clot retraction, enhanced prostacyclin release, prolonged bleeding time, raised plasma levels of β-thromboglobulin and abnormalities of platelet factor 4.

Deficiency of the vitamin K-dependent proteins may occur secondary to malnutrition, antibiotic therapy, uraemic enteritis or from an associated liver impairment. Circulating levels of fibrinogen, factor VIII and vWF often are raised as an acute phase response. The circulating level of vWF often exceeds that of factor VIII, probably reflecting damage to vascular endothelium. Multimeric analysis of vWF often reveals a loss of higher molecular weight multimers which will contribute to the impairment of platelet function. In nephrotic syndrome isolated deficiencies of factors IX, XII, ATIII and plasminogen have been described due to their selective loss in urine. A low grade compensated DIC often occurs in renal disease.

Fibrinolytic activity generally is decreased in renal failure with a reduced circulating level of urokinase and an excess of plasminogen inhibitor. Locally, however, glomerular fibrinolytic activity typically is increased, probably in response to fibrin deposition.

Treatment-associated Haemostatic Disorders

Drug-induced Disorders of Haemostasis

Anticoagulant Drugs

Anticoagulant therapy using oral anticoagulants or intravenous heparin infusion is intended to produce a controlled coagulopathy. However, complications resulting from inadequate monitoring may occur. Overdosage may result in haemorrhagic complications whereas underdosage may precipitate thomboembolic complications. Even in the presence of careful control, many other factors can influence individual responses. For example, as shown in Table 23.3, many other drugs interact with oral anticoagulants such as warfarin resulting in potentiation or inhibition of its effect. It is therefore extremely important to monitor closely patients who change medications while taking oral anticoagulants. The subject of therapeutic anticoagulation is described in more detail later in this chapter.

Potentiators	Inhibitors
Aspirin	Adrenal corticosteroids
Anabolic steroids	Barbiturates
Broad-spectrum antibiotics	Carbamazepine
Clofibrate	Griseofulvin
Indomethacin	Haloperidol
Ketoprofen	Oestrogens
Mefenamic acid	Oral contraceptives
Naproxin	Rifampin
Neomycin	
Oxyphenbutazone	
Phenylbutazone	
Phenytoin	
Quinine	
Sulphonamides	
Tetracycline	
Tricyclic antidepressants	

Table 23.3 *A small selection of drugs which interfere with oral anticoagulant therapy*

Antiplatelet Drugs

Many drugs affect platelet function but few cause bleeding complications. Those which may produce haemorrhagic problems include the **non-steroidal anti-inflammatory drugs (NSAIDs)** such as aspirin and the **semi-synthetic penicillins**. Some drugs are used specifically for their antiplatelet activity. For example, the **salicylates** act by the irreversible acetylation of the enzyme cyclo-oxygenase in platelets and endothelial cells, thereby inducing inhibition of the synthesis of thromboxane A_2 and prostacyclin. However, the effect on prostacyclin synthesis is more short-lived than that on thromboxane A_2 synthesis, so the net effect is inhibition of platelet function. Low dose aspirin (acetylsalicylic acid) is widely used as an antiplatelet agent in the prophylaxis of thrombotic strokes and myocardial infarction. **Dipyridamol** also has an antiplatelet activity, the exact nature of which is unknown. **Epoprostenol** (prostacyclin), a naturally occurring prostaglandin, exerts its antiplatelet effect by binding to specific platelet surface membrane receptors, activating adenylate cyclase thereby increasing cyclic AMP levels and by inhibiting the actions of the platelet enzymes phospolipase and cyclo-oxygenase. **Sulphinpyrazone** has been shown to act as a competitive inhibitor of cyclo-oxygenase. Its effect is slow to manifest but is irreversible.

Drug-induced Immune Thrombocytopaenia

Drug-induced immune thrombocytopaenia (DIT) has been described in association with many different drugs, but is most frequently seen following quinine and quinidine ingestion. Typically, thrombocytopaenia occurs rapidly and is most commonly seen in those who have previously been exposed to the offending drug. The mechanism involved in the induction of thrombocytopaenia is similar to the "innocent bystander" immune haemolysis described in Chapter 10 in association with rifampicin therapy.

Heparin-induced Thrombocytopaenia

The reported incidence of heparin-induced thrombocytopaenia (HIT) varies but bovine heparin preparations appear to carry a higher risk than porcine material. A mild, clinically insignificant thrombocytopaenia may occur in up to 5% of cases of intravenous heparin therapy. The acute and more severe form of HIT carries a 20% risk of arterial or venous thrombosis, a unique complication among drug-induced thrombocytopaenic disorders.

Induction of thrombocytopaenia typically occurs several days after the commencement of therapy and is mediated by the appearance in the plasma of IgG antibodies directed against repeating epitopes on the surface of the heparin molecule. When heparin-antiheparin complexes are localised at platelet surfaces, the IgG antibody binds to the platelet via its Fc receptors, thereby stimulating platelet activation and aggregation. The removal of platelet aggregates by the reticuloendothelial system results in thrombocytopaenia. The mechanisms underlying the associated thrombosis are less clear. It has been suggested that the antiheparin antibodies may bind to heparan sulphate expressed on the surface of vascular endothelial cells, resulting in the release of tissue factor. However, the absence of DIC in the majority of cases does not support this hypothesis.

Other Drug Interactions

Broad-spectrum antibiotics can cause a reduction in the activity of the vitamin K-dependent coagulation factors, either by interference with the mechanisms of γ carboxylation or by depletion of the intestinal bacteria which are responsible for vitamin K synthesis. **Cephalothin** and other cephalosporins have been associated with an impairment in fibrin polymerisation and platelet function. The anti-tumour enzyme **L-asparaginase**, used in the treatment of acute lymphoblastic leukaemia and lymphoblastic lymphoma results in impaired hepatic production of coagulation factors and is associated with intracranial haemorrhage or thrombosis. Many other anti-tumour agents interfere with haemostasis, particularly fibrin polymerisation and platelet function.

Massive Blood Transfusion

Massive blood transfusions of more than 10 units of blood are associated with the induction of a bleeding tendency. Stored whole blood contains relatively low levels of viable coagulation factors, particularly of the labile factors V and VIII. Modern transfusion practice dictates that the plasma is removed from most units of blood soon after donation and is used for the manufacture of other blood products. Because of this, more than 80% of banked blood consists of a suspension of red cells in a saline solution which is enriched with adenine, glucose and mannitol (SAGM) and is devoid of coagulation factors. Thus, replacement of the blood volume by stored blood is associated with an acquired deficiency of coagulation factors. The simultaneous use of crystalloids, human albumin solutions or artificial colloid substitutes may further dilute the coagulation factors.

The resultant bleeding tendency typically is manifest as excessive bleeding from surgical wounds or lesions. Frequently, the severity of bleeding is greater than predicted by the laboratory coagulation screening results, suggesting a multifactorial aetiology. Thrombocytopaenia and platelet dysfunction also are common following massive blood transfusion. Other factors which contribute to the bleeding tendency include shock, the administration of large volumes of blood which is below body temperature and is more acidic than normal, activation of fibrinolysis and citrate toxicity. In addition to their dilutional effect, some volume expanders exert other deleterious effects on haemostasis. For example, hydroxyethyl starch and dextran have been shown to decrease plasma vWF levels, to prolong the thrombin clotting time by inhibition of fibrin polymerisation and to coat platelets, thereby inhibiting their function. It also has been suggested that large volumes of human albumin solution may inhibit hepatic protein synthesis and stimulate fibrinolysis. In patients with pre-existing disturbances of haemostasis, such as in liver disease, a bleeding tendency may be induced by the administration of as little as 4 units of banked blood.

Avoidance of bleeding problems following massive transfusion requires active attempts to prevent the dilutional effect by replacement therapy. As a general rule, 2 units of fresh frozen plasma should be administered with each 10 units of banked blood and 5 units of platelet concentrate should be administered if the platelet count falls below $50 \times 10^9/l$.

Extracorporeal Circulation

Extracorporeal circulation is required, for example, during cardiac surgery and used to be associated with haemorrhagic complications. However, improved technology has considerably reduced the problems associated with circulatory bypass machines although, even today, the procedure inevitably results in some degree of haemostatic activation. Although this, in itself, may not cause problems, it does cause a "priming" effect which can result in acute and unexpectedly severe bleeding should any other complication occur. The treatment required for this form of bleeding essentially mirrors that for DIC.

Pregnancy and the Neonatal Period

Pregnancy and Delivery

Normal, uncomplicated pregnancy is associated with considerable changes in haemostatic function. Although there is considerable interpersonal variation, most women experience a progressive rise in the concentration of fibrinogen, factor VIII and vWF and a fall in the level of protein S and fibrinolytic activity. Some workers have suggested that the mild hypercoagulable state which results is a normal physiological preparation for the rigours of delivery and placental separation. Complications of pregnancy frequently lead to a prothrombotic or haemorrhagic state.

DIC in Pregnancy

DIC is a common complication of a number of obstetric disorders:

- *abruptio placentae* relates to premature separation of the placenta from the wall of the uterus and is a common cause of acute DIC in pregnancy. The placenta is a particularly rich source of tissue factor. Injuries to the placenta such as *abruptio placentae* stimulate release of tissue factor into the circulation and trigger DIC. In most cases, evacuation of the uterus results in rapid resolution of the DIC, without the need for massive replacement therapy. The most serious complications of this condition relate to shock, renal failure and thromboembolism. The use of heparin in obstetric DIC is highly controversial. Most obstetricians avoid the use of heparin whereas others are strong advocates of its use to prevent the accumulation of FDPs which have been shown to inhibit uterine contraction.

- **amniotic fluid embolism** occurs when a small amount of amniotic fluid is forced into the circulation and is most closely associated with difficult deliveries in older, multiparous women. It presents as an acute and severe DIC with profound respiratory distress secondary to thrombotic occlusion of the pulmonary microcirculation, and uterine haemorrhage. Treatment options include massive replacement therapy and the administration of heparin or the fibrinolytic inhibitor ε-aminocaproic acid (EACA). However, none of these options has proved to be particularly effective: the mortality rate of this complication is in excess of 80%.

- **retained dead foetus**. Prompt evacuation of the uterus following foetal death typically is not associated with haemostatic complications. However, if the death of the foetus passes unnoticed, chronic, compensated DIC typically ensues after about 4 weeks with a gradual and progressive drop in the platelet count and a rise in the level of circulating FDP. Significant bleeding typically is absent. As described above, chronic DIC occasionally may accelerate to the acute form.

- **septic abortion**. Because of the mild hypercoagulable state which accompanies pregnancy, any severe infective complication such as septic abortion threatens to trigger acute DIC with shock and acute renal failure.

- **eclampsia** describes a curious syndrome of pregnancy which is characterised by progressive hypertension, a raised blood urate level secondary to renal impairment, proteinuria, convulsions and chronic, compensated DIC. Occasionally, a hitherto relatively stable case may accelerate abruptly into acute DIC with Haemolysis, Elevated Liver enzymes and Low Platelets, a condition known as the **HELLP syndrome**. This clinical emergency threatens the life of both mother and baby and requires massive replacement therapy and rapid delivery.

Antiphospholipid Syndrome

The antiphospholipid syndrome is associated with placental thrombosis, spontaneous abortion, intrauterine foetal death and intrauterine growth retardation. This puzzling condition is described in more detail later in this chapter.

The Neonatal Period

Most normal neonates show some degree of haemostatic impairment at delivery, most notably secondary to hepatic immaturity and vitamin K deficiency. The first weeks of life are the most critical time for haemorrhage due to hereditary and acquired coagulopathies. At full term, factor VIII, vWF and factor V are at adult levels whereas factors XI, XII and particularly the vitamin K-dependent factors II, VII, IX and X are only at around 40% of adult levels and fall further during the first 5 days of life. The circulating fibrinogen level typically is normal but there may be a significant proportion of the foetal variant of fibrinogen which shows delayed aggregation of fibrin monomers.

Plasma concentrations of coagulation factors in neonates differ significantly from those in adults. A normal full-term infant attains adult levels by the age of 3 months.

II	30-40%
VII	10-45%
IX	10-15%
X	10-30%
XI	20-80%
ATIII	raised
Fibrinolytic activity	depressed

Haemorrhagic Disease of the Newborn

The K vitamins exist in two forms: vitamin K_1, known as **phylloquinone**, is synthesised by plants whereas vitamin K_2, **menaquinone**, is synthesised by microorganisms. Both forms contribute to the normal daily intake of this fat-soluble vitamin. Vitamin K is readily absorbed in the upper small intestine in the presence of bile and pancreatic juice. It has a relatively short half-life and body stores are low. Deficiency states are common in neonates and in adults secondary to poor dietary intake, biliary obstruction, malabsorption or drug interaction. One of the earliest indicators of vitamin K deficiency is the detection of non-γ-carboxylated (PIVKA) coagulation factors II, VII, IX, X, protein C and protein S in the plasma.

Haemorrhagic disease of the newborn describes an acquired bleeding tendency, sometimes severe, which develops in the first days of life and is secondary to deficiency of the vitamin K-dependent coagulation factors. In the absence of supplementation, vitamin K deficiency can be expected to develop in more than half of normal full-term babies because of low body stores at birth and the inadequacy of the dietary supply of this vitamin. Powdered baby milk is supplemented with vitamin K during manufacture and so provides a better dietary source than breast milk. Because of the considerable hazard presented by haemorrhagic disease of the newborn, it has become standard practice to administer vitamin K to all neonates within 24 hours of birth. Serious haemorrhagic disease of the newborn is rarely encountered following adequate vitamin K prophylaxis. Treatment of haemorrhagic disease of the newborn consists of the administration of vitamin K_1 and, in severe instances, replacement therapy using fresh frozen plasma.

A variant manifestation of haemorrhagic disease of the newborn occurs in premature babies secondary to hepatic immaturity with failure of production of coagulation factors and consequent poor utilisation of vitamin K. In these, circumstances, vitamin K treatment is ineffective.

A prolongation of the prothrombin time and activated partial thromboplastin time are the commonest laboratory findings in haemorrhagic disease of the newborn. Care should be taken in the interpretation of these variables as neonatal normal ranges are markedly different from adult values.

Disseminated Intravascular Coagulation

Neonatal disseminated intravascular coagulation may be triggered by birth asphyxia, respiratory distress syndrome, trauma, viral or bacterial infection, aspiration of meconium and amniotic fluid or hypothermia. Hepatic immaturity or liver disease may further exacerbate this condition. The pathophysiology of the condition is identical to that seen in adults.

Platelet Disorders

The most common acquired abnormality of platelets in neonates is thrombocytopaenia, which may be secondary to a variety of conditions including DIC, transplacental passage of maternal antiplatelet antibodies, congenital cyanotic heart disease, giant haemangioma and following exchange transfusion. Neonatal platelet dysfunction may be seen following antibiotic or other drug therapy. The pathogenesis of these disorders is described later in this chapter and elsewhere in this book.

Acquired Purpuras

The acquired purpuras are a group of disorders of primary haemostasis which are manifest as mucous membrane bleeding and a tendency to bruise spontaneously or following minimal trauma. They can be divided into the vascular purpuras and the platelet-associated purpuras, depending on which component is most affected. In most cases, however, the pathogenesis of the purpura is complex and multifactorial.

Vascular Purpuras

A number of acquired vascular lesions are associated with the development of purpura. Perhaps the most common of this group of disorders, **senile purpura,** is a benign condition of old age which is manifest as persistent purplish patches on the backs of the hands, forearms and neck which appear spontaneously and leave permanent brown stains when they fade. The condition is caused by a combination of loss of skin elasticity, atrophy of vascular collagen and loss of the cushioning effect of subcutaneous fat. Up to 40% of elderly people display this natural phenomenon for which no treatment is required or available. A similar phenomenon is associated with long-term or high dose steroid therapy.

The apparent excess of easy bruising seen in young women, for which no cause can be found, is known by the spuriously scientific title of **purpura simplex**. In cases of excessive bruising, for which no cause can be found, the possibility of self-mutilation secondary to psychiatric disturbance or physical abuse by carers must be considered.

Severe, prolonged vitamin C deficiency, or **scurvy,** is associated with defects of collagen formation and stability which may lead to a pronounced haemorrhagic tendency with gingival bleeding, haemarthroses and haemorrhagic stroke. Scurvy is associated with chronic malnourishment and, in the developed world, is most commonly seen in alcoholics, the elderly and the poor.

Henoch-Schönlein purpura (HSP), or allergic purpura, is a self-limited allergic vasculitis which is seen most commonly in young children and is manifest as a purpuric rash covering the arms, legs and buttocks, renal impairment and abdominal and joint pain. Typically, a recent history of upper respiratory tract infection, most commonly involving *Neisseria spp, Streptococci spp* or *Salmonella spp,* or of penicillin or sulphonamide therapy, is present. HSP appears to be caused by IgA immune complex-mediated vascular endothelial damage.

Thrombocytopaenic Purpuras

Thrombocytopaenia is the most common acquired platelet abnormality and can result from a variety of causes:

- **failure of thrombopoiesis** such as occurs in the aplastic anaemias, in severe vitamin B_{12} or folic acid deficiency and following suppression of thrombopoiesis secondary to bacterial or viral infection. Bacterial septicaemia may also be associated with thrombocytopaenia in the absence of significant intravascular coagulation, probably secondary to the secretion of bacterial toxins. The pathogenesis of the thrombocytopaenia which commonly accompanies protozoal infections such as malaria is immune-mediated.

- **accelerated consumption or destruction of platelets** such as occurs in immune thrombocytopaenic purpura (ITP), thrombotic thrombocytopaenic purpura (TTP) and haemolytic uraemic syndrome (HUS). These disorders are discussed later in this chapter. Mild, reversible, thrombocytopaenia is common following many surgical procedures: surgical implants such as cardiac valves and indwelling catheters and the use of extracorporeal circulation expose platelets to contact with foreign surfaces and accelerate platelet destruction, resulting in mild thrombocytopaenia although haemorrhagic complications are rare. Surgical hypothermia has also been associated with a mild, reversible thrombocytopaenia secondary to platelet clumping and splenic sequestration.

- **splenic sequestration of platelets**. Normally, about 30% of the total platelet pool is located in the spleen. This splenic platelet pool is in free exchange with the blood platelet pool. Hypersplenism or splenomegaly is associated with an increase in the size of the splenic platelet pool which may, in extreme cases, result in an apparent peripheral thrombocytopaenia.

Idiopathic or Immune Thrombocytopaenic Purpura

Immune thrombocytopaenic purpura (ITP) is characterised by antibody-mediated destruction of platelets with thrombocytopaenia, extensive petechiae, bruising and mucosal haemorrhagic complications such as epistaxis and menorrhagia. The white cell count, differential count and haemoglobin concentration typically are normal. Examination of the bone marrow reveals megakaryocytic hyperplasia with an increase in immature, hypolobulated forms. Three forms of immune thrombocytopaenic purpura are recognised:

- an acute, usually self-limited form which is most common in children between the ages of 2 and 6 years. This form of ITP often is preceded by an acute viral illness of childhood such as rubella, measles or chicken pox. At presentation, severe thrombocytopaenia typically is present with widespread petechiae, bruising and epistaxis. However, bleeding problems seldom are life-threatening. Up to 80% of cases of acute ITP remit spontaneously within a few weeks of presentation. The immune response to the viral illness is thought to result in the non-specific adsorption of viral antigen:antibody complexes onto the platelet surface with subsequent removal via Fc receptor mediated phagocytosis in the spleen. The haemorrhagic manifestations may be exacerbated by immune-complex mediated damage to vascular endothelium. Acute ITP in children may be managed conservatively or a combination of prednisone and polyvalent IgG may be administered to block macrophage Fc receptors.

- a chronic form with an insidious onset and no history of recent viral illness. This form of ITP is most common in young adults but women are affected more frequently than men. Chronic ITP is associated with slightly higher platelet counts than the acute form but seldom remits spontaneously. In common with the acute form of ITP, platelet destruction is mediated by the presence of platelet-bound immunoglobulin with subsequent Fc receptor-mediated phagocytosis by splenic macrophages. In contrast to the acute form, however, the IgG antibodies which characterise chronic ITP are directed against the platelet glycoproteins GPIIb-IIIa or, less commonly, GPIa. Remission of the thrombocytopaenia can be achieved in most cases with high dose prednisone, but long-term steroid therapy is dangerous and most cases relapse following withdrawal of this drug. Splenectomy, because it removes the most important source of anti-platelet antibody and the most important site of platelet destruction, is associated with at least partial remission of the thrombocytopaenia in up to 75% of cases. Refractory cases may be treated with high dose polyvalent IgG.

- neonatal ITP is associated with the passive transplacental transfer of maternal anti-platelet antibodies. These may be directed against GPIIb-IIIa or GPIb in cases of maternal chronic ITP or may be directed against paternal platelet antigens in a reaction analogous to haemolytic disease of the newborn. In both cases, the thrombocytopaenia is self-limited but the risk of intracranial haemorrhage is high, particularly during a traumatic birth.

Thrombotic Thrombocytopaenic Purpura

Thrombotic thrombocytopaenic purpura (TTP) is a rare but clinically serious disorder which most commonly affects young adults and is characterised by fever, erratic neurological disturbances such as convulsions, hallucinations and paralysis, renal failure, microangiopathic haemolysis and thrombocytopaenia with haemorrhagic manifestations. The haemolysis and thrombocytopaenia are secondary to the disseminated deposition of platelet-fibrin microthrombi in arterioles and capillaries. The trigger for the formation of these thrombotic lesions is unknown although endothelial cell damage with defective release of prostacyclin and abnormalities of von Willebrand factor and platelet activating factor activity have been implicated. It is increased platelet aggregation and consumption, rather than coagulation factor depletion, that is the major cause of morbidity and mortality in this condition.

Examination of the blood reveals the classical stigmata of microangiopathic haemolysis viz microspherocytes, schistocytes and poikilocytes, severe thrombocytopaenia and an increased fibrinogen turnover. However, other signs of DIC typically are absent. TTP has been described secondary to a variety of conditions including pregnancy, bacterial infection, autoimmune disease, neoplasia and drug ingestion.

The treatment for TTP involves intensive supportive care such as haemodialysis, artificial ventilation, plasmapheresis and transfusion of fresh frozen plasma. The administration of anticoagulants such as heparin or antiplatelet drugs is of dubious benefit. The mortality rate of TTP may be as high as 50%.

A closely related condition, haemolytic uraemic syndrome (HUS), most commonly affects infants and young children and is associated with the localised deposition of platelet-fibrin microthrombi in the renal vasculature with thrombocytopaenia, microangiopathic haemolysis and renal failure. In many cases, there is a recent history of bacterial infection, particularly involving *Escherichia coli, Streptococci spp, Staphylococci spp* and various other enteric pathogens. It is thought that HUS is triggered by immune-mediated damage to vascular endothelium with defective prostacyclin synthesis or release. Occasionally, adult cases of TTP have a history of relapsing HUS in childhood.

The treatment for HUS involves haemodialysis and supportive measures such as blood and platelet transfusion. In severe cases, heparin therapy and antiplatelet drugs may limit the thrombotic complications. With early recognition and prompt treatment, the mortality rate of HUS may be as low as 5%.

Thrombocytopathic Purpuras

Many of the acquired disorders of platelet function, such as those induced by drugs, uraemia and the presence of a grossly elevated concentration of fibrin(ogen) degradation products, have been discussed earlier in this chapter. In addition, the ingestion of some foods have been shown to impair platelet function including garlic, ginger, black tree fungus and some herbs.

An acquired storage pool disease is associated with the non-leukaemic myeloproliferative disorders and the myelodysplastic syndromes. These conditions are discussed in Chapters 19 and 18 respectively. Similar defects have been reported following severe burns, in association with DIC and in a variety of autoimmune disorders.

Hyperaggregable platelets have been found in hyperlipidaemia, Raynaud's disease and chronic renal failure. In the case of hyperlipidaemias the effects are normalised following lipid reducing therapy.

Acquired Inhibitors of Coagulation Factors

Factor VIII Inhibitors

In approximately 5-10% of haemophilia A patients an IgG antibody is produced which is directed against factor VIII. The mechanism of antibody production is unclear but it is not related to the degree of therapy or to the baseline plasma factor VIII concentration. In contrast to haemophilia B, there is no obvious relationship between the presence of a gross factor VIII gene deletion and inhibitor production. There does, however, appear to be a familial tendency towards inhibitor production.

Whatever the stimulatory mechanism, once the inhibitor is formed, further factor VIII infusion acts as an antigenic stimulus, markedly increasing the concentration of the inhibitor. The incidence of inhibitor production is highest in severe haemophiliacs although, rarely, they have been found in mild or moderate cases following factor VIII infusion. Factor VIII inhibitors can also occur spontaneously in non-haemophiliacs in association with pregnancy (post partum), rheumatoid arthritis, multiple sclerosis, drug sensitivity reactions, SLE, skin diseases, some tumours and also in the elderly, sometimes in the absence of obvious predisposing factors. Males and females have an equal tendency to inhibitor production.

The kinetics of the factor VIII-inhibitor reaction are highly variable. In non-haemophiliacs, complex reaction kinetics commonly are found as shown in Figure 23.3. When the inhibitor is incubated with factor VIII *in vitro*, there is a rapid initial loss of factor VIII activity which slows progressively until an equilibrium is reached. The factor VIII-inhibitor complex may dissociate spontaneously, leaving a residual factor VIII activity of about 0.03 iu/ml. Some inhibitors found in haemophiliacs show a similar reaction pattern but most show simple reaction kinetics with progressive and complete destruction of factor VIII as shown in Figure 23.2.

Recombinant factor VIIa has been used successfully to treat more than 50 patients with inhibitors to factor VIII or IX. Included in this group were both haemophiliacs with inhibitors induced by treatment and non-haemophiliacs with spontaneously acquired inhibitors. This form of treatment shows promise as an alternative approach to the treatment of this clinically challenging group of patients.

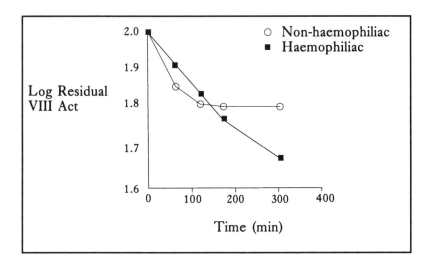

Figure 23.2 *Reaction kinetics of factor VIII inhibitors*

Acquired factor VIII inhibitors are associated with the same clinical sequelae as severe haemophilia ie spontaneous soft tissue haemorrhage and bleeding into joints. Acute haemorrhage can be treated with high dose human factor VIII which can swamp the inhibitor, with porcine factor VIII (provided that the inhibitor is not cross-reactive) or with prothrombinase complex preparations such as FEIBA (Factor Eight Inhibitor Bypassing Activity). The prothrombinase complex preparations have the ability to promote clot formation, bypassing factors VIII and IX. However, there is no way of monitoring dosage and thrombotic complications have been described during this form of therapy. In the presence of a high-titre inhibitor, factor VIII replacement therapy is relatively ineffective because of rapid clearance of factor VII-inhibitor complexes.

The long-term treatment of factor VIII inhibitors is fraught with difficulty but treatment options include the use of immunosuppressive drugs; the use of anti-idiotype antibodies or attempting to induce immune tolerance using long-term continuous infusion of factor VIII. All have been tried with varying degrees of success.

vWF Inhibitors

Inhibitors directed against vWF are less common than factor VIII inhibitors but have been found in association with severe von Willebrand's disease following treatment, autoimmune disease, malignant paraproteinaemia, hypothyroidism, myeloproliferative disorders and lymphoproliferative disorders. The inhibitors tend to react with the high molecular weight multimers of vWF and reduce ristocetin cofactor activity. The observed reduction in VIII activity is variable. In contrast to factor VIII inhibitors, these antibodies can be either IgG or IgM immunoglobulins. The treatment of choice remains DDAVP, but the benefit gained typically is much shorter lived than in uncomplicated vWD. In previously normal individuals, spontaneous remission commonly occurs.

Factor IX Inhibitors

Factor IX inhibitors are associated with treatment of haemophilia B, particularly where a gross deletion of the factor IX gene is present. They also occur, very rarely, as a spontaneous event in non-haemophiliacs, usually in association with autoimmune disease or in the post partum period. In contrast to factor VIII inhibitors, these antibodies act immediately.

Factor V Inhibitors

Inhibitors directed against factor V are rare but have occurred spontaneously, following blood transfusion, in association with streptomycin treatment and in the presence of IgA and IgM paraproteinaemias. Both IgG and IgM polyclonal inhibitors have been reported. These inhibitors are seldom associated with significant haemorrhage and frequently disappear spontaneously. The most effective therapy involves the administration of platelet concentrates, both as a source of factor V and as a means of clearing the inhibitor through binding to surface bound factor V.

Miscellaneous Coagulation Factor Inhibitors

Acquired inhibitors directed against most coagulation factors have been described as rare events, including:

- fibrinogen inhibitors which interfere with fibrinopeptide A release and fibrin monomer polymerisation. These are associated with systemic lupus erythematosus

- a factor VII inhibitor, found in association with bronchogenic carcinoma

- inhibitors directed against factors XI and XII, in association with autoimmune disease or chlorpromazine therapy

- IgM antibodies with generalised contact factor specificity, resulting in depletion of factors XI and XII

- inhibitors directed against prothrombin. These are very rare and need to be distinguished from lupus-type antibodies with prothrombin involvement

- inhibitors directed against factor XIII which interfere with fibrin cross-linking in the presence of activated factor XIII. These are found in association with isoniazid therapy

Single Factor Deficiencies in the Absence of Inhibitors

A number of acquired single coagulation factor deficiency states have been described which cannot be traced to the presence of a specific inhibitor:

- factor X deficiency has been described in association with multiple myeloma secondary to adsorption of the coagulation factor onto amyloid deposits. Rarely, factors IX and VII also have been depleted via this means

- deficiency of antithrombin III and factor XII have been described due to excessive excretion in the urine in nephrotic syndrome

- factor IX and vWF deficiency have been described in association with Gaucher's disease

- isolated factor XII and factor XIII deficiencies have been reported in association with leukaemia

Acquired Thrombophilia

Thromboembolic disease is a major cause of morbidity and mortality in developed countries, rivalling malignancy as the most important cause of non-accidental death. Thrombosis can be defined as the deposition of a semi-solid mass of blood constituents, a thrombus, on a blood vessel wall, and essentially represents an abnormal manifestation of a normal mechanism. In 1856 Virchow suggested that three factors could determine the site and extent of thrombus formation:

- **mechanical effects** of which blood flow characteristics are the most important

- **constituents of the blood** ie the balance between the opposing coagulant and anticoagulant forces

- **blood vessel walls** ie the balance between the clot-promoting and inhibitory activities of normal or damaged vascular endothelium

There are two main types of thrombi found in the body. **White thrombi** consist mainly of platelets and fibrin and form in arteries where the rate of blood flow and shear forces are such that red cells do not tend to be involved. White thrombi only form at sites of endothelial damage such as atheromatous plaques. In contrast, **red thrombi** consist mainly of fibrin and trapped red cells and are found in the slower blood flow of the venous system, particularly near venous valves. An **occlusive thrombus** occurs when the entire lumen of the blood vessel is occupied by coagulated material and blood flow is obstructed. When the thrombus adheres to one side of the blood vessel only and blood flow is restricted but not arrested, a **mural thrombus** is present.

Arterial Thrombosis

Thromboembolic events within the arterial circulation almost always are secondary to vascular endothelial injury. For example, rupture of a pre-existing atheromatous plaque in one of the coronary arteries prompts the localised formation of a white thrombus which may propagate sufficiently to cause occlusion of the artery. This results in severe oxygen starvation of the left ventricle of the heart which is manifest as acute myocardial ischaemia and may progress to **myocardial infarction** or **ischaemic left ventricular fibrillation** with sudden death. Similar episodes involving the cerebral circulation result in **transient ischaemic attacks** and **thrombotic stroke**.

Myocardial infarction presents as crushing tightness of the chest with sweating, nausea, breathlessness and collapse. The chest pain frequently radiates to the arms, throat and jaw but may, in its early stages be confused with severe indigestion. Transient ischaemic attacks are accompanied by fleeting neurological dysfunction or loss of vision. Completed thrombotic stroke is accompanied by similar symptoms which persist for more than 24 hours and may be severely and permanently disabling.

Venous Thrombosis

The most common thromboembolic event is a **deep vein thrombosis** of the lower limbs. The main site for this thrombus formation is within a valve pocket where there is maximum stasis and vortex-type blood flow. Because of the low shear rates experienced in such locations, propagation of the thrombus is associated with red cell entrapment and results in the formation of a red thrombus. Vascular endothelial damage usually is absent. Venous thrombi may become dislodged or may fragment, resulting in the formation of circulating **emboli**, which frequently lodge in the pulmonary microcirculation, resulting in a **pulmonary embolism**. Spontaneous thrombus formation most commonly is associated with the venous circulation.

Venous thrombosis typically presents with pain, swelling, discolouration and warmth in the affected area. However, symptoms may be absent and none of these symptoms are specific for this condition. Pulmonary embolism presents as acute chest pain and breathlessness with shock, cough and haemoptysis and may be rapidly fatal.

Risk Factors for Arterial and Venous Thrombosis

A number of risk factors have been identified which are associated with an increased incidence of thromboembolic disease as shown in Table 23.4. Certain procedures such as hip replacement surgery with reduced leg mobility are known to carry high thromboembolic risk. In these procedures, or in surgical patients with other predisposing factors, prophylactic therapy with the anticoagulant heparin may be given. Thrombosis becomes more common with increasing age and many acquired disorders can result in increased risk of thromboembolism.

Venous Thrombosis	Arterial Thrombosis
Increasing age	Increasing age
Obesity	Obesity
Immobility	Lack of exercise
Pregnancy (post partum)	High saturated fat, low fibre diet
Oral contraceptive use	Smoking
Malignancy	Stress
Lupus anticoagulant	Hyperlipidaemia
Nephrotic syndrome	Hypertension
Post-operative period	Polycythaemia
Homocystinaemia	Elevated factor VII concentration
Diabetes mellitus	Elevated fibrinogen concentration
Gout	Probable genetic factors
Polycythaemia	

Table 23.4 *Risk factors for arterial and venous thrombosis*

Although the nature and interaction of the factors which predispose to thrombosis are still incompletely understood, Virchow's triad provides a useful conceptual framework for their discussion.

Mechanical Effects

Any condition which leads to a reduction in the rate of blood flow will promote venous stasis and the formation of venous thrombi. For example, the thrombotic tendency seen in cases of primary proliferative polycythaemia is partly explained by the increase in blood viscosity (and hence reduction in the rate of blood flow) which accompanies an increased haematocrit. Similarly, one of the most important risk factors for venous thrombosis in the post-operative period is prolonged immobility which promotes stasis, particularly in the lower limbs. It is for this reason that post-operative patients are encouraged to get out of bed and walk about as soon as possible.

Constituents of the Blood

Any change in the constituents of the blood which tilts the haemostatic balance in favour of procoagulant activities will promote thrombosis. For example, the marked increase in platelet numbers which accompanies primary proliferative polycythaemia and thrombocythaemia is prothrombotic. Paradoxically, a coincident bleeding tendency may be present in these conditions because platelets frequently are dysfunctional in the haematological malignancies.

Nephrotic syndrome is accompanied by a thrombotic tendency because of an increase in the circulating concentration of the acute phase proteins factor VIII and fibrinogen and, more importantly, by an acquired deficiency of ATIII secondary to urinary losses. Acquired deficiency of ATIII is also seen in association with oral contraceptive use, liver disease, renal failure, in premature infants and following liver transplantation. Acquired deficiency of proteins C and S accompany deficiency of vitamin K and liver disease. The plasma concentration of protein S also falls in pregnancy.

Epidemiological studies have shown an association between an increased plasma concentration of factor VII and fibrinogen and an increased incidence of arterial thrombosis. Fibrinogen concentration has a major influence on plasma viscosity and hence on blood flow characteristics. Certain abnormal forms of fibrinogen are resistant to fibrinolytic breakdown and so promote thrombosis.

Deficiency of factor XII is associated with a thrombotic tendency, probably because of the failure of factor XII-mediated activation of fibrinolysis. Abnormalities associated with poor tissue plasminogen activator (tPA) release following venous occlusion and elevated plasma concentrations of plasminogen activator inhibitor (PAI) have been demonstrated in association with thrombotic events. Whether these findings predispose to thrombosis or are secondary to the event is unknown. In the majority of cases, repeat investigations six months later show normal results. Family studies have largely failed to demonstrate any familial link between these fibrinolytic abnormalities and thrombosis.

Blood Vessel Walls

Vascular endothelial cells provide a continuous protective layer which prevents the blood from contacting subendothelial substances such as collagen and elastin and also are responsible for the synthesis and secretion of a variety of haemostatically active substances such as prostacyclin and vWF. Disruption of vascular endothelial structure or function may be powerfully prothrombotic. For example, in elastic and muscular arteries the force and turbulence of the blood flow damages the endothelial layer and promotes the formation of **atheromatous plaques**. These consist of fatty infiltration and collagenous overgrowth of the vascular intima and lead to narrowing of the arterial lumen. The resultant impairment of blood flow prejudices oxygen delivery to the tissues supplied by the artery and may result in **ischaemia**. For example, atheroma in the coronary arteries leads to oxygen debt in the heart during exertion which is manifest as **angina**. Further, exposure of subendothelial structures during plaque formation results in platelet and fibrin deposition and may lead to the formation of an arterial thrombus which may occlude the artery completely. When this occurs in the coronary arteries, oxygen starvation of the heart ensues and **myocardial infarction** results. In advanced cases, atheroma may extend into the arterial media with progressive loss of arterial elasticity and the formation of a permanently dilated, thin-walled **aneurysm** which is liable to sudden and catastrophic rupture.

Although the above discussion of the predisposing factors for thrombosis is conceptually useful, it is grossly simplistic. In most cases of thrombosis, multiple prothrombotic factors are present and it is difficult to ascribe blame to a single risk factor. For example, the thrombotic risk which accompanies hip replacement surgery is high because of the advanced age of the subject, the extensive tissue damage caused by the procedure and the inevitable post-operative immobility. These factors may be compounded by other variables such as obesity, smoking, hypertension and gout all of which are relatively common in the elderly.

The Anti-phospholipid Syndrome

The anti-phospholipid syndrome (APS) is caused by the spontaneous production of IgG or, more rarely, IgM antibodies which are directed against anionic phospholipids. This is manifest *in vitro* as prolongation of phospholipid-dependent coagulation screening tests which usually is indicative of a bleeding tendency. However, these antibodies seldom are associated with a bleeding tendency *in vivo*. Rather, binding of the anti-phospholipid antibodies to platelet and vascular endothelial cell membranes promotes platelet adhesion and suppresses the synthesis and release of prostacyclin and tissue plasminogen activator: the result is a thrombotic tendency. The range of thrombotic manifestations is extremely wide: both arterial and venous thromboses have been described and diffuse renal thrombosis and thrombophlebitis with ulceration and gangrene are common.

The anti-phospholipid antibodies which characterise the APS sometimes are known as **lupus anticoagulants** but use of this term is discouraged for three reasons:

- the antibodies do not function as anticoagulants *in vivo*

- most cases of APS are not associated with systemic lupus erythematosus (SLE)

- fewer than one in ten SLE patients develop APS

A number of conditions have been associated with APS and screening for anti-phospholipid antibodies should be considered in the categories listed in Table 23.5. The condition also occurs occasionally in otherwise healthy individuals and may be detected as a chance finding as part of routine pre-operative screening.

Conditions where screening for APS is indicated

First thrombotic event below the age of 40
History of recurrent thromboembolic disease
Recurrent foetal loss in the 1st or 2nd trimester
Patients with SLE
Pre hormone-replacement therapy

Table 23.5 *Conditions where screening for APS is indicated*

Detection of APS is particularly important in pregnancy where it is responsible for repeated and progressive thrombotic infarction of the placental circulation, leading to foetal loss. Up to 50% of women with a history of recurrent foetal loss in the first and second trimester of pregnancy can be shown to have circulating antiphospholipid antibodies. In most cases, there are no other reasons to suspect the presence of APS. Prophylactic administration of prednisone to suppress antibody production and aspirin to inhibit platelet function has resulted in a successful outcome of pregnancy in some of these cases.

Prophylaxis and Treatment of Thrombosis

As alluded to in the previous chapter, one of the most important approaches to the prevention of thrombosis is reduction or even removal of risk factors such as smoking, obesity, lack of exercise and poor diet. Only when this proves to be impossible, impractical or ineffective is pharmacologic intervention required.

Anti-platelet Drugs

The deposition of platelets at sites of arterial vascular endothelial damage is an important step in the pathogenesis of atheroma and arterial thrombosis. This is certain because arterial thrombi typically are rich in platelets and also because the prophylactic administration of anti-platelet drugs such as **aspirin (acetylsalicylic acid)** has been shown to be effective in reducing the rate of reinfarction and sudden death in those who have survived myocardial infarctions. The major risk associated with any form of anti-thrombotic therapy is that of inducing haemorrhagic complications. Indeed, early clinical trials of prophylactic aspirin therapy showed a significant reduction in death due to infarction but this was balanced to a large extent by an increased incidence of death due to haemorrhagic stroke. Since then, several large-scale clinical trials have been conducted to define the optimal dose of aspirin and have shown conclusively that the daily administration of 50-100 mg of aspirin (1 standard adult aspirin tablet typically contains 300 mg) retains the antithrombotic effect while minimising the risk of haemorrhagic complications.

Oral Anticoagulants

Oral anticoagulants have the advantage that they are suitable for self-administration and so can be used outside of the hospital setting. The most widely prescribed oral anticoagulants, including **warfarin**, are coumarin analogues which act by inhibiting the normal recycling of vitamin K within hepatocytes thereby preventing the γ-carboxylation of the terminal glutamate residues of the vitamin K-dependent coagulation factors. Briefly, the carboxylation of these coagulation factors requires the coincident conversion of vitamin K hydroquinone to vitamin K epoxide under the influence of a carboxylase enzyme. The newly-formed vitamin K epoxide normally is rapidly converted back to vitamin K hydroquinone via an intermediate quinone form. These reactions are catalysed by warfarin-sensitive reductase enzymes. Thus, warfarin therapy induces an artificial deficiency of vitamin K hydroquinone with the result that the haemostatically inactive PIVKA forms of the vitamin K-dependent coagulation factors accumulate.

Because the action of warfarin relies on the inhibition of the synthesis of new coagulation factors, its anticoagulant effect is not fully expressed for some hours after commencement of therapy. Factor VII has the shortest *in vivo* half-life (about 6 hours) and so its plasma concentration is the first to fall. It is soon joined by the other vitamin K-dependent coagulation factors which have *in vivo* half-lives of between 24 hours (factor IX) and 60 hours (prothrombin). Thus the anticoagulant effect of warfarin is not fully expressed for about 3 days after the commencement of therapy. The required degree of anticoagulation typically is maintained by heparin therapy during this period.

The search for new anti-thrombotic agents with improved safety and clinical effectiveness represents a major challenge for bio-medical research. Several new anticoagulants have been developed which show early promise and currently are undergoing clinical trials to assess their efficacy and safety. Among these is **hirudin**, a direct inhibitor of thrombin which originally was extracted from the medicinal leech but is now available in recombinant form. Hirudin has been shown to inhibit fibrin-bound thrombin more effectively than heparin:ATIII complexes and may prove to be a suitable alternative to heparin therapy, particularly where heparin is contraindicated. In contrast to heparin, hirudin and its analogues are consumed by their antithrombotic activities.

Therapeutic anticoagulation requires the induction of a controlled coagulopathy and therefore is fraught with dangers. Successful therapy involves treading the fine line between haemorrhagic and prothrombotic states. It is essential that the required degree of anticoagulation is established early and subsequently is closely controlled. The degree of anticoagulation required differs widely in different clinical conditions and a full discussion of the intricacies of dosage and therapeutic monitoring is beyond the scope of this book. A major complicating factor in the use of oral anticoagulants is the wide range of commonly encountered drugs which either antagonise or potentiate their anticoagulant effect, with potentially catastrophic consequences. A list of some of the drugs which are known to interfere with the action of warfarin is shown earlier in Table 23.3.

Heparin

Heparin is a naturally-occurring sulphated mucopolysaccharide which is purified for clinical use from bovine lung or porcine intestinal mucosa. Clinical preparations of heparin consist of a mixture of polymeric forms ranging in molecular weight between 2,000 and 40,000. Heparin is ineffective as an oral anticoagulant because it cannot be absorbed from the intestine: it must therefore be administered via intravenous or subcutaneous routes. The anticoagulant effect of heparin is instantaneous, making it the treatment of choice for acute thrombotic episodes. Heparin exerts its anticoagulant effect by binding to ATIII and potentiating its action against thrombin, X_a and other activated serine proteases.

For the treatment of established thrombosis, high-dose heparin is administered by continuous intravenous infusion, following a bolus loading dose. The bolus dose is intended to clear the relatively large amounts of activated coagulation factors which are present in the circulation immediately following thrombosis. Once this has been achieved, the continuous infusion maintains a constant protective anticoagulant effect and is designed to prevent a subsequent thrombotic event. The desired degree of anticoagulation is achieved by adjustment of the rate of the continuous infusion. The short *in vivo* half-life of heparin (of the order of one hour) facilitates fine adjustment of the anticoagulant effect.

Heparin therapy is associated with a number of clinical problems, including a severe risk of haemorrhage which may be exacerbated by the induction of immune-mediated, heparin-dependent thrombocytopaenia in some cases and, following long-term treatment, osteoporosis. Low molecular weight preparations of heparin have been shown to retain much of their anticoagulant activity but to pose significantly less risk of severe thrombocytopaenia and haemorrhage. The *in vivo* half-life of low molecular weight heparin is about twice as long as the conventional preparation and therefore the dose-response curve is more predictable.

Low doses of heparin administered subcutaneously have been shown to offer effective post-operative prophylaxis for those undergoing abdominal surgery. When administered via this route, the plasma concentration of heparin slowly increases to reach a peak after about 4 hours, before gradually clearing by about 8 hours. To maintain the anticoagulant effect, repeated injections at 8 or 12 hour intervals are required. The incidence of significant bleeding problems is much lower than for intravenous heparin therapy, although the problems of thrombocytopaenia and osteoporosis persist.

Thrombolytic Drugs

The therapeutic anticoagulants described above are effective prophylactic antithrombotic agents and can also be used at higher dose to prevent the propagation of an established thrombus. However, they do not promote lysis of thrombi and so cannot help to prevent, for example, the ischaemic tissue damage which accompanies occlusive thrombi. This is the role of the thrombolytic agents such as **streptokinase (SK), tissue plasminogen activator (tPA)** and **acylated plasminogen streptokinase activated complex (APSAC)**.

SK is synthesised by β-haemolytic streptococci and activates both free and fibrin-bound plasminogen *in vivo* to release the powerful proteolytic enzyme, plasmin. The resultant systemic fibrinolysis shows no specificity for the site of the thrombus and so induces a profound hypocoagulable state which is accompanied by a severe risk of bleeding, for example, from surgical wounds. However, when administered quickly after the onset of chest pain in acute myocardial infarction, SK therapy is associated with a highly significant reduction in morbidity due to ischaemic muscle damage and also in the incidence of reinfarction. The *in vivo* half-life of SK is less than 10 minutes. The repeated use of SK is limited by its immunogenicity and its tendency to induce febrile reactions.

Recombinant human tPA is currently a very expensive product but is highly fibrin-specific and so exerts its lytic action directly on the formed thrombus and does not induce systemic fibrinolysis. The rate of success in achieving recanalisation of an occluded coronary artery following tPA therapy is higher than that for SK therapy but the rate of reinfarction may be higher. Further, although tPA is fibrin-specific, it is not thrombus-specific. Digestion of multiple small haemostatic plugs which form part of the normal defence against wear and tear may result in serious haemorrhage. Overall, the incidence of haemorrhagic complications during tPA therapy is similar to that for SK therapy. The *in vivo* half-life of tPA is less than 10 minutes.

APSAC is prepared by acylation of the serine active site on the plasminogen molecule, rendering it temporarily inactive. In vivo, this complex binds to both fibrin and fibrinogen. However, deacylation occurs relatively quickly at sites of fibrin formation but much more slowly in plasma. This property confers a degree of fibrin-specificity and also results in a more sustained fibrinolytic effect. The *in vivo* half-life of APSAC is about 90 minutes.

Suggested Further Reading

Bloom, A.L. and Thomas, D.P (eds). *Haemostasis and Thrombosis*. (3rd ed). Edinburgh: Churchill Livingstone.

Verstraete, M. and Collen, D. (1986). Thrombolytic therapy in the eighties. *Blood* **67**:1529.

BCSH Haemostasis and Thrombosis Task Force (1990). BSH Guidelines on Oral Anticoagulation. 2nd ed. *Journal of Clinical Pathology* **43**:177-183.

Index